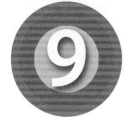

Edition 9

Medical Dosage Calculations

June L. Olsen, MS, RN
Professor of Nursing (Emeritus)
College of Staten Island
Staten Island, NY

Dolores M. Shrimpton, MA, RN
Professor of Nursing
Chairperson, Department of Nursing
Kingsborough Community College
Brooklyn, NY

Anthony Patrick Giangrasso, PhD
Professor of Mathematics
LaGuardia Community College
Long Island City, NY

Patricia M. Dillon MA, RN
Professor of Nursing
Deputy ChairPerson, Department of Natural
and Applied Science
LaGuardia Community College
Long Island City, NY

PEARSON
Prentice Hall

Upper Saddle River, New Jersey, 07458

Library of Congress Cataloging-in-Publication Data
Olsen, June Looby.
  Medical dosage calculations / June Looby Olsen, Anthony Patrick Giangrasso, Dolores M. Shrimpton. -- 9th ed.
    p. ; cm.
  Includes index.
  ISBN 0-13-238470-1
  1. Pharmaceutical arithmetic. 2. Pharmaceutical arithmetic--Problems, exercises, etc. I. Giangrasso, Anthony Patrick. II. Shrimpton, Dolores M. III. Title.
  [DNLM: 1. Pharmaceutical Preparations--administration & dosage--Nurses' Instruction. 2. Mathematics--Nurses' Instruction. QV 748 O52m 2007]
  RS57.M425 2007 615'.14--dc22

Publisher: Julie Levin Alexander
Publisher's Assistant: Regina Bruno
Editor-in-Chief: Maura Connor
Acquisitions Editor: Kelly Trakalo
Editorial Assistant: JulieAnn Oliveros
Development Editor: Michael Giacobbe
Managing Editor, Development: Marilyn Meserve
Managing Production Editor: Patrick Walsh
Production Liaison: Yagnesh Jani
Production Editor/Comp: Preparè Inc.
Manufacturing Manager: Ilene Sanford

Manufacturing Buyer: Pat Brown
Design Director: Maria Guglielmo-Walsh
Interior Designer/Cover Designer: Wanda España
Director of Marketing: Karen Allman
Senior Marketing Manager: Francisco Del Castillo
Marketing Coordinator: Michael Sirinides
Media Development Editor: John J. Jordan
New Media Project Manager: Tina Rudowski
Printer/Binder: Courier Kendallville
Cover Printer: Phoenix Color
Unit Openers and Chapter Openers: Photodisk/Getty Images

Notice: Care has been taken to confirm the accuracy of information presented in this book. The authors, editors, and the publisher, however, cannot accept any responsibility for errors or omissions or for consequences from application of the information in this book and make no warranty, express or implied, with respect to its contents. The authors and publisher have exerted every effort to ensure that drug selections and dosages set forth in this text are in accord with current recommendations and practice at time of publication. However, in view of ongoing research, changes in government regulations, and the constant flow of information relating to drug therapy and drug reactions, the reader is urged to check the package inserts of all drugs for any change in indications of dosage and for added warnings and precautions. This is particularly important when the recommended agent is a new and/or infrequently employed drug.

Pearson Education Ltd.
Pearson Education Singapore Pte. Ltd.
Pearson Education Canada, Ltd.
Pearson Education—Japan
Pearson Education Australia Pty. Limited

Pearson Education North Asia Ltd.
Pearson Educación de Mexico, S.A. de C.V.
Pearson Education Malaysia Pte. Ltd.
Pearson Education Inc., Upper Saddle River, New Jersey

10 9 8 7 6 5 4 3 2 1

Isbn 10:   0-13-238470-1
Isbn 13: 978-0-13-238470-4

Dedications

For my three girls, with love: Larissa, Michelle, and Taylor.

—June Looby Olsen

To Carlos Arevalo, James Kwee, and George Rivara: good tennis buddies, great physicians, and even better human beings.

—Anthony Giangrasso

To my son, Shawn, daughter-in-law, Kim, granddaughters, Brooke Elizabeth and Paige Dolores, and our newest addition Jack Paul for all the love and happiness they have brought into my life.

—Dolores M. Shrimpton

To my husband, Patrick, and daughters Leigh Ann and Katie, for their enduring patience and loving support, and to my colleague, Sheila Acheson, for inspiration.

—Patricia M. Dillon

About the Authors

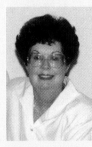

JUNE LOOBY OLSEN began her nursing career in Burlington, Vermont, at Bishop De Goesbriand Memorial Hospital, where she graduated from its Nursing Program. She obtained her BS and MS degrees in nursing from St. John's University, New York. She was a staff nurse, nurse supervisor, and became Head Nurse at the Veterans Administration Hospital in Brooklyn, New York.

Her teaching career began at Staten Island Community College, and she retired as Full Professor Emeritus from the College of Staten Island of the City University of New York. In addition to this textbook, Professor Olsen has written, *Fundamentals of Nursing Review* and *Dosage Calculation* both published by Springhouse. She was a recipient of the Mu Epsilon Leadership in Nursing award.

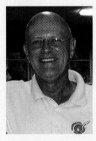

ANTHONY GIANGRASSO was born and raised in Maspeth, NY. He attended Rice High School on a scholarship, and in his senior year was named in a citywide contest by the *New York Journal-American* newspaper as New York City's most outstanding high school scholar-athlete. He was also awarded a full-tuition scholarship to Iona College, from which he obtained a BA in mathematics, magna cum laude, with a ranking of sixth in his graduating class.

Anthony began his teaching career as a fifth-grade teacher in Manhattan as a member of the Christian Brothers of Ireland, and taught high school mathematics and physics in Harlem and Newark, NJ. He possesses an MS and PhD from New York University, and has taught at all levels from elementary school through graduate school. He is currently teaching at Adelphi University and LaGuardia Community College, where he was chairman of the mathematics department. He has authored seven college textbooks.

Anthony's community service has included membership on the Boards of Directors of the Polish-American Museum Foundation, Catholic Adoptive Parents Association, and Family Focus Adoptive Services. He was the president of the Italian-American Faculty Association of the City University of New York, and the founding Chairman of the Board of the Italian-American Legal Defense and Higher Education Fund, Inc. He and his wife, Susan, are proud parents of three children Anthony, Michael, and Jennifer. He enjoys tennis, and in 2002 was ranked #1 for his age group in the Eastern Section by the United States Tennis Association.

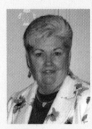

DOLORES M. SHRIMPTON is a professor and chairperson of the Department of Nursing at Kingsborough Community College of the City University of New York. She has been a nurse for more than 35 years and received a diploma in nursing from the Kings County Hospital Center School of Nursing. She obtained a BS degree from C. W. Post College and an MA degree in nursing administration from New York University. She also has a post-Master's certificate in nursing education from Adelphi University. She is a member of the Upsilon and Mu Upsilon Chapters of Sigma Theta Tau.

Dolores is the immediate past president of the New York State Associate Degree Nursing Council, where she also served as the vice president and member of its board of directors. She is the cochair of the CUNY Nursing Discipline Council and an active member of the Nurses Association of the Counties of Long Island (NACLI), D 14 of the New York State Nurses Association. She serves on a number of advisory boards of LPN, associate degree, and baccalaureate degree nursing programs. She is also the project codirector of the New York State Coalition for Nursing Educational Mobility (NYSCNEM).

Dolores has received many awards for her achievements in nursing. She is a recipient of the Presidential Award in Nursing Leadership from NACLI, the Mu Upsilon award for Excellence in Nursing Education, and the 2006 Mu Upsilon award for Excellence in Nursing Leadership. Dolores has taught a wide variety of courses in practical nursing, diploma, and associate degree nursing programs. Her area of clinical practice is maternity, with a focus on labor and delivery.

Dolores lives in Brooklyn, NY, and especially enjoys spending time with her grandchildren, Brooke Elizabeth, Paige Dolores, and Jack Paul, and their parents, Kim and Shawn.

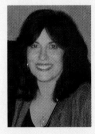

PATRICIA M. DILLON As far back as she can remember, Pat always loved math and science, and after getting a Regents Scholarship in Nursing, she decided that fate wanted her to choose that career. She obtained her BS in Nursing, from Lehman College and MA from New York University.

Pediatric surgery became Pat's specialty at New York University Medical Center, where she also worked in neurosurgery, and finally in maternity. Her 22 years of experience in education began at Molloy College, followed by 4 years at Interfaith School of Nursing in Brooklyn, and to her longest position of 16 years in the Nursing Program at LaGuardia Community College. While there, she moved through the ranks from Assistant Professor of Nursing to her present position as Professor and Natural Applied Sciences Deputy Chair of Nursing. During her earlier years, she created a medical dosages video for Dimensional Analysis, which the nursing students found to be a very valuable learning supplement.

Pat has always been deeply involved in professional nursing organizations. Her numerous positions have included vice chairperson of the Parent-Child Health Nursing Clinical Practice Unit of New York State Nurses Association (NYSNA), as well as a 4-year term as chair of the same NYSNA PCHN-CPU Committee. She was later appointed chair of NYSNA's Council on Nursing Practice and an auxiliary member of the NY State Board of Nursing. Her awards include the Ruth W. Harper Distinguished Service Award for Commitment to Professional Excellence and Leadership from the Nurses Association of Long Island (NACLI), NYSNA Local District 14, as well as the NYSNA 2004 Student's Choice Award. In 2006, she was inducted into the New York State Nurses Association Leadership Institute.

Preface

Dimensional Analysis is a simple approach to drug calculations that frees the student from the need to memorize formulas. Once this technique is mastered, you will be able to calculate drug dosages quickly and safely. It is the method most commonly employed in the physical sciences. In courses such as chemistry and physics, students learn to routinely change a quantity in one unit of measurement to an equivalent quantity in a different unit of measurement by cancelling matching units of measurement. In the first edition of this book (1974) we introduced this method; we called this method by the name *Dimensional Analysis*. We coined this phrase because the units of measure (for example, feet and inches) are called *dimensions*, and the problems have to be *analyzed* in order to solve them.

In a growing range of healthcare settings, nursing and allied health professionals are assuming increasing responsibilities in every aspect of medication administration. The first step in assuming this responsibility is learning to calculate drug dosages accurately. Dosage calculation is not just about math skills; it is an introduction to the **professional context** of drug administration. Calculation skills and the reason for their application—this is what *Medical Dosage Calculations* has taught generations of students with unmatched success through eight editions.

Medical Dosage Calculations is a combined text and workbook designed for the student of dosage calculations. Its consistent focus on safety, accuracy, and professionalism make it a valuable part of a dosage calculation course for nursing or allied health programs. It is also highly effective for independent study and may be used as a refresher to dosage calculation skills or as a professional reference.

Medical Dosage Calculations is arranged into four basic learning units:

Unit 1: Basic Calculation Skills and Introduction to Medication Administration
Chapters 1 and 2 review basic mathematics skills and introduce the essentials of drug administration. Chapter 3 introduces Dimensional Analysis using a friendly, common sense approach.

Unit 2: Systems of Measurement
Chapters 4 and 5 present the three systems of measurement that nurses and other allied health professionals must understand to interpret medication orders and calculate dosages. Students learn to convert measurements between and within measurement systems.

Unit 3: Oral and Parenteral Medications
Chapters 6, 7, 8, and 9 prepare students to calculate oral and parenteral dosages and introduce them to the essential equipment needed for administration and preparation of solutions.

Unit 4: Infusions and Pediatric Dosages
This important final unit provides a solid foundation for calculating intravenous and enteral flow rates, intravenous piggyback infusions, and duration of infusions (Chapters 10 and 11).
Pediatric dosages and daily fluid maintenance needs are discussed in Chapter 12.

Topics introduced and developed in *Medical Dosage Calculations* include:

- Basic arithmetic skills
- Systems of measurement
- Dosage calculations for all common forms of drug preparations
- IV and specialized calculations

In addition to these topics, the ninth edition includes substantially more information about safety in medication administration and follows the National Patient Safety Goals of the Joint Commission on Accreditation of Health Care Organizations (JCAHO) recommendations. Readers will learn how to interpret actual drug labels, package inserts, and various forms of medication orders, as well as how to select the appropriate equipment to administer the prescribed dose.

Benefits of Using *Medical Dosage Calculations*

- Constant skill reinforcement through frequent practice opportunities.
- More than 1,000 problems for students to solve.
- Actual drug labels, syringes, drug package inserts, prescriptions, medication administration records (MARs), are illustrated throughout the text.
- Ample work space on every page for note taking and problem solving.
- Completely worked out solutions to problems are found in Appendix A.

Acknowledgments

Our special thanks to the nursing and mathematics faculty and the students at the College of Staten Island, La Guardia Community College, and Kingsborough Community College. Also, a thank you to our editor, Kelly Trakalo; media editor John Jordan; associate editor Michael Giacobbe; and the production and marketing teams at Prentice Hall. Also thanks to Patricia M. Dillon for supplying the basis of the art program used in this edition.

Thank you also to the following for supplying art work for this edition:

Abbot Laboratories

American Pharmaceutical Partners

Amgen, Inc.

Astra-Zeneca LP

Baxter

Bayer Pharmaceutical Corporation

Eisai Inc.

Eli Lilly and Company

Forrest Pharmaceuticals Inc.

GlaxoSmithKline

Merck and Company, Inc.

Novartis Pharmaceuticals

Pfizer, Inc

Purdue Pharma

Roxane Laboratories

Teva Pharmaceutical Industries Ltd.

Reviewers

Dr. Mandyam A. Tirumalachar, MD FRCP
Allied Health Sciences
Austin Community College
Austin, TX

Leonard Lichtblau, PhD
Assistant Professor
School of Nursing
University of Minnesota
Minneapolis, MN

Linda Walter, RN, MSN, FNP
Health Occupations Nursing
Northwestern Michigan College
Kalkaska, MI.

Susan Randol, BSN, MSN
Nursing Coordinator
University of Louisiana—Lafayette
Lafayette, LA

Rebecca Raimann, MA
Mathematics Instructor
Inver Hills Community College
Inver Grove Heights, MN

Katherine Conrad, RN, MN, CNS
Nursing Instructor
Mt. Hood Community College
Gresham, OR

Kathleen Buhler, BSN
Nursing Instructor
Mt. Hood Community College
Gresham, OR

Regina Janoski, BSN, MSN
Nursing Instructor
Montgomery County Community College
Blue Bell, PA

Margaret Freede, RN, JD
Nursing Professor
University of Oklahoma
Oklahoma City, OK

Kathy Cooper, RN, MS
College of Nursing Instructor
The University of Oklahoma
P.O. Box 26901
Oklahoma City, OK. 73190

Laura Hodgson, RN, BSN
Nursing Laboratory Instructor
Illinois Valley Community College
Oglesby, Illinois

Contents

Learn to Calculate Dosages Safely and Accurately!

The Ease of Learning With Dimensional Analysis

Medical Dosage Calculations provides the ease of learning dimensional analysis with a building block approach of the basics.

The Diagnostic Test of Arithmetic helps you rediscover your understanding of basic math concepts and guides you in identifying areas for review.

Learn by Example!
Each chapter unfolds basic concepts and skills through completely worked out questions with solutions.

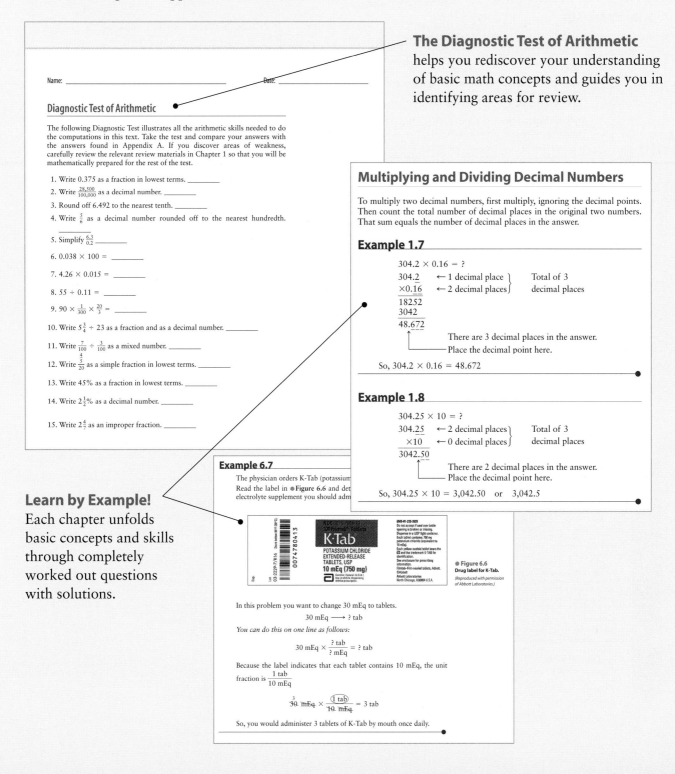

Name: _____ Date: _____

Diagnostic Test of Arithmetic

The following Diagnostic Test illustrates all the arithmetic skills needed to do the computations in this text. Take the test and compare your answers with the answers found in Appendix A. If you discover areas of weakness, carefully review the relevant review materials in Chapter 1 so that you will be mathematically prepared for the rest of the test.

1. Write 0.375 as a fraction in lowest terms. _____
2. Write $\frac{28,500}{100,000}$ as a decimal number. _____
3. Round off 6.492 to the nearest tenth. _____
4. Write $\frac{5}{6}$ as a decimal number rounded off to the nearest hundredth. _____
5. Simplify $\frac{6.3}{0.2}$ _____
6. $0.038 \times 100 =$ _____
7. $4.26 \times 0.015 =$ _____
8. $55 \div 0.11 =$ _____
9. $90 \times \frac{1}{300} \times \frac{20}{3} =$ _____
10. Write $5\frac{3}{4} \div 23$ as a fraction and as a decimal number. _____
11. Write $\frac{7}{100} \div \frac{3}{100}$ as a mixed number. _____
12. Write $\frac{\frac{4}{5}}{20}$ as a simple fraction in lowest terms. _____
13. Write 45% as a fraction in lowest terms. _____
14. Write $2\frac{1}{2}\%$ as a decimal number. _____
15. Write $2\frac{4}{7}$ as an improper fraction. _____

Multiplying and Dividing Decimal Numbers

To multiply two decimal numbers, first multiply, ignoring the decimal points. Then count the total number of decimal places in the original two numbers. That sum equals the number of decimal places in the answer.

Example 1.7

$304.2 \times 0.16 = ?$

$304.\underline{2}$ ← 1 decimal place } Total of 3
$\times 0.\underline{16}$ ← 2 decimal places } decimal places
$\overline{18252}$
3042
$\overline{48.672}$

There are 3 decimal places in the answer.
Place the decimal point here.

So, $304.2 \times 0.16 = 48.672$

Example 1.8

$304.25 \times 10 = ?$

$304.\underline{25}$ ← 2 decimal places } Total of 3
$\times 10$ ← 0 decimal places } decimal places
$\overline{3042.50}$

There are 2 decimal places in the answer.
Place the decimal point here.

So, $304.25 \times 10 = 3,042.50$ or $3,042.5$

Example 6.7

The physician orders K-Tab (potassium _____
Read the label in ● **Figure 6.6** and det _____
electrolyte supplement you should adm _____

K-Tab
POTASSIUM CHLORIDE
EXTENDED-RELEASE
TABLETS, USP
10 mEq (750 mg)

● Figure 6.6
Drug label for K-Tab.
(Reproduced with permission of Abbott Laboratories.)

In this problem you want to change 30 mEq to tablets.

$$30 \text{ mEq} \longrightarrow ? \text{ tab}$$

You can do this on one line as follows:

$$30 \text{ mEq} \times \frac{? \text{ tab}}{? \text{ mEq}} = ? \text{ tab}$$

Because the label indicates that each tablet contains 10 mEq, the unit fraction is $\frac{1 \text{ tab}}{10 \text{ mEq}}$

$$\overset{3}{\cancel{30}} \text{ mEq} \times \frac{(1 \text{ tab})}{\cancel{10} \text{ mEq}} = 3 \text{ tab}$$

So, you would administer 3 tablets of K-Tab by mouth once daily.

Safe and Accurate Medical Dosage Calculation

Safe and accurate medical dosage calculation comes from practice and critical thinking.

Try These For Practice, Exercises, and Additional Exercises, found in every chapter, test your comprehension of material.

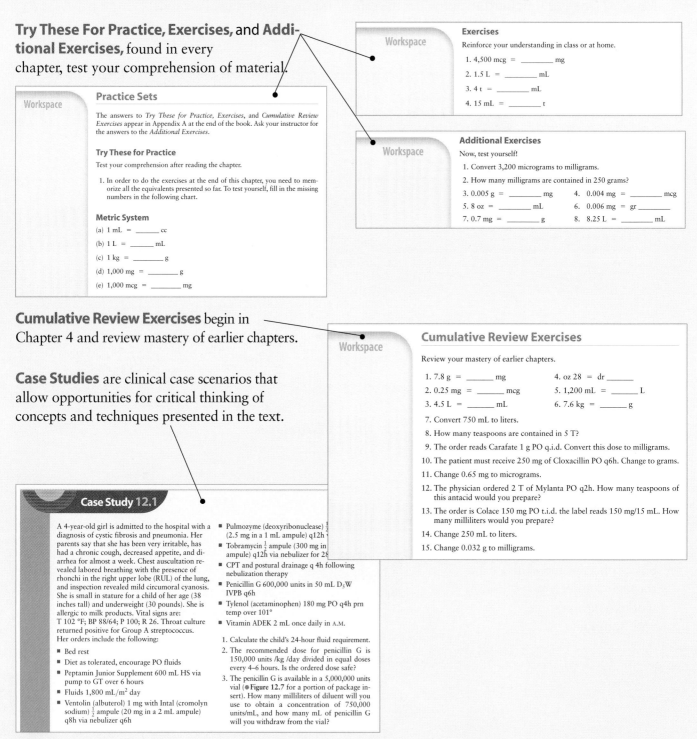

Workspace

Practice Sets

The answers to *Try These for Practice*, *Exercises*, and *Cumulative Review Exercises* appear in Appendix A at the end of the book. Ask your instructor for the answers to the *Additional Exercises*.

Try These for Practice

Test your comprehension after reading the chapter.

1. In order to do the exercises at the end of this chapter, you need to memorize all the equivalents presented so far. To test yourself, fill in the missing numbers in the following chart.

Metric System

(a) 1 mL = _____ cc

(b) 1 L = _____ mL

(c) 1 kg = _____ g

(d) 1,000 mg = _____ g

(e) 1,000 mcg = _____ mg

Workspace

Exercises

Reinforce your understanding in class or at home.

1. 4,500 mcg = _____ mg

2. 1.5 L = _____ mL

3. 4 t = _____ mL

4. 15 mL = _____ t

Workspace

Additional Exercises

Now, test yourself!

1. Convert 3,200 micrograms to milligrams.

2. How many milligrams are contained in 250 grams?

3. 0.005 g = _____ mg   4. 0.004 mg = _____ mcg

5. 8 oz = _____ mL   6. 0.006 mg = gr _____

7. 0.7 mg = _____ g   8. 8.25 L = _____ mL

Cumulative Review Exercises begin in Chapter 4 and review mastery of earlier chapters.

Workspace

Cumulative Review Exercises

Review your mastery of earlier chapters.

1. 7.8 g = _____ mg   4. oz 28 = dr _____

2. 0.25 mg = _____ mcg   5. 1,200 mL = _____ L

3. 4.5 L = _____ mL   6. 7.6 kg = _____ g

7. Convert 750 mL to liters.

8. How many teaspoons are contained in 5 T?

9. The order reads Carafate 1 g PO q.i.d. Convert this dose to milligrams.

10. The patient must receive 250 mg of Cloxacillin PO q6h. Change to grams.

11. Change 0.65 mg to micrograms.

12. The physician ordered 2 T of Mylanta PO q2h. How many teaspoons of this antacid would you prepare?

13. The order is Colace 150 mg PO t.i.d. the label reads 150 mg/15 mL. How many milliliters would you prepare?

14. Change 250 mL to liters.

15. Change 0.032 g to milligrams.

Case Studies are clinical case scenarios that allow opportunities for critical thinking of concepts and techniques presented in the text.

Case Study 12.1

A 4-year-old girl is admitted to the hospital with a diagnosis of cystic fibrosis and pneumonia. Her parents say that she has been very irritable, has had a chronic cough, decreased appetite, and diarrhea for almost a week. Chest auscultation revealed labored breathing with the presence of rhonchi in the right upper lobe (RUL) of the lung, and inspection revealed mild circumoral cyanosis. She is small in stature for a child of her age (38 inches tall) and underweight (30 pounds). She is allergic to milk products. Vital signs are: T 102 °F; BP 88/64; P 100; R 26. Throat culture returned positive for Group A streptococcus. Her orders include the following:

- Bed rest
- Diet as tolerated, encourage PO fluids
- Peptamin Junior Supplement 600 mL HS via pump to GT over 6 hours
- Fluids 1,800 mL/m² day
- Ventolin (albuterol) 1 mg with Intal (cromolyn sodium) ½ ampule (20 mg in a 2 mL ampule) q8h via nebulizer q6h

- Pulmozyme (deoxyribonuclease) ½ (2.5 mg in a 1 mL ampule) q12h
- Tobramycin ½ ampule (300 mg in ampule) q12h via nebulizer for 28
- CPT and postural drainage q 4h following nebulization therapy
- Penicillin G 600,000 units in 50 mL D₅W IVPB q6h
- Tylenol (acetaminophen) 180 mg PO q4h prn temp over 101°
- Vitamin ADEK 2 mL once daily in A.M.

1. Calculate the child's 24-hour fluid requirement.

2. The recommended dose for penicillin G is 150,000 units /kg /day divided in equal doses every 4–6 hours. Is the ordered dose safe?

3. The penicillin G is available in a 5,000,000 units vial (● **Figure 12.7** for a portion of package insert). How many milliliters of diluent will you use to obtain a concentration of 750,000 units/mL, and how many mL of penicillin G will you withdraw from the vial?

Notes and **Alerts** highlight concepts and principles for safe medication calculation and administration.

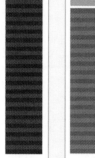

NDC 0173-0712-04

2
0173-0712-04
N 3

AVODART®
(dutasteride)
Soft Gelatin Capsules
0.5 mg

R only

GX CE2

90 Capsules

Each capsule contains 0.5 mg dutasteride.

Usual Dosage: 0.5 mg once a day.
See prescribing information for further dosing information.

Store at 25° C (77° F); excursions permitted to 15-30° C (59-86° F) [see USP Controlled Room Temperature].

Dispense in a well-closed container as defined in the USP.

Do not use if printed safety seal under cap is broken or missing.

LOT **APRIL**
EXP **2008**

gsk GlaxoSmithKline

Manufactured by Cardinal Health
Beinheim, France for
GlaxoSmithKline
Research Triangle Park, NC 27709
Made in France

WARNING: AVODART should not be used by women or children. Women who are or may potentially be pregnant should not use or handle AVODART Soft Gelatin Capsules (see prescribing information). If contact is made with leaking capsule, wash immediately with soap and

Realistic Illustrations!
Real drug labels and realistic syringes aid students in identifying what they will see in the real world.

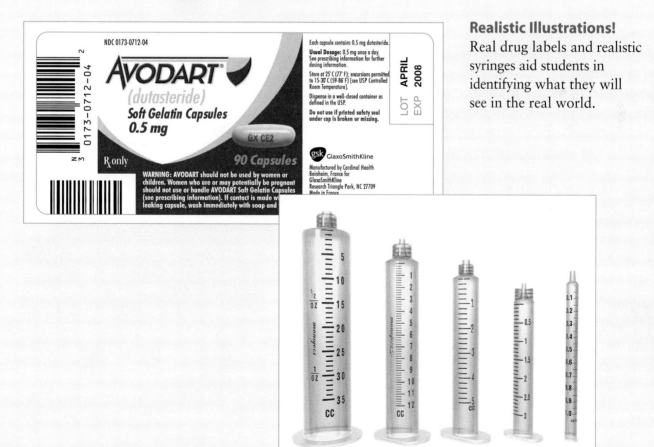

Additional Student Resources!

Prentice Hall's Dosage Calculation Tutor. New to this edition!
This CD-ROM comes packaged with every textbook. A unique interface guides you through animated examples of chapter topics, provides practice questions, chapter challenge tests and a comprehensive final test.

Companion Website. Go to *www.prenhall.com/olsen* for your online study guide. The Companion Website provides even more review and practice questions!

Pocket Reminder Card!
Use this handy reference for examples and equivalency charts so you can accurately calculate medical dosages wherever and whenever you need to!

Additional Instructor Resources!

Instructor's Resource Manual. The instructor's manual that accompanies this book provides extra test questions and answers, answers to the additional exercises that are found in the book, a list of key terms, possible teaching approaches relevant to each chapter, an overview of learning outcomes for each chapter and comprehensive examinations with answers. This instructor's manual helps instructors prepare lectures and examinations quickly.

Instructor's Resource CD-ROM. This CD-ROM resource contains a TestGen test item file, and PowerPoint slides to help guide lectures.

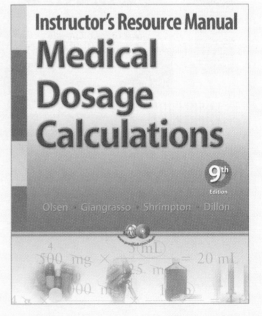

Instructor's Resource Manual
Medical Dosage Calculations

9th Edition

Olsen · Giangrasso · Shrimpton · Dillon

Basic Calculation Skills and Introduction to Medication Administration

Chapter 1

Review of Arithmetic for Medical Dosage Calculations

Chapter 2

Safe and Accurate Drug Administration

Chapter 3

Dimensional Analysis

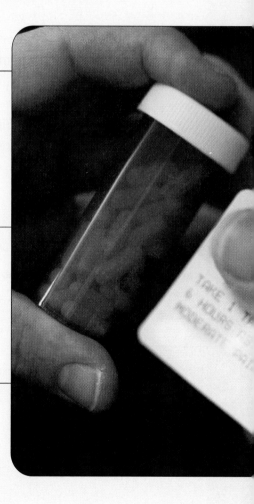

Review of Arithmetic for Medical Dosage Calculations

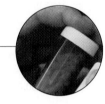

Learning Outcomes

After completing this chapter, you will be able to

1. Convert decimal numbers to fractions.
2. Convert fractions to decimal numbers.
3. Round decimal numbers to a desired number of places.
4. Multiply and divide decimal numbers.
5. Multiply and divide fractions.
6. Simplify complex fractions.
7. Write percentages as decimal numbers.
8. Write percentages as fractions.

Medical dosage calculations can involve whole numbers, fractions, decimal numbers, and percentages. Your results on the *Diagnostic Test of Arithmetic*, found on the next page, will identify your areas of strength and weakness. You can use Chapter 1 to improve your math skills or simply to review the kinds of calculations you will encounter in this text.

Diagnostic Test of Arithmetic

The following Diagnostic Test illustrates all the arithmetic skills needed to do the computations in this text. Take the test and compare your answers with the answers found in Appendix A. If you discover areas of weakness, carefully review the relevant review materials in Chapter 1 so that you will be mathematically prepared for the rest of the test.

1. Write 0.375 as a fraction in lowest terms. _____

2. Write $\frac{28,500}{100,000}$ as a decimal number. _____

3. Round off 6.492 to the nearest tenth. _____

4. Write $\frac{5}{6}$ as a decimal number rounded off to the nearest hundredth. _____

5. Simplify $\frac{6.3}{0.2}$ _____

6. $0.038 \times 100 =$ _____

7. $4.26 \times 0.015 =$ _____

8. $55 \div 0.11 =$ _____

9. $90 \times \frac{1}{300} \times \frac{20}{3} =$ _____

10. Write $5\frac{3}{4} \div 23$ as a fraction and as a decimal number. _____

11. Write $\frac{7}{100} \div \frac{3}{100}$ as a mixed number. _____

12. Write $\frac{\frac{4}{5}}{20}$ as a simple fraction in lowest terms. _____

13. Write 45% as a fraction in lowest terms. _____

14. Write $2\frac{1}{2}\%$ as a decimal number. _____

15. Write $2\frac{4}{7}$ as an improper fraction. _____

Changing Decimal Numbers and Whole Numbers to Fractions

A decimal number represents a fraction with a denominator of 10, 100, 1,000, and so on. Each decimal number has three parts: the whole-number part, the decimal point, and the fraction part. Table 1.1 shows the names of the decimal positions.

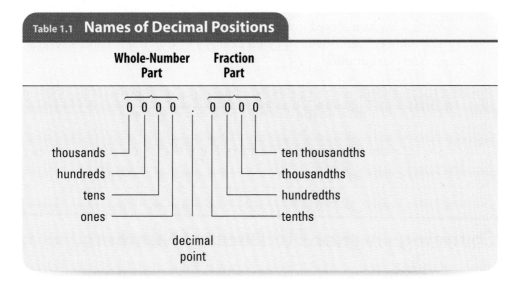

Table 1.1 Names of Decimal Positions

Reading a decimal number will help you write it as a fraction.

Decimal Number	$\longrightarrow$	Read	$\longrightarrow$	Fraction
4.1	$\longrightarrow$	four and one tenth	$\longrightarrow$	$4\dfrac{1}{10}$
0.3	$\longrightarrow$	three tenths	$\longrightarrow$	$\dfrac{3}{10}$
6.07	$\longrightarrow$	six and seven hundredths	$\longrightarrow$	$6\dfrac{7}{100}$
0.231	$\longrightarrow$	two hundred thirty-one thousandths	$\longrightarrow$	$\dfrac{231}{1,000}$
0.0025	$\longrightarrow$	twenty-five ten thousandths	$\longrightarrow$	$\dfrac{25}{10,000}$

A number can be written in different forms. A decimal number *less than 1*, such as 0.9, is read as *nine tenths* and can also be written as the *proper fraction* $\frac{9}{10}$. In a **proper fraction**, the numerator (the number on the top) of the fraction is smaller than its denominator (the number on the bottom).

A decimal number *greater than 1*, such as 3.5, is read as *three and five tenths* and can also be written as the *mixed number* $3\frac{5}{10}$ or $3\frac{1}{2}$. A **mixed number** combines a whole number and a proper fraction. The *mixed number* $3\frac{1}{2}$, can be changed to an *improper fraction* as follows:

$$3\frac{1}{2} = \frac{3 \times 2 + 1}{2} = \frac{7}{2}$$

The numerator (top number) of an **improper fraction** is larger than or equal to its denominator (bottom number).

Any number can be written as a fraction by writing it over 1. For example, 9 can be written as the improper fraction $\frac{9}{1}$.

Example 1.1

NOTE

In Example 1.1, $\frac{25}{100}$ was simplified by dividing both numerator and denominator by 25.

$$\frac{25 \div 25}{100 \div 25} = \frac{1}{4}$$

This process is called *cancelling*.

Write 2.25 as a mixed number and as an improper fraction.

The number 2.25 is read *two and twenty-five hundredths* and is written $2\frac{25}{100}$. You can simplify:

$$2\frac{25}{100} = 2\frac{\overset{1}{\cancel{25}}}{\underset{4}{\cancel{100}}} = 2\frac{1}{4} = \frac{2 \times 4 + 1}{4} = \frac{9}{4}$$

So, 2.25 can be written as the mixed number $2\frac{1}{4}$ or as the improper fraction $\frac{9}{4}$.

Changing Fractions to Decimal Numbers

To change a fraction to a decimal, think of the fraction as a division problem. For example:

$$\frac{2}{5} \quad \text{means} \quad 2 \div 5 \quad \text{or} \quad 5\overline{)2}$$

Here are the steps for this division.

Step 1 Replace 2 with 2.0 and then place a decimal point directly above the decimal point in 2.0

$$5\overline{)2.0}^{\,.}$$

Step 2 Perform the division.

$$\begin{array}{r} 0.4 \\ 5\overline{)2.0} \\ \underline{2\,0} \\ 0 \end{array}$$

So, $\frac{2}{5} = 0.4$

Example 1.2

Write $\frac{2}{5}$ as a decimal number.

$$\frac{5}{2} \quad \text{means} \quad 5 \div 2 \quad \text{or} \quad 2\overline{)5}$$

Step 1 $2\overline{)5.0}$

Step 2
$$\begin{array}{r} 2.5 \\ 2\overline{)5.0} \\ \underline{4} \\ 1\,0 \\ \underline{1\,0} \end{array}$$

So, $\dfrac{5}{2} = 2.5$

Example 1.3

Write $\frac{193}{10}$ as a decimal number.

$$\frac{193}{10} \quad \text{means} \quad 193 \div 10 \quad \text{or} \quad 10\overline{)193}$$

Step 1 $10\overline{)193.0}$

Step 2
$$\begin{array}{r} 19.3 \\ 10\overline{)193.0} \\ \underline{10} \\ 93 \\ \underline{90} \\ 30 \\ \underline{30} \\ 0 \end{array}$$

So, $\dfrac{193}{10} = 19.3$

There is a quicker way to do this problem. To divide a *decimal number by 10*, you *move* the decimal point in the number *one place to the left*. Notice that there is one zero in 10.

$$\frac{193}{10} = \frac{193.}{10} = 193. = 19.3$$

To *divide a number by 100, move* the decimal point in the number *two places to the left* because there are two zeros in 100. So, the quick way to divide by 10, 100, 1,000, and so on is to count the zeros and then move the decimal point to the left the same number of places. The answer should always be a smaller number than the original number. Check your answer to be sure.

Example 1.4

Write $\frac{9.25}{100}$ as a decimal number.

There are two zeros in 100, so move the decimal point in 9.25 two places to the left, and fill the empty position with a zero.

$$\frac{9.25}{100} = 9.25 = 0.0925$$

Rounding Decimal Numbers

Sometimes it is convenient to round an answer—that is, to use an approximate answer rather than an exact one.

Rounding Off

To round off 1.267 to the *nearest tenth*—that is, to round off the number to one decimal place—do the following:

Look at the digit after the tenths place (the hundredths place digit). Because this digit (6) is 5 or more, round off 1.267 by adding 1 to the tenths *place digit. Finally, drop all the digits after the tenths place. So, 1.267 is approximated by 1.3 when rounded off to the nearest tenth.*

To round off 0.8345 to the *nearest hundredth*—that is, to round off the number to two decimal places—do the following:

Look at the digit after the hundredths place (the thousandths place digit). Because this digit (4) is less than 5, round off 0.8345 by leaving the hundredths digit alone. Finally, drop all the digits after the hundredths place. So, 0.8345 is approximated by 0.83 when rounded off to the nearest hundredth.

Example 1.5

Round off 4.8075 to the nearest hundredth, tenth, and whole number.

4.8075 rounded off to the nearest: hundredth = 4.81

tenth = 4.8

whole number = 5

Rounding *off* numbers produces results, which can be either larger or smaller than the given numbers. When numbers are rounded *down*, however, the results cannot be larger than the given numbers.

Rounding Down

To round *down* a number to a particular place, merely *drop all the digits after that place*. In particular, to round *down* to the tenths place, merely drop all the digits after the tenths place.

Example 1.6

Round down 4.8075 to the nearest hundredth, tenth and whole number.

4.8075 rounded *down* to the nearest   hundredth = 4.80

tenth = 4.8

whole number = 4

ALERT

The danger of an overdose must always be guarded against. Therefore, the amount of medication to be administered is often rounded *down* instead of rounded *off*. This rounding down is done routinely in pediatrics and when administering high-alert drugs to adults.

Multiplying and Dividing Decimal Numbers

To multiply two decimal numbers, first multiply, ignoring the decimal points. Then count the total number of decimal places in the original two numbers. That sum equals the number of decimal places in the answer.

Example 1.7

$304.2 \times 0.16 = ?$

$$
\begin{array}{r}
304.2 \quad \leftarrow 1 \text{ decimal place} \\
\times 0.16 \quad \leftarrow 2 \text{ decimal places} \\
\hline
18252 \\
3042 \\
\hline
48.672
\end{array}
$$

Total of 3 decimal places

There are 3 decimal places in the answer.
Place the decimal point here.

So, $304.2 \times 0.16 = 48.672$

NOTE

Unless otherwise specified, quantities *less than 1* will generally be rounded to the *nearest hundredth*, whereas quantities *greater than 1* will generally be rounded to the *nearest tenth*. For the sake of uniformity, when rounding numbers in this book, rounding *off* will be used rather than rounding *down*. However, in Chapter 12 *all pediatric dosages will be rounded down*.

Example 1.8

$304.25 \times 10 = ?$

$$
\begin{array}{r}
304.25 \quad \leftarrow 2 \text{ decimal places} \\
\times 10 \quad \leftarrow 0 \text{ decimal places} \\
\hline
3042.50
\end{array}
$$

Total of 3 decimal places

There are 2 decimal places in the answer.
Place the decimal point here.

So, $304.25 \times 10 = 3,042.50$ or $3,042.5$

There is a quicker way to do this problem. To *multiply any decimal number by 10, move* the decimal point in the number being multiplied *one place to the right*. Notice that there is one zero in 10.

$$304.25 \times 10 = 304.25 \quad \text{or} \quad 3,042.5$$

To *multiply a number by 100, move* the decimal point in the number *two places to the right* because there are two zeros in 100. So, the quick way to multiply by 10, 100, 1,000, and so on is to count the zeros and then move the decimal point to the right the same number of places. The answer should always be a larger number than the original. Check your answer to be sure.

Example 1.9

$$23.597 \times 1{,}000 = ?$$

There are three zeros in 1,000, so move the decimal point in 23.597 three places to the right.

$$23.597 \times 1{,}000 = 23.597 \quad \text{or} \quad 23{,}597$$

So, $23.597 \times 1{,}000 = 23{,}597$

Example 1.10

Write $\frac{106.8}{15}$ as a decimal number to the nearest tenth; that is, round off the answer to one decimal place.

$$\frac{106.8}{15} \quad \text{means} \quad 15\overline{)106.8}$$

Step 1 $15\overline{)106.8}$

Step 2   Because you want the answer to the nearest tenth (one decimal place), do the division to two decimal places and then round off the answer. Because the second place digit in the answer is *less than* 5, leave the first decimal place digit alone. Finally, drop the digit in the second (hundredths) decimal place.

$$
\begin{array}{r}
7.12 \\
15\overline{)106.80} \\
\underline{105} \\
1\ 8 \\
\underline{1\ 5} \\
30 \\
\underline{30} \\
0
\end{array}
$$

So, $\frac{106.8}{15}$ is 7.1 to the nearest tenth.

Example 1.11

Simplify $\frac{48}{0.002}$.

Since there are three decimal places in 0.002, move the decimal points in both numbers three places to the right.

$$\frac{48}{0.002} \quad \text{means} \quad 0.002\overline{)48.} \quad \text{or} \quad 0.002\overline{)48.000}$$

$$
\begin{array}{r}
24{,}000. \\
2\overline{)48{,}000.} \\
\underline{4} \\
08 \\
\underline{8} \\
0
\end{array}
$$

So, $\dfrac{48}{0.002} = 24{,}000$

Multiplying and Dividing Fractions

To *multiply fractions*, multiply the numerators to get the new numerator and multiply the denominators to get the new denominator.

Example 1.12

$$\frac{3}{5} \times 6 \times \frac{1}{5} = ?$$

A whole number can be written as a fraction with 1 in the denominator. So, in this example, write 6 as $\frac{6}{1}$ to make all the numbers fractions.

$$\frac{3}{5} \times \frac{6}{1} \times \frac{1}{5} = \frac{3 \times 6 \times 1}{5 \times 1 \times 5} = \frac{18}{25}$$

Example 1.13

$$\frac{4}{5} \times \frac{3}{10} \times \frac{20}{7} = ?$$

It is often convenient to cancel before you multiply.

$$\frac{4}{5} \times \frac{3}{\cancel{10}_{1}} \times \frac{\cancel{20}^{2}}{7} = \frac{24}{35}$$

To *divide fractions*, change the division problem to an equivalent multiplication problem by inverting the second fraction.

Example 1.14

$$1\frac{2}{5} \div \frac{7}{9} = ?$$

Write $1\frac{2}{5}$ as the improper fraction $\frac{7}{5}$.

The *Division* problem

$$\frac{7}{5} \div \frac{7}{9}$$

Becomes the *Multiplication* problem by inverting the second fraction.

$$\frac{7}{5} \times \frac{9}{7}$$

$$\frac{\cancel{7}^{1}}{5} \times \frac{9}{\cancel{7}_{1}} = \frac{9}{5} = 1\frac{4}{5}$$

Sometimes you must deal with whole numbers, fractions, and decimal numbers in the same multiplication and division problems.

NOTE

Avoid cancelling decimal numbers. It is a possible source of error.

Example 1.15

Give the answer to the following problem in simplified fractional form.

$$\frac{1}{300} \times 60 \times \frac{1}{0.4} = ?$$

Write 60 as a fraction and cancel.

$$\frac{1}{\overset{}{\underset{5}{\cancel{300}}}} \times \frac{\overset{1}{\cancel{60}}}{1} \times \frac{1}{0.4} = \frac{1}{5 \times 0.4} = \frac{1}{2}$$

Sometimes you will need to simplify *fractions that contain decimal numbers.*

Example 1.16

Give the answer to the following problem in simplified fractional form.

$$0.35 \times \frac{1}{60} = ?$$

Write 0.35 as the fraction $\frac{0.35}{1}$.

$$\frac{0.35}{1} \times \frac{1}{60} = \frac{0.35}{60}$$

The numerator of this fraction is 0.35, a decimal number. You can write an equivalent form of the fraction by multiplying the numerator and denominator by 100.

$$\frac{0.35}{60} \times \frac{100}{100} = \frac{0.35}{60.00} = \frac{35}{6,000} = \frac{7}{1,200}$$

Example 1.17

Give the answer to the following problem in simplified fractional form.

$$0.88 \times \frac{1}{2.2} = ?$$

$$\frac{0.88}{1} \times \frac{1}{2.2} = \frac{0.88}{2.2}$$

Multiply the numerator and the denominator of this fraction by 100 to eliminate both decimal numbers.

$$\frac{0.88}{2.2} \times \frac{100}{100} = \frac{0.88}{2.2} = \frac{88}{220} = \frac{2}{5}$$

You can simplify $\frac{0.88}{2.2}$ a different way by dividing 0.88 by 2.2.

$$2.2\overline{)0.88}^{\,0.4} \quad \text{and} \quad 0.4 = \frac{4}{10} \quad \text{or} \quad \frac{2}{5}$$

Complex Fractions

Fractions that have numerators or denominators that are themselves fractions are called *complex fractions*.

The longest line in the complex fraction separates the numerator (top) from the denominator (bottom) of the complex fraction. As with any fraction, you can write the complex fraction as a division problem [*Top ÷ Bottom*].

In the complex fraction $\frac{1}{\frac{2}{5}}$, the numerator is 1 and the denominator is $\frac{2}{5}$.

You can simplify this complex fraction as follows:

$$\frac{1}{\frac{2}{5}} \quad \text{means } 1 \div \frac{2}{5} \quad \text{or} \quad 1 \times \frac{5}{2}, \quad \text{which is} \quad \frac{5}{2}$$

In the complex fraction $\frac{\frac{1}{2}}{5}$, the numerator is $\frac{1}{2}$ and the denominator is 5.

You can simplify this complex fraction as follows:

$$\frac{\frac{1}{2}}{5} \quad \text{means} \quad \frac{1}{2} \div 5 \quad \text{or} \quad \frac{1}{2} \times \frac{1}{5}, \quad \text{which is} \quad \frac{1}{10}$$

In the complex fraction $\frac{\frac{3}{5}}{\frac{2}{5}}$, the numerator is $\frac{3}{5}$ and the denominator is $\frac{2}{5}$.

You can simplify this complex fraction as follows:

$$\frac{\frac{3}{5}}{\frac{2}{5}} \quad \text{means} \quad \frac{3}{5} \div \frac{2}{5} \quad \text{or} \quad \frac{3}{\overset{}{\underset{1}{5}}} \times \frac{\overset{1}{5}}{2}, \quad \text{which is} \quad \frac{3}{2}$$

Example 1.18

$$\frac{\frac{1}{25} \times 500}{\frac{1}{4}} = ?$$

In this complex fraction, the numerator is $(\frac{1}{25} \times 500)$ and the denominator is $\frac{1}{4}$. So, you can write the following:

$$\left(\frac{1}{25} \times \frac{500}{1} \right) \div \frac{1}{4} = ?$$

Do the multiplication inside the parentheses.

$$\left(\frac{1}{\underset{1}{25}} \times \frac{\overset{20}{500}}{1} \right) \div \frac{1}{4} =$$

$$\frac{20}{1} \div \frac{1}{4} =$$

$$\frac{20}{1} \times \frac{4}{1} = 80$$

Example 1.19

$$\frac{2}{3} \times \frac{1}{\frac{3}{4}} = ?$$

You can multiply the numerators to get the new numerator and multiply the denominators to get the new denominator, as follows:

$$\frac{2}{3} \times \frac{1}{\frac{3}{4}} = \frac{2 \times 1}{3 \times \frac{3}{4}} = \frac{2}{\frac{9}{4}}$$

Now, the numerator is 2 and the denominator is $\frac{9}{4}$, so you get

$$\frac{2}{1} \div \frac{9}{4}$$

which becomes

$$\frac{2}{1} \times \frac{4}{9} = \frac{8}{9}$$

This problem could have been done another way by simplifying $\frac{1}{\frac{3}{4}}$ first.

You can write $\frac{1}{\frac{3}{4}}$ as $1 \div \frac{3}{4}$

Then

$$\frac{2}{3} \times \frac{1}{\frac{3}{4}} = \frac{2}{3} \times \left(1 \div \frac{3}{4}\right)$$

$$\frac{2}{3} \times \left(1 \times \frac{4}{3}\right)$$

$$\frac{2}{3} \times \left(\frac{4}{3}\right) = \frac{8}{9}$$

Percentages

Percent (%) means *parts per 100* or *divided by 100*. Thus 50% means 50 *parts per hundred* or 50 *divided by 100*, which can also be written as the fraction $\frac{50}{100}$. The fraction $\frac{50}{100}$ can be changed to the decimal numbers 0.50 and 0.5 or reduced to the fraction $\frac{1}{2}$.

13%   means $\frac{13}{100}$ or   0.13

100%   means $\frac{100}{100}$ or   1

12.3% means $\frac{12.3}{100}$ or   0.123

$6\frac{1}{2}$%   means   6.5%   or $\frac{6.5}{100}$ or   0.065

Example 1.20

Write 0.5% as a fraction in lowest terms.

$$0.5\% = \frac{0.5}{100} = \frac{5}{1,000} = \frac{1}{200}$$

There is another way to get the answer. Because you understand that $0.5 = \frac{1}{2}$, then

$$0.5\% = \frac{1}{2}\% = \frac{1}{2} \div 100 = \frac{1}{2} \div \frac{100}{1} = \frac{1}{2} \times \frac{1}{100} = \frac{1}{200}$$

Summary

In this chapter, all the essential mathematical skills that are used in this textbook were reviewed.

When working with fractions:
- Proper fractions have smaller numbers in the numerator than in the denominator.
- Improper fractions have numerators that are larger than or equal to their denominators.
- Improper fractions can be changed to mixed numbers, and vice versa.
- Any number can be changed into a fraction by writing the number over 1.
- Cancel first when you multiply fractions.
- Change a fraction to a decimal number by dividing the numerator by the denominator.

- Simplify complex fractions by dividing the numerator by the denominator.

When working with decimals:
- Move the decimal point 3 places to the right when multiplying a decimal number by 1,000.
- Move the decimal point 3 places to the left when dividing a decimal number by 1,000.
- Count the total number of places in the numbers you are multiplying to determine the number of decimal places in the answer.
- Avoid cancelling with decimal numbers.

When working with percentages:
- Change to fractions or decimal numbers before doing any calculations.

Practice Sets

The answers to *Try These for Practice* and *Exercises* appear in Appendix A at the back of the book. Ask your instructor for the answers to the *Additional Exercises*.

Try These for Practice

Test your comprehension after reading the chapter.

1. Write $\frac{5}{16}$ as a decimal number. _____

2. Write $\frac{6.47 \times 2.3}{0.2}$ as a decimal number rounded off to the nearest tenth.

_____

3. Write 40% as a decimal number and as a fraction in lowest terms.

_____

4. $\frac{3}{7} \times \frac{14}{15} \times \frac{5}{6} =$ _____

5. Simplify: $\dfrac{\frac{5}{6}}{\frac{5}{12}}$ _____

Workspace

Exercises

Reinforce your understanding in class or at home.

Convert to proper fractions or mixed numbers.

1. $0.85 = $ _____

2. $2.7 = $ _____

3. $40 \times \dfrac{1}{2} \times \dfrac{9}{16} = $ _____

4. $2\dfrac{3}{5} \div 2 = $ _____

5. $15 \div 3\dfrac{2}{3} = $ _____

6. $9.6 \div \dfrac{3}{7} = $ _____

7. $42 \times \dfrac{1}{9,450} \times \dfrac{3}{0.02} = $ _____

Convert to decimal numbers.

8. $\dfrac{1}{8} = $ _____
   (round down to the nearest hundredth)

9. $\dfrac{14}{25} = $ _____

10. $5\dfrac{3}{10} = $ _____

11. $\dfrac{1}{200} = $ _____

12. $\dfrac{1}{75} = $ _____
    (round off to the nearest hundredth)

13. $\dfrac{870}{1,000} = $ _____

14. $\dfrac{2.73}{100} = $ _____

15. $\dfrac{14.36}{7} = $ _____
    (round down to the nearest tenth)

16. $\dfrac{0.63}{0.9} = $ _____

17. $\dfrac{0.063}{0.09} = $ _____

18. $5\dfrac{1}{2}\% = $ _____

19. $55\% = $ _____

Simplify and write the answer in decimal form.

20. $4.63 \times 6.21 = $ _____
    (round off to the nearest hundredth)

21. $0.004 \times 100 = $ _____

22. $2.3456 \times 1,000 = $ _____

23. $850 \div 0.03 = $ _____
    (round off to the nearest tenth)

24. $8.5 \div 0.12 = $ _____
    (round down to the nearest hundredth)

Simplify and write the answer in fractional form and in decimal form rounded off to the nearest tenth.

25. $0.72 \times \dfrac{1}{0.7} = $ _____

26. $\dfrac{\frac{2}{3}}{8} = $ _____

27. $\dfrac{\frac{2}{5}}{100} \times \dfrac{500}{6} =$ _____

28. $\dfrac{26 \times \frac{5}{13}}{\frac{9}{100}} =$ _____

29. $10.3\% =$ _____

30. $99.5\% =$ _____

Additional Exercises

Now, test yourself!

Convert the decimal numbers to proper fractions or mixed numbers.

1. $0.62 =$ _____

2. $5.75 =$ _____

Convert the fraction to decimal numbers.

3. $\dfrac{3}{8} =$ _____

4. $\dfrac{7}{25} =$ _____

5. $\dfrac{1}{5} =$ _____

6. $\dfrac{1}{400} =$ _____

7. $\dfrac{1}{150} =$ _____
(round down to the nearest thousandth)

8. $\dfrac{92}{100} =$ _____

9. $\dfrac{3.75}{1,000} =$ _____

10. $\dfrac{193.4}{7} =$ _____
(round off to the nearest tenth)

Convert to decimal numbers.

11. $\dfrac{0.36}{0.4} =$ _____

12. $\dfrac{0.036}{0.04} =$ _____

Multiply the decimal numbers.

13. $278.2 \times 100 =$ _____

14. $10.075 \times 10.3 =$ _____

15. $64.73 \times 1,000 =$ _____

Divide the decimal numbers.

16. $95 \div 0.05 =$ _____

17. $9.5 \div 0.05 =$ _____

Write the answers to Problems 18 through 22 in fractional form.

18. $\dfrac{7}{15} \times 20 \times \dfrac{1}{2} =$ _____

19. $3\dfrac{1}{2} \div 6 =$ _____

20. $13 \div 2\dfrac{1}{3} =$ _____

21. $6.35 \times \dfrac{1}{5} =$ _____

22. $\dfrac{1}{500} \times 1.75 \times \dfrac{1}{0.5} =$ _____

Write the answers to Problems 23 through 26 in fractional form and in decimal form rounded off to the nearest tenth.

23. $7.75 \times \dfrac{1}{0.5} =$ _____

24. $\dfrac{7}{\frac{3}{8}} =$ _____

25. $\dfrac{\frac{1}{5}}{4} \times 9 =$ _____

26. $\dfrac{\frac{2}{3} \times 170}{\frac{3}{8}} =$ _____

Write the percentages as decimal numbers.

27. $24\dfrac{3}{5}\% =$ _____

28. $63\% =$ _____

Write the percentages as fractions.

29. $2.75\% =$ _____

30. $7.5\% =$ _____

MediaLink
www.prenhall.com/olsen

Animated examples, interactive practice questions with animated solutions, and challenge tests for this chapter can be found on the Prentice Hall Dosage Calculation Tutor that accompanies this text. Additional, unique, interactive resources and activities can be found on the Companion Website.

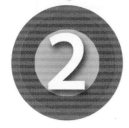
Safe and Accurate Drug Administration

Learning Outcomes

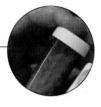

After completing this chapter you will be able to

1. Describe the six "rights" of safe medication administration.
2. Explain the legal implications of medication administration.
3. Describe the routes of medication administration.
4. Identify common abbreviations used in medication administration.
5. Compare the trade name and generic name of drugs.
6. Describe the forms in which medications are supplied.
7. Identify and interpret the components of a Drug Prescription, Physician's Order, and Medication Administration Record.
8. Interpret information found on drug labels and drug package inserts.

This chapter introduces the process of safe and accurate medication administration. The rights of the patients and the responsibilities of the people involved in the administration of medication are described.

The various forms and routes of drugs are presented as well as abbreviations used in prescribing and documenting the administration of medications. You will learn how to interpret drug orders, drug prescriptions, drug labels, medication administration records, and package inserts.

A generic drug may be manufactured by different companies under different trade names. For example, the generic drug ibuprofen is manufactured by McNeil PPC under the trade name Motrin, and by Wyeth pharmaceuticals under the trade name Advil. The active ingredients in Motrin and Advil are the same, but the size, shape, color, or fillers may be different. Be aware that patients may become confused and worried about receiving a medication that has a different name or appears to be dissimilar from their usual medication. State and federal governments now permit, encourage, and in some states mandate that the consumer be given the generic form when buying prescription drugs.

The person who administers the drug has the last opportunity to identify an error before a patient might be injured.

The Drug Administration Process

Drug administration is a process involving a chain of healthcare professionals. The **prescriber writes** the drug order, the **pharmacist fills** the order, and the **nurse administers** the drug to the patient; each is responsible for the accuracy of the order. To ensure patient safety, they must understand how a patient's drugs act and interact.

Drugs can be life-saving or life-threatening. Every year, thousands of deaths occur because of medication errors. Errors can occur at any point in the medication process.

Who Administers Drugs?

Physicians can legally prescribe medications. In many states, **physician's assistants**, **certified nurse midwives**, and **nurse practitioners** can also prescribe a range of medications related to their areas of practice.

Although prescribers may administer drugs to patients, the **registered professional nurse (RN)**, **licensed practical nurse (LPN)**, and **licensed vocational nurse (LVN)** are usually responsible for administering drugs ordered by the prescriber.

Personnel who administer medications must be familiar with applicable state laws, policies, and procedures relative to the administration of medications, and they have a legal and ethical responsibility to report medication errors. There are many organizations and groups that are striving to reduce medication errors.

Six Rights of Medication Administration

In order to prepare and administer drugs, it is imperative that you understand and follow the *Six Rights of Medication Administration*:

- Right drug
- Right dose
- Right route
- Right time
- Right patient
- Right documentation

These six "rights" should be checked before administering any medications. Failure to achieve any of these rights constitutes a medication error.

Some institutions recognize additional rights, such as the *right to know* and the *right to refuse*. Patients need to be educated about their medications, and if a patient refuses a medication, the reason must be documented and reported.

The Right Drug

A drug is a chemical substance that acts on the physiological processes in the human body. For example, the drug insulin is given to patients whose bodies do not manufacture sufficient insulin. Some drugs have more than one action. Aspirin, for example, is an antipyretic (fever-reducing), analgesic (pain-relieving), and anti-inflammatory drug that also has anticoagulant properties (keeps the blood from clotting). A drug may be taken for one, some, or all its therapeutic properties.

The *generic* name is the official accepted name of a drug, as listed in the United States Pharmacopeia (USP). The designation of USP after a drug name indicates that the drug meets government standards. A drug has only one generic name, but can have many trade names. By law, generic names must be identified on all drug labels.

Many companies may manufacture the same drug using different **trade** (patented, brand, or proprietary) names. The drug's trade name is followed by the

trademark symbol ™ or the **registration** symbol ®. For example, **Avodart**® is the trade name and **dutasteride** is the generic name for the drug shown in ● **Figure 2.1**.

Dosage strength indicates the amount of drug in a specific unit of measurement. The dosage strength of Avodart is 0.5 mg per capsule.

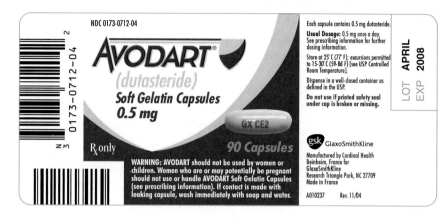

● **Figure 2.1**
Drug label for Avodart.

(Reproduced with permission of GlaxoSmithKline.)

Each drug has a unique identification number. This number is called the **National Drug Code (NDC) number**. The NDC number for Avodart is 0173-0712-04. It is printed in two places on the label and is also encoded in the bar code.

To help avoid errors, drugs should be prescribed using only the generic name or by using both the generic and trade names. *Many drugs have names that sound alike, or have names or packaging that look alike.* A healthcare organization must develop its own list of "look-alike/sound-alike drugs" in order to meet The Joint Commission on Accreditation of Healthcare Organizations (JCAHO) National Patient Safety Goals. Table 2.1 includes a sample list of drugs whose names may be confused.

Table 2.1   Look-Alike/Sound-Alike Drugs

Drug Name	Look-Alike/Sound-Alike Drug Name*
Acetazolamide*	acetohexamide
ceftazidime (Tazidime)	ceftizoxime sodium (Cefizox)
ceftin (cefuroxime axetil)	Cefzil (cefprozil)
cephalexin hydrochloride (Keftab)	cephalexin monohydrate (Keflex)
dactinomycin	daptomycin
DiaBeta*	Zebeta
ephedrine*	epinephrine
Evista*	Avinza
fluconazole (Diflucan)	fluorouracil (Adrucil)
folic acid*	folinic acid (leucovorin calcium)
glipizide (Glucotrol)	glyburide (Micronase)
heparin*	Hespan
Humalog*	Humulin
hydralazine hydrochloride (Apresoline)	hydroxyzine embonate (Atarax)
indarubicin*	daunorubicin
Inderal (propanolol hydrochloride)	Inderide (propanolol hydrochlorothiazide)
nizatidine (Axid)	nifedipine (Procardia)
Novolin 70/30*	Novolog Mix 70/30
Protapam Chloride (pralidoxime chloride)	protamine sulfate
Retrovir*	ritonvair
vinblastine*	vincristine

* These drug names are included on the JCAHO's list of look-alike or sound-alike drug names.

ALERT

The calibrated dropper *supplied with a medication* should be used ONLY for that medication. For example, the dropper that is supplied with digoxin (Lanoxin) can not be used to measure furosemide (Lasix)

The Right Dose

A person prescribing or administering medications has the *legal responsibility* of knowing the correct dose. Since no two people are exactly alike, and no drug affects every human body in exactly the same way, drug doses must be individualized. Responses to drug actions differ according to the gender, race, genetics, nutritional and health status, age, and weight of the patient (especially children and the elderly), as well as the route and time of administration.

Body surface area (BSA) is an estimate of the total skin area of a person measured in meters squared (m^2). Body surface area is determined by formulas based on height and weight or by the use of a BSA nomogram (See Chapter 6). Many drug doses administered to children or used for cancer therapy are calculated based on BSA.

Carefully read the drug label to determine the **dosage strength**. Perform and **check calculations** and pay special attention to decimal points. When giving an IV drug to a pediatric patient or giving a high-alert drug (one that has a high risk of causing injury), always **double check the dosage and pump settings**, and confirm these with a colleague. Be sure to check for the recommended **safe dosage range** based on the patient's age, BSA or weight. After you have calculated the dose, be certain to administer using standard measuring devices such as calibrated medicine droppers, syringes or cups.

The Right Route

Medications must be administered *in the form* and *via the route specified by the prescriber*. Medications are manufactured in the form of tablets, capsules, liquids, suppositories, creams, patches, or injectable medications (which are supplied in solution or in a powdered form to be reconstituted). The route indicates the site of the body and method of drug delivery.

Oral Medications. Oral medications are administered **by mouth** (PO). Oral drugs are supplied in both solid and liquid form. The most common solid forms are *tablets* (tab), *capsules* (cap), and *caplets* (●**Figure 2.2**). **Scored** tablets have a groove down the center so that the tablet can be easily broken in half. To avoid an incorrect dose, unscored tablets should never be broken. **Enteric-coated** tablets are meant to dissolve in the intestine rather than in the stomach. Therefore, they should neither be chewed nor crushed. A **capsule** contains a powder, liquid or granules in a gelatin case. *Sustained-release* (SR) or *extended-release* (XL) tablets or capsules slowly release a controlled amount of medication into the body over a period of time. Therefore, these drugs should not be opened, chewed, or crushed. Tablets for *buccal* administration (absorbed by the mucosa of

●**Figure 2.2**
Forms of oral medications.

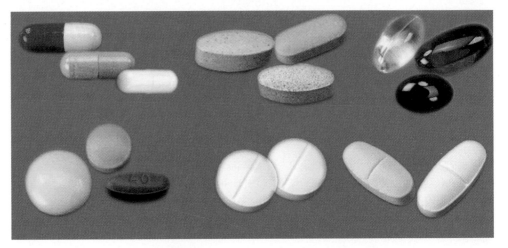

the mouth) and tablets for *sublingual* (SL) administration (absorbed under the tongue) should never be swallowed. Oral drugs also come in liquid forms: *elixir, syrup* and *suspension*. An **elixir** is an alcohol solution, a **syrup** is a medication dissolved in a sugar and water solution, and a **suspension** consists of an insoluble drug in a liquid base.

Parenteral Medications. Parenteral medications are those that are injected (via needle) into the body by various routes. Drug forms for parenteral use are sterile and must be administered using aseptic (sterile) technique.

The most common parenteral sites are the following:

- **Intramuscular (IM):** into the muscle
- **Subcutaneous (subcut):** into the subcutaneous tissue
- **Intravenous (IV):** into the vein
- **Intradermal (ID):** beneath the skin
- **Intracardiac (IC):** into the cardiac muscle

Cutaneous Medications. Cutaneous medications are those that are administered through the skin or mucous membrane. Cutaneous routes include the following:

- **Topical:** administered on the skin surface
- **Transdermal:** contained in a patch or disk and applied to the skin
- **Inhalation:** breathed into the respiratory tract through the nose or mouth
- **Solutions and ointments:** applied to the mucosa of the eyes (optic), nose (nasal), ears (otic), and mouth
- **Suppositories:** are shaped for insertion into a body cavity (vagina, rectum, or urethra) and dissolve at body temperature

Some drugs are supplied in multiple forms and therefore can be administered by a variety of routes. For example, Tigan (trimethobenzamide HCl) is supplied as a capsule, suppository, or solution for injection.

The Right Time

The prescriber will indicate when and how often a medication should be administered. Oral medications can be given either before or after meals, depending on the action of the drug. Medications can be ordered *once a day* (daily), *twice a day* (b.i.d.), *three times a day* (t.i.d.), and *four times a day* (q.i.d). Most healthcare facilities designate specific times for these administrations. To maintain a more stable level of the drug in the patient, the period between administrations of the drug should be prescribed at regular intervals, such as q4h (every four hours), q6h, q8h, or q12h.

Be aware that b.i.d. is not necessarily the same as q12h. B.i.d. may mean *administer at 10 A.M. and 6 P.M.*, whereas q12h may mean *administer at 10 A.M. and 10 P.M.* (depending on the particular facility's policy). Drugs can also be ordered to be administered as needed (prn).

The Right Patient

Before administering any medication, it is essential to determine the identity of the recipient. Know the identifiers recognized and required by your agency. JCAHO requires the use of at least two identifiers, such as the patient identification bracelet information, verbalization of the patient's name by the patient or parent, patient's hospital number, or patient's home telephone number. *Never use the patient's bed number or room number.* After identifying the patient, match the drug order, patient's name, and age to the Medication Administration Record (MAR). Some agencies use a scanner to match a bar code on the patient's ID bracelet to a bar code on the MAR.

The Right Documentation

Always document the name and dosage of the drug, as well as the route and time of administration on the MAR. Sign your initials *immediately after, but never before*, the dose is given. It is important to include any relevant information. For example, document patient allergies to medications, heart rate (when giving digoxin), and blood pressure (when giving antihypertensive drugs). All documentation must be legible. Remember the axiom, "If it's not documented, it's not done."

Anticipate side effects! A side effect is an undesired physiologic response to a drug. For example, codeine relieves pain, but its side effects include constipation, nausea, drowsiness, and itching. Be sure to record any observed side effects and discuss them with the prescriber.

Safe drug administration requires a knowledge of common abbreviations. For instance, when the prescriber writes **"Demerol 75 mg IM q4h prn pain,"** the person administering the drug reads this as **"Demerol, 75 milligrams, intramuscular, every four hours, as needed for pain."** Only approved abbreviations should be used (Table 2.2).

Table 2.2 Common Abbreviations Used for Medication Administration

Abbreviation	Meaning	Abbreviation	Meaning
Route:		q12h	every twelve hours
ID	intradermal	Q.I.D., q.i.d.	four times per day
IM	intramuscular	Stat	immediately
IV	intravenous	T.I.D., t.i.d.	three times per day
IVP	intravenous push		
IVPB	intravenous piggyback	**General:**	
NG	nasogastric tube	cap	capsule
PEG	percutaneous endoscopic gastrostomy	d.a.w.	dispense as written
		ER	extended release
PO	by mouth	g	gram
PR	by rectum	gr	grain
SL	sublingual	gtt	drop
Supp	suppository	kg	kilogram
		L	liter
Frequency:		mcg	microgram
ac	before meals	mg	milligram
ad lib	as desired	mL	milliliter
B.I.D., b.i.d.	two times a day	NKA	no known allergies
h, hr	hour	NPO	nothing by mouth
pc	after meals	Sig	directions to patient
prn	whenever needed or necessary	Susp	suspension
q	every	SR	sustained release
q2h	every two hours	t or tsp	teaspoon
q4h	every four hours	T or tbs	tablespoon
q6h	every six hours	tab	tablet
q8h	every eight hours	XL	extended release

JCAHO requires healthcare organizations to follow its official *"Do Not Use List"* that applies to all medication orders and all medication documentation. See Table 2.3.

Table 2.3   JCAHO Official "Do Not Use List"[1]

Do Not Use	Potential Problem	Use Instead
U (for unit)	Mistaken for "0" (zero), the number "4" (four) or "cc"	Write "unit"
IU (International Unit)	Mistaken for IV (intravenous) or the number 10 (ten)	Write "International Unit"
Q.D., QD, q.d., qd (daily)	Mistaken for each other	Write "daily"
Q.O.D., QOD, q.o.d, qod (every other day)	Period after the Q mistaken for "I" and the "O" mistaken for "I"	Write "every other day"
Trailing zero (X.0 mg)[2]	Decimal point is missed	Write X mg
Lack of leading zero (.X mg)		Write 0.X mg
MS	Can mean morphine sulfate or magnesium sulfate	Write "morphine sulfate"
		Write "magnesium sulfate"
MSO_4 and $MgSO_4$	Confused for one another	

[1] Applies to all orders and all medication-related documentation that is handwritten (including free-text computer entry) or on preprinted forms.

[2] **Exception:** A "trailing zero" may be used only where required to demonstrate the level of precision of the value being reported, such as for laboratory results, imaging studies that report size of lesions, or catheter/tube sizes. It may not be used in medication orders or other medication-related documentation.

Additional Abbreviations, Acronyms, and Symbols
(For *possible* future inclusion in the Official "Do Not Use" List)

Do Not Use	Potential Problem	Use Instead
> (greater than)	Misinterpreted as the number "7" (seven) or the letter "L"	Write "greater than"
< (less than)		Write "less than"
	Confused for one another	
Abbreviations for drug names	Misinterpreted due to similar abbreviations for multiple drugs	Write drug names in full
Apothecary units	Unfamiliar to many practitioners	Use metric units
	Confused with metric units	
@	Mistaken for the number "2" (two)	Write "at"
cc	Mistaken for U (units) when poorly written	Write "mL" or "milliliters"
μg	Mistaken for mg (milligrams) resulting in one thousand-fold overdose	Write "mcg" or "micrograms"

Drug Prescriptions

Before anyone can administer any medication, there must be a legal order or prescription for the medication.

A *drug prescription* is a directive to the pharmacist for a drug to be given to a patient who is being seen in a medical office or clinic, or is being discharged from a healthcare facility. A prescription can be written, faxed, phoned, or emailed from a secure encrypted computer system to a pharmacist.

There are many varieties of prescription forms. All prescriptions should contain the following:

■ Prescriber's full name, address, telephone number, and (when the prescription is given for a controlled substance), the Drug Enforcement Administration (DEA) number

■ Date the prescription is written

■ Patient's full name, address, and age or date of birth

■ Drug name (generic name should be included), dosage, route, frequency, and amount to be dispensed

■ When only the trade name is written, the prescriber must indicate whether it is acceptable to substitute a generic form

■ Directions to the patient that must appear on the drug container

■ Number of refills permitted

Every state has a drug substitution law that either mandates or may permit a less-expensive generic drug substitution by the pharmacist. If the prescriber has an objection to a generic drug substitute, the prescriber will write "do not substitute," "dispense as written," "no generic substitution," or "medically necessary." (●**Figure 2.3**).

Adam Smith, M.D.
100 Main Street
Utopia, New York, 10000

Phone (212) 345- 6789   License # 123456

Name: *Joan Soto*   Date: *November 24, 2007*

Address: *4205 Main Street*   Age/DOB: *04/20/48*
Utopia, NY

Rx   *Glucotrol 5 mg tablets*
Sig: *1 tablet PO, daily, 30 minutes before breakfast*

Dispense: *90*
Refills: *1*

THIS PRESCRIPTION WILL BE FILLED GENERICALLY UNLESS THE PRESCRIBER WRITES "d a w" IN THE BOX BELOW.

	d a w	
	Adam Smith MD	

●**Figure 2.3**
Drug prescription for Glucotrol.

This prescription is interpreted as follows:

■ Prescriber: Adam Smith, M.D.
■ Prescriber address: 100 Main Street., Utopia, NY
■ Prescriber phone number: (212) 345-6789
■ Date prescription written: November 24, 2007
■ Patient's full name: Joan Soto

- Patient address: 4205 Main Street, Utopia NY
- Patient date of birth: April 20, 1948
- Drug name: Glucotrol (trade name)
- Dosage: 5 mg
- Route: by mouth (PO)
- Frequency: once a day
- Amount to be dispensed: 90 tablets
- Acceptable to substitute a   no, the prescriber has written "d a w"
  generic form?
- Directions to the patient: take 1 tablet daily 30 minutes before breakfast
- Refill instructions: one refill permitted

Read the prescription in ● **Figure 2.4** and complete the following information.

- Date prescription written: _____
- Patient full name: _____
- Patient address: _____
- Patient date of birth: _____
- Generic drug name: _____
- Dosage: _____
- Route: _____
- Frequency: _____
- Amount to be dispensed: _____
- Acceptable to substitute a generic form? _____
- Directions to the patient: _____
- Refill instructions: _____

Primary Care Associates
1234 Spring Street, Kansas
(913) 999-5678

Name: _Mary Moral_   Date: _10/22/07_
Address: _124 Winding Lane_   Date of Birth: _4/29/52_
Manhattan, Kansas

Rx   _doxycycline (Vibra-Tabs) 100 mg_
Disp # 14
Sig: Take 1 capsule PO b.i.d. for 7 days

Refills: _0_

Alicia Rodriguez, ARNP
Alicia Rodriguez, Adult Registered Nurse Practitioner

_____

Substitution is mandatory
unless the words "no substitution" appear in the box above.

● **Figure 2.4**
**Drug prescription
for doxycycline.**

This is what you should have found:

- Date prescription written: 10/22/07
- Patient full name: Mary Moral
- Patient address: 124 Winding Lane, Manhattan, Kansas
- Patient date of birth: 4/29/52
- Generic drug name: doxycycline
- Dosage: 100 mg
- Route: by mouth
- Frequency: two times a day
- Amount to be dispensed: 14 capsules
- Acceptable to substitute a generic form?   yes
- Directions to the patient: take one capsule twice a day for 7 days
- Refill instructions: cannot be refilled

Medication Orders and Administration Records

Medication Orders

Medication orders are directives to the pharmacist for the drugs used in a hospital or other healthcare facility. The terms **medication orders, drug orders,** and **physician's orders** are used interchangeably; and the forms used will vary from agency to agency. No medication should be given without a medication order. Medication orders can be **written** or **verbal.**

Written medication orders are stated in a special book for doctor's orders, on a physician's order sheet in the patient's chart, or in a computer.

A *verbal* order must contain the same components as a written order or else it is invalid. In order to provide for the safety of the patient generally verbal orders may be taken only in an emergency. Each medication order should follow a specific sequence: drug name, dose, route, and frequency. The verbal order must eventually be written and signed by the physician.

Types of Medication Orders

The most common type of medication order is the *routine order*, which indicates that the ordered drug is administered until a discontinuation order is written or until a specified date is reached.

A *standing order* is prescribed in anticipation of sudden changes in a patient's condition. Standing orders are used frequently in critical care units, where a patient's condition may change rapidly, and immediate action would be required. Standing orders may also be used in long-term care facilities where a physician may not be readily available; for example, "*Tylenol (acetaminophen) 650 mg PO q4h for temperature of 101 °F or higher.*"

A *prn order* is written by the prescriber for a drug to be given when a patient needs it; for example, "*Codeine 30 mg PO q4h prn mild–moderate pain.*"

A *stat order* is an order that is to be administered immediately. Stat orders are usually written for emergencies or when a patient's condition suddenly changes; for example, "*Lasix 80 mg IV stat.*"

ALERT

If persons administering medications have difficulty understanding or interpreting the orders, they must clarify the orders with the prescribers.

Components of a Medication Order

The essential components of a medication order are the following:

- **Patient's full name and date of birth:** Often this information is stamped or imprinted on the medication order form. Additional information may include the patient's admission number, religion, type of insurance, and physician's name.

- **Date and time the order was written:** This includes the month, day, year, and time of day. Many institutions use military time, which is based on a "24 hour clock" that does not use A.M. or P.M. (●**Figure 2.5**). Military times are written as four-digit numbers. Thus, 2:00 A.M. in military time is 0200h (pronounced "Oh two hundred hours"), 12 noon is 1200h (pronounced twelve hundred hours), 2:00 P.M. is 1400h (pronounced *fourteen hundred hours*), and midnight is 2400h, also written as 0000h.

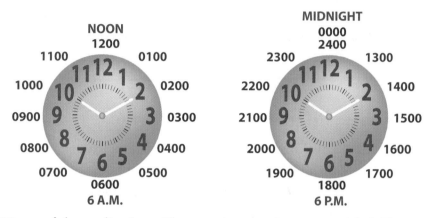

●**Figure 2.5**
Clocks Showing 10:10 A.M. (1010h) and 10:10 P.M. (2210h).

- **Name of the medication:** The generic name is recommended. If a prescriber desires to prescribe a trade name drug, "no generic substitution" must be specified.

- **Dosage of the medication:** The amount of the drug.

- **Route of administration.**

- **Time and frequency of administration.**

- **Signature of the prescriber:** The medication order is not legal without the signature of the prescriber.

- **Signature of the person transcribing the order:** This may be the responsibility of a nurse or others identified by agency policy.

The physician's order in ●**Figure 2.6** can be interpreted as follows:
Name of patient: John Camden
Birth date: Feb. 11, 1955
Date of admission: Nov. 20, 2007
Admission number: 602412
Religion: Roman Catholic (RC)
Insurance: Blue Cross Blue Shield (BCBS)
Date and time the order was written: 11/20/2007 at 0800h or 8:00 A.M.
Name of the medication: captopril
Dosage: 25 mg
Route of administration: PO (by mouth)
Frequency of administration: t.i.d., three times a day for 7 days
Signature of person writing the order: I. Patel, M.D.
Person who transcribed the order: Mary Jones, RN

⊙ GENERAL HOSPITAL ⊙

PRESS HARD WITH BALLPOINT PEN. WRITE DATE & TIME AND SIGN EACH ORDER

DATE	TIME	A.M.
11/20/2007	0800h	P.M.

IMPRINT
602412   11/20/07
John Camden   2/11/55
23 Jones Ave.   RC
New York, NY 10024   BCBS

I. Patel, M.D.

Captopril 25 mg PO t.i.d. for 7 days

ORDERS NOTED
DATE *11/20/07* TIME *0830*   A.M.
                                 P.M.

NURSE'S SIG. *Mary Jones RN*

SIGNATURE   *I. Patel*   M.D.

FILLED BY   DATE

PHYSICIAN'S ORDERS

● **Figure 2.6**
Physician's order for captopril.

Example 2.1

Interpret the physician's order sheet shown in ● **Figure 2.7** and record the following information:

⊙ GENERAL HOSPITAL ⊙

PRESS HARD WITH BALLPOINT PEN. WRITE DATE & TIME AND SIGN EACH ORDER

DATE	TIME	A.M.
11/22/2007	1800h	P.M.

IMPRINT
422934   11/22/07
Catherine Rodriguez   12/01/62
40 Addison Avenue
Rutlans, VT 06701   Prot

M. Ling, M.D.   GHI-CPB

Cipro (ciprofloxacin) 500 mg

PO q12h

ORDERS NOTED
DATE *11/22/07* TIME *1830h*   A.M.
                                  P.M.

NURSE'S SIG. *Sara Gordon RN*

SIGNATURE   *Mae Ling*   M.D.

FILLED BY   DATE

PHYSICIAN'S ORDERS

● **Figure 2.7**
Physician's order for Cipro.

Date order written: _____

Time order written: _____

Name of drug: _____

Dosage: _____

Route of administration: _____

Frequency of administration: _____

Name of prescriber: _____

Name of patient: _____

Birth date: _____

Religion: _____

Type of insurance: _____

Person who transcribed the order: _____

This is what you should have found:

■ **Date order written:**	11/22/2007
■ **Time order written:**	1800h or 6:00 P.M.
■ **Name of drug:**	Cipro (ciprofloxacin)
■ **Dosage:**	500 mg
■ **Route:**	by mouth
■ **Frequency of administration:**	every 12 hours
■ **Name of prescriber:**	Mae Ling, M.D.
■ **Name of patient:**	Catherine Rodriguez
■ **Birth date:**	December 1, 1962
■ **Religion:**	Protestant
■ **Type of insurance:**	GHI-CBP
■ **Person who transcribed the order:**	Sara Gordon, RN

Medication Administration Records

A Medication Administration Record (MAR) is a form that healthcare facilities use to document all the drugs administered to a patient.

Routine, PRN, and STAT medications all may be written in separate locations on the MAR. PRN and STAT medications may also have a separate form. If a medication is to be given regularly, a complete schedule is written for all administration times. Each time a dose is administered, the healthcare worker initials the time of administration. The full name, title, and initials of the person who gave the medication must be recorded on the MAR.

After a prescriber's order has been verified, a nurse or other healthcare provider transcribes the order to the MAR. This record is used to check the medication order; prepare the correct medication dose; and record the date, time, and route of administration.

The essential components of the MAR include the following:

- **Patient information:** a stamp or printed label with patient identification (name, date of birth, medical record number).
- **Dates:** when the order was written, when to start the medication, and when to discontinue it.
- **Medication information:** full name of the drug, dose, route, and frequency of administration.
- **Time of administration:** frequency as stated in the prescriber's order; for example, t.i.d. Times for PRN and *one-time doses* are recorded *precisely* at the time they are administered.
- **Initials:** the initials and the signature of the person who administered the medication are recorded.
- **Special instructions:** instructions relating to the medication; for example, "Hold if systolic BP is less than 100."

Example 2.2

Study the MAR in ●Figure 2.8; then complete the following chart and answer the questions.

UNIVERSITY HOSPITAL	789652 Wendy Kim 44 Chester Avenue New York, N.Y. 10003	7/3/07 12/20/60 RC Medicaid
DAILY MEDICATION ADMNISTRATION RECORD	Dr. Juan Rodriguez, M.D.	

PATIENT NAME _____ *Wendy Kim* _____

ROOM # _____ *422* _____   IF ANOTHER RECORDS IS IN USE ☐

ALLERGIC TO (RECORD IN RED): _____ *tomato, codeine* _____

DATES GIVEN ⋮ ↓   DATE DISCHARGED:

RED CHECK INITIAL	ORDER DATE	INITIAL	EXP DATE	MEDICATION, DOSAGE, FREQUENCY AND ROUTE	HOURS	12	13	14	15											
	9/12	JY	9/19	Pepcid (famotidine) 20 mg	0600	/	MC	MC												
				IVPB q12h for 7 days begin at 1800h	1800	MJ	SG	SG												
	9/12	JY	9/18	digoxin 0.125 mg PO daily	0900	JY	JY	JY												
	9/12	JY	9/18	Lotensin (benazepril hydrochloride)	0900	JY	JY	JY												
				20 mg PO q12h	2100	MJ	SG	SG												
	9/12	JY	9/18	Ticlid (ticlopidine hydrocholoride)	0900	JY	JY	JY												
				250 mg PO daily																
	9/12	JY	9/18	Xanax (alprazolam) 0.5 mg PO HS	2100	MJ	SG	SG												

INT.	NURSES' FULL SIGNATURE AND TITLE	INT.	NURSES' FULL SIGNATURE AND TITLE
JY	Jim Young R.N.		
MC	Marie Colon R.N.		
MJ	Mary Jones L.P.N.		
SG	Sara Gordon R.N.		

●**Figure 2.8**
MAR for Wendy Kim.

Name of Drug	Dose	Route of Administration	Time of Administration

1. Identify the drugs and their doses administered at 9:00 A.M.

   _____

2. Identify the drugs and their doses administered at 9:00 P.M.

   _____

3. Who administered the ticlopidine hydrochloride on 9/14?

   _____

4. What is the route of administration for famotidine?

   _____

5. What is the time of administration for Pepcid?

   _____

This is what you should have found:

Name of Drug	Dose	Route of Administration	Time of Administration
Pepcid (famotidine)	20 mg	IVPB	0600h (6 A.M.) & 1800h (6 P.M.)
digoxin	0.125 mg	PO	0900h (9 A.M.)
Lotensin(benazepril hydrochloride)	20 mg	PO	0900h (9 A.M.) and 2100h (9 P.M.)
Ticlid (ticlopidine hydrochloride)	250 mg	PO	0900h (9 A.M.)
Xanax (alprazolam)	0.5 mg	PO	2100h (9 P.M.)

1. Digoxin 0.125 mg; Lotensin 20 mg; Ticlid 250 mg
2. Lotensin 20 mg, Xanax 0.5mg
3. Jim Young, RN
4. IVPB
5. 0600h (6 A.M.) and 1800h (6 P.M.)

Example 2.3

Study the MAR in ●Figures 2.9a and 2.9b; then fill in the following chart and answer the questions.

Name of Routine Drug	Dose	Route of Administration	Time of Administration

1. Which drugs were administered at 10:00 A.M. on 11/23?

   _____

2. Which drug was given stat and what was the route; date and time?

   _____

3. Who administered the captopril at 2:00 P.M. on 11/21?

   _____

4. What is the route of administration for Epogen?

   _____

5. How many doses of Capoten did the patient receive by 7:00 P.M. on 11/24?

   _____

UNIVERSITY HOSPITAL	659204 Mohammad Kamal 4103 Ely Avenue Bronx, N.Y. 10466	11/20/07 10/2/52 Musl GHI-CBP
DAILY MEDICATION ADMNISTRATION RECORD	Dr. Indu Patel, M.D.	

PATIENT NAME _____Mohammad Kamal_____

ROOM # _____302_____   ☐ IF ANOTHER RECORDS IS IN USE

ALLERGIC TO (RECORD IN RED): _____sulfa, fish_____

DATES GIVEN MONTH/DAY   YEAR: _2007_

RED CHECK INITIAL	ORDER DATE	INITIAL	EXP DATE	MEDICATION, DOSAGE, FREQUENCY AND ROUTE	TIME	11/20	11/21	11/22	11/23	11/24	11/25	11/26
	11/20	MC	11/26	Coumadin (warfarin sodium) 10 mg PO daily	10AM	—	MC	MC	MC	MJ	MJ	JY
	11/20	MC	11/26	Capoten (captopril) 25 mg PO t.i.d.	10AM	—	MC	MC	MC	MJ	MJ	JY
					BP	—	160/110	150/70	160/110	138/86	130/80	130/80
					2PM	MC	MC	MC	MC	MJ	MJ	JY
					BP	150/90	140/80	140/90	140/80	130/84	130/82	128/76
					6PM	MC	MC	MC	MC	MJ	MJ	JY
					BP	160/100	150/90	160/100	140/80	130/80	128/80	128/80
	11/20	MC	11/26	Lasix (furosemide) 20 mg PO daily	10AM	—	MC	MC	MC	MJ	MJ	JY
	11/20	SG	11/27	Maxipime (cefepime hydrochloride) 1g IVBP q12hr for 7 days	10AM	—	MC	MC	MC	MJ	MJ	JY
					10PM	—	SG	SG	SG	SG	SG	SG
	11/21	MC	11/27	Epogen (erythropoietin) 3,000 units subcutaneous, three times per week, start on 11/21	10AM	—	MC		MC		MJ	
	11/21	MC	11/27	digoxin, 0.125 mg PO daily	10AM	—	MC	MC	MC	MJ	MJ	JY
					HR		72	70	96	76	80	80

INT.	NURSES' FULL SIGNATURE AND TITLE	INT.	NURSES' FULL SIGNATURE AND TITLE
MC	Marie Colon R.N.		
SG	Sara Gordon R.N.		
MJ	Mary Jones L.P.N.		
JY	Jim Young R.N.		

● **Figure 2.9a**
MAR for Mohammad Kamal.

UNIVERSITY HOSPITAL

659204	11/20/07
Mohammad Kamal	10/2/52
4103 Ely Avenue	Musl
Bronx, N.Y. 10466	GHI-CBP

DAILY MEDICATION ADMINSTRATION RECORD

Dr. Indu Patel, M.D.

PATIENT NAME ___Mohammad Kamal___

ROOM # ___302___

IF ANOTHER RECORDS IS IN USE ☐

ALLERGIC TO (RECORD IN RED): ___sulfa, fish___

DATES GIVEN ⬇ MONTH/DAY   YEAR: ___2007___

PRN MEDICATION

ORDER DATE	EXPIRATION DATE/TIME	MEDICATION, DOSAGE, FREQUENCY AND ROUTE		DOSES GIVEN						
11/20	11/27	Tylenol (acetaminophen) 650 mg PO q 3-4 h prn pain	DATE	11/20	11/20	11/20				
			TIME	6 PM	10 AM	6 PM				
			INIT	MJ	MC	6 PM				
11/20	11/27	Robitussin DM 10 ml	DATE	11/20	11/21					
			TIME	10 AM	10 PM					
			INIT	MJ	SG					
		PO q12h prn	DATE							
			TIME							
			INIT							
11/20	11/27	Tylenol (acetaminophen) 325 mg PO q 3-4 h prn	DATE							
			TIME							
			INIT							
		Temp above 101° F	DATE							
			TIME							
			INIT							

STAT-ONE DOSE-PRE-OPERATIVE MEDICATIONS   ⬭ Check here if additional sheet in use.

ORDER DATE	MEDICATION-DOSAGE ROUTE	DATE	TIME	INIT	ORDER DATE	MEDICATION-DOSAGE ROUTE	DATE	TIME	INIT
11/23	Dilaudid (hydromorphone) 2 mg IV now	11/23	10AM	MC					

INT.	NURSES' FULL SIGNATURE AND TITLE	INT.	NURSES' FULL SIGNATURE AND TITLE
MJ	Mary Jones R.N.		
MC	Marie Colon R.N.		
SG	Sara Gordon R.N.		

● **Figure 2.9b**
MAR for Mohammad Kamal.

Here is what you should have found:

Name of Routine Drug	Dose	Route of Administration	Time of Administration
Coumadin (warfarin sodium)	10 mg	PO	10:00 A.M.
Capoten (captopril)	25 mg	PO	10:00 A.M., 2:00 P.M., 6:00 P.M.
Lasix (furosemide)	20 mg	PO	10:00 A.M.
Maxipime (cefepime hydrochloride)	1 g	IVPB	10:00 A.M. and 10:00 P.M.
Epogen (erythropoietin)	3,000 units	subcutaneously	three times a week at 10:00 A.M.
digoxin	0.125 mg	PO	10:00 A.M.

1. Coumadin 10 mg; Capoten 25 mg; Lasix 20 mg; Maxipime 1g, Epogen 3,000 units, digoxin 0.125 mg, Dilaudid 2 mg.
2. Dilaudid IV on 11/23 at 10:00 A.M.
3. Marie Colon, RN
4. subcutaneous
5. 14

Computerized Recordkeeping

Many healthcare agencies computerize the medication process. Those who prescribe or administer medications must use security codes and passwords to access the computer system. Prescribers input orders and all other essential patient information directly into a computer terminal. The order is received in the pharmacy, where a patient's drug profile (list of drugs) is maintained. The nurse verifies the order in the computer and inputs his/her digital ID after the medication is administered. A computer printout replaces the handwritten MAR.

One advantage of a computerized system is that handwritten orders do not need to be deciphered or transcribed. The computer program can also identify possible interactions among the patient's medications and automatically alert the pharmacist and persons administering the drugs.

Example 2.4

The MAR in ●**Figure 2.10** breaks the day into "shifts:" 11 P.M. to 7 A.M., 7 A.M. to 3 P.M., and 3 P.M. to 11 P.M. . Use this computerized MAR to answer the following questions:

●**Figure 2.10**
A portion of a computerized MAR.

SCHEDULED	12/06/07–12/07/07 2301–0700	12/07/07 0701–1500	12/07/07 1501–2300
℞ Cefepime (Maxipime)		0840 2 g TVPB MAB	2015
℞ Emoxaparin Na (Lovenox)		1026 40 mg subcutaneous MAB	
℞ Furosemide (Lasix)	0611 20 mg TVP DJS		
℞ Hetastarch (he SPAN)		0920 250 mL IVPB MAB	
℞ KCl (Potassium chloride)		1026 20 mEq ER tab PO MAB	
℞ Metoprolol XL (Toprol XL)		1000 CANCEL MAB	2200
℞ Metronidazole (Flagyl)	0611 500 mg IVPB DJS	1324 500 mg IVPB MAB	2200
℞ NTG (Nitroglycerin)	0110 15 mg oint topical DJS 0611 15 mg oint topical DJS	1231 15 oint topical MAB	1800
℞ Pantoprazole (Protonix) 40 mg IVPB		1026 40 mg IVPB MAB	
PRN	12/06/07–12/07/07 2301–0700	12/07/07 0701–1500	12/07/07 1501–2300
℞ Saline flush	0110 2 mL IV flush DJS	0829 2 mL IV flush MAB	1600
℞ Morphine	0115 4 mg IVP DJS 0439 4 mg IVP DJS	1306 2 mg IVP MAB	
IV	12/06/07–12/07/07 2301–0700	12/07/07 0701–1500	12/07/07 1501–2300
℞ NS (NaCl, 0.9%, 1 L)		0810	2130
PRN ORDERS			
Hydrocodone 5 mg and Acetaminophen 500 mg	x 1–2 tab PO q4h prn process if pain		
Saline flush	2 mL IV flush q8 at 0000/0800/1600 and prn		
Insulin, human regular sliding scale {Novolin R SS}	See scale prn if BS 200–249 mg/dL give 4 Units of Reg Insulin		

1. Identify the extended-release drug administered on 12/07/07.

   _____

2. What drugs were administered at 6:11 A.M. on 12/06/07?

   _____

3. Identify the dosage, route, and time that Flagyl was administered before noon on 12/07/07.

   _____

4. Identify the name, dosage, route, and time of administration of the PRN drugs administered after noon on 12/07/07.

   _____

5. How many times did the patient receive NTG (Nitroglycerin) on 12/07/07?

   _____

This is what you should have found:

1. KCl (Potassium chloride)

2. Furosemide (Lasix), Metronidazole (Flagyl), and NTG (Nitroglycerin)

3. 500 mg, IVPB at 0611h (6:11 A.M.)

4. Saline flush 2 mL IV flush was given at 0829h (8:29 A.M.) and Morphine 2 mg IVP was given at 1306h (1:06 P.M.)

5. Three times

Drug Labels

You will need to understand the information found on drug labels in order to calculate drug dosages. The important features of a drug label are identified in ● Figure 2.11.

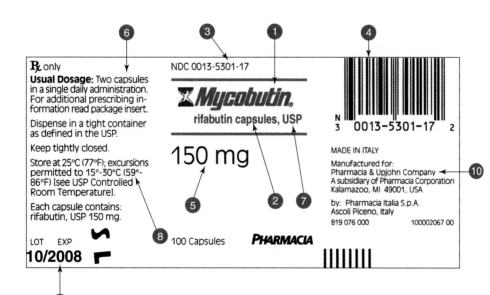

● **Figure 2.11**
Drug label for Mycobutin.

1. **Name of drug:** Mycobutin is the trade name. In this case, the name begins with an uppercase letter, is in large type, and is boldly visible on the label. The generic name is rifabutin, written in lowercase letters.

2. **Form of drug:** The drug is in the form of a capsule.

3. **National Drug Code (NDC) number:** 0013-5301-17.

4. **Bar code:** Has the NDC number encoded in it.

5. **Dosage strength:** 150 mg of the drug are contained in one capsule.

6. **Dosage recommendations:** 2 capsules in a single daily administration. **Note that the manufacturer informs you to read the package insert.**

7. **USP:** This drug meets the standards of the United States Pharmacopeia.

8. **Storage directions:** Some drugs have to be stored under controlled conditions if they are to retain their effectiveness. This drug should be stored at 25°C (77°F).

9. **Expiration date:** The expiration date specifies when the drug should be discarded. After 10/2008 (October 31, 2008), the drug cannot be dispensed and should be discarded. For the sake of simplicity, not every drug label in this textbook will have an expiration date.

10. **Manufacturer:** Pharmacia & Upjohn.

ALERT

Always read the expiration date! After the expiration date, the drug may lose its potency or act differently in a patient's body. Discard expired drugs. Never give expired drugs to patients!

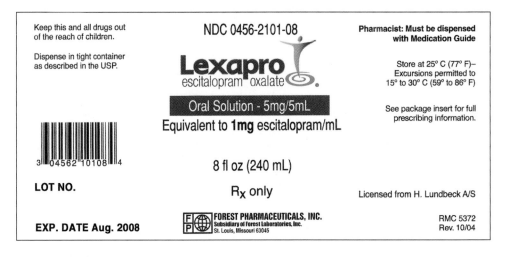

● **Figure 2.12**
Drug label for Lexapro.

(Courtesy of Forest Pharmaceuticals, Inc.)

The label in ● **Figure 2.12** indicates the following information:

1. **Trade name:** Lexapro

2. **Generic name:** escitalopram oxalate

3. **Form:** oral solution

4. **Dosage strength:** 5 mg/5 mL, equivalent to 1 mg of escitalopram/mL

5. **Dosage recommendations:** See package insert for full prescribing information

6. **NDC number:** 0456-2101-08

7. **Expiration date:** August 2008

8. **Total volume in container:** 8 fl oz (240 mL)

9. **Manufacturer:** Forest Pharmaceuticals, Inc.

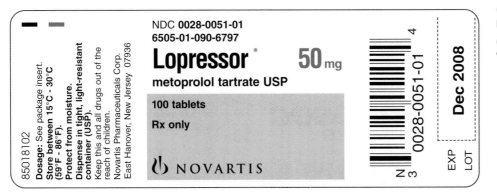

● **Figure 2.13**
Drug label for Lopressor.

(Reproduced with the permission of Novartis Pharmaceuticals.)

The label for the antihypertensive drug Lopressor in ●**Figure 2.13** indicates the following:

1. **Trade name:** Lopressor
2. **Generic name:** metoprolol tartrate
3. **Form:** Tablets
4. **Dosage strength:** 50 mg per tablet
5. **NDC number:** 0028-0051-01
6. **Expiration:** Discard after December 31, 2008
7. **Instructions for dispensing:** Protect from moisture and dispense in tight, light-resistant container

Example 2.5

Examine the label shown in ●**Figure 2.14** and record the following information:

1. Trade name: _____
2. Generic name: _____
3. Form: _____
4. Dosage strength: _____
5. Amount of drug in container: _____
6. Storage temperature: _____
7. Special instructions: _____

This is what you should have found:

1. **Trade name:** Norvir
2. **Generic name:** ritonavir
3. **Form:** Oral solution
4. **Dosage strength:** 80 mg per mL
5. **Amount of drug in container:** 240 mL
6. **Storage temperature:** Do not refrigerate
7. **Special instructions:** Shake well before use. ALERT: Find out about medicines that should NOT be taken with Norvir.

NDC 0074-1940-63
240 mL

NORVIR®

(RITONAVIR ORAL SOLUTION)

80 mg per mL

Shake well before each use.
DO NOT REFRIGERATE
Use by product expiration date.

Ⓐ   ℞ only   02-8410-2/R4

ALERT
Find out about medicines
that should NOT be taken
with NORVIR.

Note to Pharmacist: Do not cover ALERT
box with pharmacy label.

EXP. MARCH 2008
LOT

● **Figure 2.14**
Drug label for Norvir.

(Reproduced with permission of Abbott Laboratories.)

Example 2.6

Examine the label shown in ● **Figure 2.15** and record the following information:

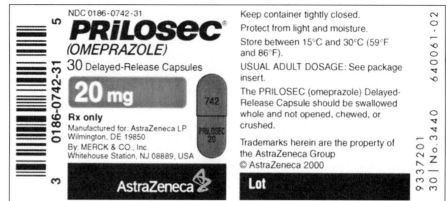

● **Figure 2.15**
Drug label for Prilosec.
(Courtesy of AstraZeneca Pharmaceuticals LP.)

1. Trade name: _____

2. Generic name: _____

3. Form: _____

4. Dosage strength: _____

5. Amount of drug in container: _____

6. Usual adult dosage: _____

7. Storage temperature: _____

8. Special instructions: _____

This is what you should have found:

1. **Trade name:** Prilosec

2. **Generic name:** omeprazole

3. **Form:** Delayed-Release capsules

4. **Dosage strength:** 20 mg per capsule

5. **Amount of drug in container:** 30 capsules

6. **Usual adult dosage:** See package insert

7. **Storage temperature:** Store between 15 °C and 30 °C (59°F to 86°F)

8. **Special instructions:** Capsule should be swallowed whole and not opened, chewed, or crushed

Some medications are a combination of two or more generic drugs in one form. Both names and strength of each drug are on the label. Two such medication labels follow.

Examine the label shown in ●**Figure 2.16**. The label for this anti-hypertensive combination drug Lotrel 5/10 indicates that each capsule contains 5 mg of amlodipine and 10 mg of benazepril.

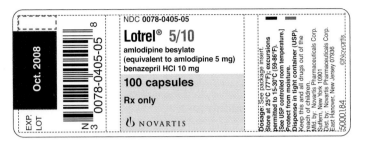

●**Figure 2.16**
Drug label for Lotrel.

(Reproduced with the permission of Novartis Pharmaceuticals.)

Example 2.7

Examine the label shown in ● Figure 2.17 and answer the following questions:

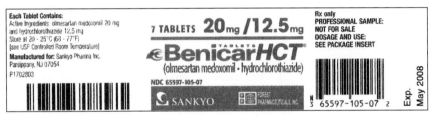

●**Figure 2.17**
Drug label for Benicar HCT.

(Courtesy of Forest Pharmaceutical, Inc.)

1. What is the trade name and dosage strength of the drug?

   _____

2. What is the dosage strength of hydrochlorothiazide?

   _____

3. What is the route of administration?

   _____

4. What is the amount of drug in the container?

   _____

5. What is the usual dosage?

   _____

   This is what you should have found:

1. Benicar HCT is the trade name, and the dosage strength is 20 mg/12.5mg per tab
2. 12.5 mg of hydrochlorothiazide per tablet
3. by mouth
4. 7 tablets
5. See package insert

Drug Package Inserts

Sometimes information needed to safely prepare, administer, and store medications is not located on the drug label. In such cases, you may need to read the **package insert**. The pharmaceutical company includes a package insert with each container of a prescription drug. The information on a drug package insert is intended for the prescriber, pharmacist, and the person who administers the drug. It contains descriptions of a drug's chemistry and how it acts in the body. ● **Figure 2.18** shows an excerpt from a drug package insert for Avodart. Always consult the package insert when you need information about

- mixing and storing a drug
- preparing a drug dose
- recommended safe dose and range
- indications, contraindications, and warnings
- side effects and adverse reactions

AVODART®
(dutasteride)
Soft Gelatin Capsules

DESCRIPTION
AVODART (dutasteride) is a synthetic 4-azasteroid compound that is a selective inhibitor of both the type 1 and type 2 isoforms of steroid 5α-reductase (5AR), an intracellular enzyme that converts testosterone to 5α-dihydrotestosterone (DHT).

Dutasteride is chemically designated as $(5\alpha,17\beta)$-N-{2,5 bis(trifluoromethyl)phenyl}-3-oxo-4-azaandrost-1-ene-17-carboxamide. The empirical formula of dutasteride is $C_{27}H_{30}F_6N_2O_2$, representing a molecular weight of 528.5 with the following structural formula:

$$NOHHHHNOHCF_3HCF_3**$$

Dutasteride is a white to pale yellow powder with a melting point of 242° to 250°C. It is soluble in ethanol (44 mg/mL), methanol (64 mg/mL), and polyethylene glycol 400 (3 mg/mL), but it is insoluble in water.

AVODART Soft Gelatin Capsules for oral administration contain 0.5 mg of the active ingredient dutasteride in yellow capsules with red print. Each capsule contains 0.5 mg of dutasteride dissolved in a mixture of mono-diglycerides of caprylic/capric acid and butylated hydroxytoluene. The inactive excipients in the capsule shell are gelatin (from certified BSE-free bovine sources), glycerin, and ferric oxide (yellow). The soft gelatin capsules are printed with edible red ink.

INDICATIONS AND USAGE
AVODART is indicated for the treatment of symptomatic benign prostatic hyperplasia (BPH) in men with an enlarged prostate to:
- Improve symptoms
- Reduce the risk of acute urinary retention
- Reduce the risk of the need for BPH-related surgery

CONTRAINDICATIONS
AVODART is contraindicated for use in women and children.

AVODART is contraindicated for patients with known hypersensitivity to dutasteride, other 5a-reductase inhibitors, or any component of the preparation.

PRECAUTIONS
General: Lower urinary tract symptoms of BPH can be indicative of other urological diseases, including prostate cancer. Patients should be assessed to rule out other urological diseases prior to treatment with AVODART. Patients with a large residual urinary volume and/or severely diminished urinary flow may not be good candidates for 5α-reductase inhibitor therapy and should be carefully monitored for obstructive uropathy.

Blood Donation: Men being treated with dutasteride should not donate blood until at least 6 months have passed following their last dose. The purpose of this deferred period is to prevent administration of dutasteride to a pregnant female transfusion recipient.

Use in Hepatic Impairment: The effect of hepatic impairment on dutasteride pharmacokinetics has not been studied. Because dutasteride is extensively metabolized and has a half-life of approximately 5 weeks at steady state, caution should be used in the administration of dutasteride to patients with liver disease.

Use with Potent CYP3A4 Inhibitors: Although dutasteride is extensively metabolized, no metabolically based drug interaction studies have been conducted. The effect of potent CYP3A4 inhibitors has not been studied. Because of the potential for drug-drug interactions, care should be taken when administering dutasteride to patients taking potent, chronic CYP3A4 enzyme inhibitors (e.g., ritonavir).

Effects on Prostate-Specific Antigen and Prostate Cancer Detection: Digital rectal examinations, as well as other evaluations for prostate cancer, should be performed on patients with BPH prior to initiating therapy with AVODART and periodically thereafter.

Dutasteride reduces total serum PSA concentration by approximately 40% following 3 months of treatment and approximately 50% following 6, 12, and 24 months of treatment. This decrease is predictable over the entire range of PSA values, although it may vary in individual patients. Therefore, for interpretation of serial PSAs in a man taking AVODART, a new baseline PSA concentration should be established after 3 to 6 months of treatment, and this new value should be used to assess potentially cancer-related changes in PSA. To interpret an isolated PSA value in a man treated with AVODART for 6 months or more, the PSA value should be doubled for comparison with normal values in untreated men.

The free-to-total PSA ratio (percent free PSA) remains constant at Month 12, even under the influence of AVODART. If clinicians elect to use percent free PSA as an aid in the detection of prostate cancer in men receiving AVODART, no adjustment to its value appears necessary.

DOSAGE AND ADMINISTRATION
The recommended dose of AVODART is 1 capsule (0.5 mg) taken orally once a day. The capsules should be swallowed whole. AVODART may be administered with or without food. No dosage adjustment is necessary for subjects with renal impairment or for the elderly (see CLINICAL PHARMACOLOGY: Pharmacokinetics: Special Populations: Geriatric and Renal Impairment). Due to the absence of data in patients with hepatic impairment, no dosage recommendation can be made (see PRECAUTIONS: General).

HOW SUPPLIED
AVODART Soft Gelatin Capsules 0.5 mg are oblong, opaque, dull yellow, gelatin capsules imprinted with "GX CE2" in red ink on one side packaged in bottles of 30 (NDC 0173-0712-15) and 90 (NDC 0173-0712-04) with child-resistant closures.

Storage and Handling: Store at 25°C(77°F); excursions permitted to 15-30°C(59-86°F) [see USP Controlled Room Temperature].

Dutasteride is absorbed through the skin. AVODART Soft Gelatin capsules should not be handled by women who are pregnant or who may become pregnant because of the potential for absorption of dutasteride and the subsequent potential risk to a developing male fetus (see CLINICAL PHARMACOLOGY: Pharmacokinetics, WARNINGS: Exposure of Women—Risk to Male Fetus, and PRECAUTIONS: Information for Patients and Pregnancy).

Manufactured by Cardinal Health
Beinheim, France for
GlaxoSmithKline
Research Triangle Park, NC 27709
©2005, GlaxoSmithKline. All rights reserved.
May 2005 RL-2188

● **Figure 2.18**
Excerpts of Avodart package insert.

(Reproduced with permission of GlaxoSmithKline.)

Example 2.8

Read the package insert in Figure 2.18 and fill in the requested information.

1. What is the generic name of the drug?

_____

2. For what condition is Avodart used?

_____

3. How long after Avodart has been discontinued can a patient donate blood?

_____

4. What is the recommended dose of the drug?

_____

5. What is the drug form?

_____

This is what you should have found:

1. Dutasteride.
2. Benign prostatic hyperplasia (BPH).
3. Men being treated with dutasteride should not donate blood until at least 6 months have passed following their last dose.
4. The recommended dose of Avodart is 1 capsule (0.5 mg) orally once a day.
5. The drug is supplied in the form of soft gelatin capsules.

Summary

In this chapter, the Medication Administration Process was discussed, including those who may administer drugs; the "six rights" and "three checks" of medication administration; and how to interpret prescriptions, and medication orders, medication administration records, drug labels, and drug package inserts.

- The six rights of medication administration serve as a guide for *safe* administration of medications to patients.
- Failure to achieve any of the six rights constitutes a medication error.
- A person administering medications has a legal and ethical responsibility to report medication errors.
- Medication errors can occur at any point in the medication process.
- A drug should be prescribed using its generic name.
- Understanding drug orders requires the interpretation of common abbreviations.
- Never use any abbreviations on the JCAHO "Official Do Not Use" list.

- Read drug labels carefully; many drugs have look-alike/sound-alike names.
- Carefully read the label to determine dosage strength and check calculations, paying special attention to decimal points.
- Medications must be administered in the form and via the route specified by the prescriber.
- Before administering any medication, it is essential to identify the patient.
- Medications should be documented immediately after, but never before, they are administered.
- No medication should be given without a legal order.
- If persons administering medications have difficulty understanding or interpreting the order, they must clarify the order with the prescriber.
- Medication administration is rapidly becoming computerized.
- Drug package inserts contain detailed information about the drug, including mixing, storing a drug, preparing a drug dose, indications, contraindications, warnings, side effects, adverse reactions, and the recommended safe dose range.

Practice Sets

The answers to *Try These for Practice* and *Exercises* appear in Appendix A at the end of the book. Ask your instructor for answers to the *Additional Exercises*.

Try These for Practice

Test your comprehension after reading the chapter.

Study the drug labels in ● **Figures 2.19** to **2.23** and answer the following five questions.

1. What is the route of administration for montelukast sodium?

2. How many tablets are contained in the container for Zocor?

3. What is the quantity of drug in each 5 mL of Omnicef?

4. What is the trade name for imatinib mesylate?

5. What is contained in 1 mL of the drug Kaletra?

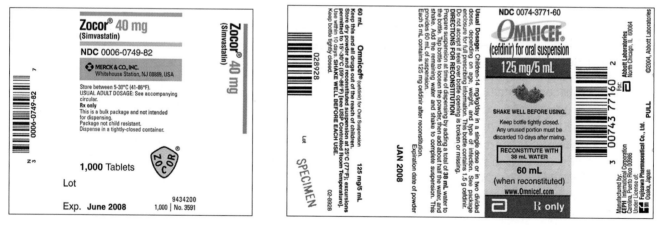

● **Figure 2.19**
Drug label for Zocor.

(The labels for the products Zocor 40mg are reproduced with permission of Merck & Co., Inc., copyright owner.)

● **Figure 2.20**
Drug label for Omnicef.

(Reproduced with permission of Abbott Laboratories.)

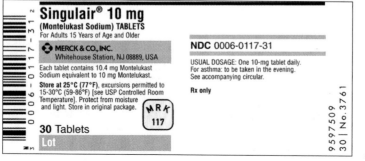

● **Figure 2.21**
Drug label for Singulair.

(The labels for the products Singulair 10mg are reproduced with permission of Merck & Co., Inc., copyright owner.)

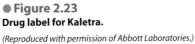

● Figure 2.22
Drug label for Gleevec.

(Reproduced with the permission of Novartis Pharmaceuticals.)

NDC 0074-3956-46
160 mL   Oral Solution

KALETRA™
(lopinavir/ritonavir) oral solution

Each mL contains:
lopinavir .... 80 mg
ritonavir .... 20 mg

a   **℞ only**   02-8413-2/R3

ALERT
Find out about medicines that
should **NOT** be taken with **KALETRA**

**Note to Pharmacist: Do not cover
ALERT box with pharmacy label.**

Exp. 7/2008

● Figure 2.23
Drug label for Kaletra.

(Reproduced with permission of Abbott Laboratories.)

Exercises

Reinforce your understanding in class or at home.

Use the information from drug labels in Figures 2.19 to 2.23 to complete Exercises 1 to 5.

1. Write the generic name for Kaletra.

   _____

2. Write the trade name for the drug whose NDC number is 0006-0117-31.

   _____

3. What is the total amount of solution in the bottle of Omnicef?

   _____

4. What is the dosage strength of imatinib mesylate?

   _____

5. What is the dosage strength of the drug whose NDC number is 0006-0749-82?

   _____

Workspace

6. Study the MAR in ●**Figures 2.24a** and **2.24b.** Fill in the following chart and answer the questions.

UNIVERSITY HOSPITAL

324689	12/7/07
Jane Ambery	5/01/47
2336 17th Avenue	Protestant
Brooklyn, N.Y.	HIP

DAILY MEDICATION ADMNISTRATION RECORD

Dr. Mae Ling

PATIENT NAME ___Jane Ambery___

ROOM # ___112___

ALLERGIC TO (RECORD IN RED): ___sulfa, fish___

IF ANOTHER RECORDS IS IN USE ☐

DATES GIVEN ⋮ MONTH/DAY   YEAR: ___2007___

RED CHECK INITIAL	ORDER DATE	INITIAL	EXP DATE	MEDICATION, DOSAGE, FREQUENCY AND ROUTE	TIME	12/7	12/8	12/9	12/10	12/11	12/12	12/13
	12/7	MC	12/13	Dilantin (phenytoin) 100 mg	10AM	MC	MC	MC	MC			
				PO t.i.d.	2PM	MC	MC	MC	MC			
					6PM	JY	JY	JY	JY			
	12/7	SG	12/16	Bactrim DS 2tabs PO q12h	8AM	SG	SG	SG	SG			
				for 10 days	8PM	JY	JY	JY	JY			
	12/7	SG	12/13	Bonivar (ibandronate sodium)	6AM	SG	SG	SG	SG			
				2.5 mg PO daily. Take 60 minutes								
				before first food or drink of day								
				(except plain water)								
	12/7	SG	12/13	Humulin N insulin 15 units	7:30AM	SG	SG	SG	SG			
				every morning								
				30 minutes before breakfast								
	12/7	SG	12/13	Humulin R insulin 8 units every morning	7:30AM	SG	SG	SG	SG			
				30 minutes before breakfast								

INT.	NURSES' FULL SIGNATURE AND TITLE	INT.	NURSES' FULL SIGNATURE AND TITLE
SG	Sara Gordon R.N.		
MC	Marie Colon R.N.		
JY	Jim Young R.N.		

● **Figure 2.24a**
Medication Administration Record for Jane Ambery.

UNIVERSITY HOSPITAL

DAILY MEDICATION ADMNISTRATION RECORD

324689
Jane Ambery
2336 17th Avenue
Brooklyn, N.Y.

12/7/07
5/01/47
Protestant
HIP

Dr. Mae Ling, M.D.

PATIENT NAME ___Jane Ambery___

ROOM # ___112___

IF ANOTHER RECORDS IS IN USE ☐

ALLERGIC TO (RECORD IN RED): ___sulfa, fish___

DATES GIVEN ┊ MONTH/DAY   YEAR: ___2007___

PRN MEDICATION

ORDER DATE	EXPIRATION DATE/TIME	MEDICATION, DOSAGE, FREQUENCY AND ROUTE	DOSES GIVEN						
12/10	12/17	*Anusol supp 1 PR q4–6h prn*	DATE	12/10					
			TIME	10 PM					
			INIT	JY					
			DATE						
			TIME						
			INIT						

STAT-ONE DOSE-PRE-OPERATIVE MEDICATIONS   ◯ Check here if additional sheet in use.

ORDER DATE	MEDICATION–DOSAGE ROUTE	DATE	TIME	INIT	ORDER DATE	MEDICATION–DOSAGE ROUTE	DATE	TIME	INIT

INT.	NURSES' FULL SIGNATURE AND TITLE	INT.	NURSES' FULL SIGNATURE AND TITLE
JY	*Jim Young R.N.*		

● **Figure 2.24b**
Medication Administration Record for Jane Ambery.

(a) Which drugs were administered at 10 P.M. on 12/10/07?

___

(b) Designate the time of the day the patient received ibandronate sodium.

___

(c) How many doses of Dilantin were administered to the patient by nurse Young?

___

(d) What drugs must be taken before breakfast?

___

(e) What is the last date on which the patient will receive Bactrim?

___

7. Study the physician's order sheet in ●**Figure 2.25** and then answer the following questions.

(a) Which drugs are ordered to be given once daily?

___

(b) Which drug should be given four times a day?

___

(c) What is the dose and route of administration of metoclopramide?

___

(d) What is the route of administration for Duragesic?

___

PHYSICIAN'S ORDERS

ORDER DATE	DATE DISC	
4/20/07	4/30/07	Omnicef (cefdinir) 300 mg PO q12h for 10 days
4/20/07	4/27/07	digoxin 0.125 mg PO daily
4/20/07	4/27/07	Glucophage (metformin HCl) 850 mg PO b.i.d. with breakfast and dinner
4/20/07	4/27/07	Reglan (metoclopramide) 10 mg PO 30 minutes before meals and at bedtime
4/20/07	4/23/07	Duragesic transdermal film ER 25 mg per hour. Remove in 72 hours.
4/20/07	4/27/07	Lasix 40 mg PO daily
PLEASE INDICATE BEEPER # →		222

2/28/52
Episcopal
Aetna

4/20/07

Jane Myers
23 College Ave
Salt Lake City
Utah 46022

Dr. Juan Rodriguez
#212332

● **Figure 2.25**
Physician's order sheet for patient Jane Myers.

   (e) Which drug is given every 12 hours?

   _____

8. Use the package insert shown in ● **Figure 2.26** to answer the following questions.

   (a) What is an appropriate dose for relief of skeletal muscle spasm?

   _____

   (b) What tests are advisable during long-term therapy?

   _____

   (c) What is the dosage strength of the Diazepam Oral Solution?

   _____

   (d) What is the NDC number of the Intensol Oral Solution (Concentrate)?

   _____

9. Fill in the following table with the equivalent times.

Standard Time	Military Time
9 A.M.	_____
_____	1500h
_____	1200h
6 P.M.	_____
_____	2015h
2:30 A.M.	_____
_____	1645h
6 A.M.	_____
_____	0000h

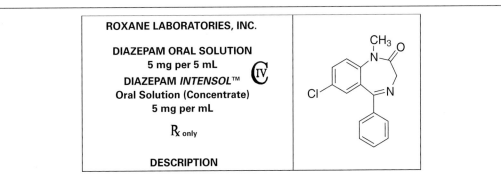

ROXANE LABORATORIES, INC.

DIAZEPAM ORAL SOLUTION
5 mg per 5 mL
DIAZEPAM *INTENSOL*™ C IV
Oral Solution (Concentrate)
5 mg per mL

R only

DESCRIPTION

INDICATIONS AND USAGE

Diazepam is indicated for the management of anxiety disorders or for the short-term relief of the symptoms of anxiety.

CONTRAINDICATIONS

Diazepam is contraindicated in patients with a known hypersensitivity to this drug and, because of lack of sufficient clinical experience, in children under 6 months of age. It may be used in patients with open angle glaucoma who are receiving appropriate therapy, but is contraindicated in acute narrow angle glaucoma.

ADVERSE REACTIONS

Side effects most commonly reported were drowsiness, fatigue and ataxia. Infrequently encountered were confusion, constipation, depression, diplopia, dysarthria, headache, hypotension, incontinence, jaundice, changes in libido, nausea, changes in salivation, skin rash, slurred speech, tremor, urinary retention, vertigo and blurred vision. Paradoxical reactions
such as acute hyperexcited states, anxiety, hallucinations, increased muscle spasticity, insomnia, rage, sleep disturbances and stimulation have been reported; should these occur, use of the drug should be discontinued.

Because of isolated reports of neutropenia and jaundice, periodic blood counts and liver function tests are advisable during long-term therapy. Minor changes in EEG patterns, usually low-voltage fast activity, have been observed in patients during and after diazepam therapy and are of no known significance.

DOSAGE AND ADMINISTRATION

Dosage should be individualized for maximum beneficial effect. While the usual daily dosages given below will meet the needs of most patients, there will be some who may require higher doses. In such cases dosage should be increased cautiously to avoid adverse effects.

Adults:	Usual Daily Dosage
Management of Anxiety Disorders and Relief of of Symptoms of Anxiety.	Depending upon severity symptoms -2 mg to 10 mg, 2 to 4 times daily.
Symptomatic Relief in Acute Alcohol Withdrawal.	10 mg, 3 or 4 times during the first 24 hours, reducing to 5 mg, 3 or 4 times daily as needed.
Adjunctively for Relief of Skeletal Muscle Spasm.	2 mg to 10 mg, 3 or 4 times daily.
Adjunctively in Convulsive Disorders.	2 mg to 10 mg, 2 to 4 times daily.

HOW SUPPLIED
5 mg per 5 mL Oral Solution (Orange-colored, wintergreen-spice flavored solution)

NDC 0054-8207-16: Unit dose Patient CupTM filled to deliver 5 mL (Diazepam 5 mg), ten 5 mL Patient CupsTM per shelf pack, 4 shelf packs per shipper. **NDC 0054-8208-16:** Unit dose Patient CupTM filled to deliver 10 mL (Diazepam 10 mg), ten 10 mL Patient CupsTM per shelf pack, 4 shelf packs per shipper. **NDC 0054-3188-63:** Bottle of 500 mL.

5 mg per mL IntensolTM Oral Solution (Concentrate)

NDC 0054-3185-44: Bottles of 30 mL with calibrated dropper [graduations of 0.2 mL (1 mg), 0.4 mL (2 mg), 0.6 mL (3 mg), 0.8 mL (4 mg), and 1 mL (5 mg) on the dropper]. Store at Controlled Room Temperature 15ϒ-30ϒC (59ϒ-86ϒF). **PROTECT FROM MOISTURE.**

● **Figure 2.26**
Excerpts from package insert for Diazepam.

(Courtesy of Roxane Laboratories Inc.)

● **Figure 2.27**
Drug labels.

2-27a (Courtesy of Rox-ane Laboratories Inc.)
2-27b (Reg. Trademark of Pfizer Inc. Reproduced with permission.)
2-27c (Reg. Trademark of Pfizer Inc. Reproduced with permission.)
2-27d (Copyright Eli Lilly and Company. Used with permission.)

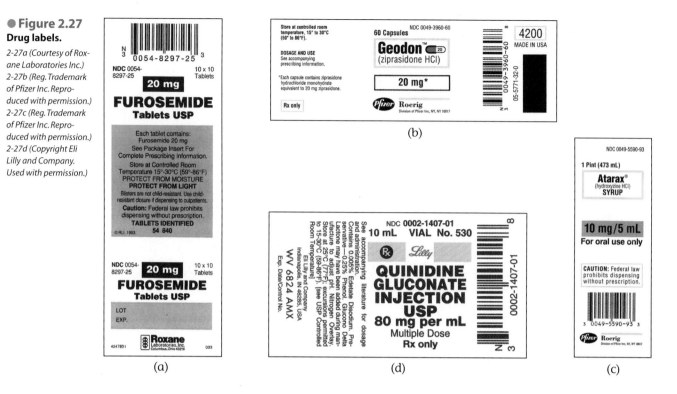

(a)   (d)   (c)

(b)

Workspace

Additional Exercises

Now, test yourself!

Study the drug labels shown in ● **Figure 2.27** to answer questions 1–5.

1. Write the generic name for Atarax.

   _____

2. Write the trade name for ziprasidone HCl.

   _____

3. Which drug can be administered by injection?

   _____

4. What is the route of administration for furosemide?

   _____

5. Write a trade name for the drug whose NDC number is 0049-5590-93.

   _____

6. Study the MAR in ● **Figure 2.28.** Fill in the following chart and answer the questions.

Name of Drug	Dose	Route of Administration	Time of Administration	Date Started	Expiration Date
Celebrex					
Flomax					
Ditropan					
Zoloft					
Seroquel					
Valium					
fluconazole					

MEDICATION RECORD

DIAGNOSIS urinary tract infection cronic depression osteoarthritis	Jim Ellington 2335 15ᵃ Ave Queens, NY 10221 12/20/20 Protestant BCBS

ALLERGIES
(LIST IN RED)

KNOWN ALLERGIES Yes ☐ No ☒ WEIGHT ___104 lb___

Mae Ling, MD   12/07/07
#324689

ORDER DATE	EXP. DATE	MEDICATION, DOSAGE, FREQUENCY & ROUTE	HOURS	December DATES GIVEN														DO NOT WRITE IN THIS COLUMN
				7	8	9	10	11	12	13	14	15	16	17	18	19	20	
12/7	12/18	Celebrex 100 mg PO	8AM	RG	RG	RG	RG	RG	MD	MD								
		b.i.d. q12h	8PM	TK	TK	TK	TK	TK	JO	JO								
12/7	12/13	Flomax 0.4 mg	5PM	RD	RD	RD	RD	RD	JO	JO								
		PO 30 min AC dinner																
12/7	12/13	Ditropan 5 mg	8AM	RG	RG	RG	RG	RG	MD	MD								
		PO daily																
12/8	12/14	Zoloft 0.1g PO	8AM	✗	RG	RG	RG	RG	MD	MD								
		q AM																
12/7	12/13	Seroquel 100 mg	9PM	RD	RD	RD	RD	RD	JO	JO								
		PO hs																
12/9	12/16	Valium 10 mg PO																
		prn q hs	9PM	✗	✗	RD	✗	RD	JO	JO								
12/8	12/15	100 ml D5/NS with	8AM	✗	✗	RG	RG	RG	MD	MD								
		fluconazole 400 mg	8PM	✗	RD	RD	RD	RD	JO	JO								
		IV q12h																

INIT.	NURSES' FULL SIGNATURE & TITLE	INIT.	NURSES' FULL SIGNATURE & TITLE	INIT.	NURSES' FULL SIGNATURE & TITLE
RG	Robert Graham	JO	Joan Olsen		
MD	Martha Daly				
TK	Taylore Keife				
RD	Rachel Dugas				

● **Figure 2.28**
Medication record.

(a) Which drug(s) was administered at 8 P.M. on 12/7/07?

_____

(b) How many doses of Valium did the patient receive in seven days?

_____

(c) What is the name of the drug administered IV?

_____

(d) How many medications were administered at 5 P.M.? Name the medication(s).

_____

(e) Designate the time of day the patient received Ditropan.

_____

(f) Identify the nurse who administered the medication on 12/7/07 at 8 A.M.

_____

(g) Identify the medication(s) administered at 9 P.M. on 12/08/07.

_____

(h) What is the name of the patient's physician?

_____

7. Study the physician's order sheet in ●**Figure 2.29**; then answer the following questions.

PHYSICIAN'S ORDERS   CHART COPY

FORM 01 109

ORDER DATE	DATE DISC		
4/20/07	4/27/07	Cefaclor 250 mg q8h PO for 7 days	
4/20/07	4/27/07	nitroglycerin transdermal 10 cm² daily	
		remove from 10 PM –7 AM daily	
4/20/07	4/27/07	Diabenase 0.1g daily PO AC breakfast	
4/22/07	4/29/07	furosemide 80 mg PO b.i.d	
4/23/07	4/30/07	Monopril 20 mg PO daily	

PLEASE INDICATE BEEPER # → 222

PATIENT CERTIFICATION

2/28/52
Episcopal
Aetna

4/20/07

Jane Myers
23 College Ave
Salt Lake City
Utah 46022

Dr. D. Looby
#212332

●**Figure 2.29**
Physician's order sheet.

(a) What is the route of administration for nitroglycerin?

_____

(b) How many doses of Cefaclor would the patient receive in 1 week?

_____

(c) Which drugs are to be given daily?

_____

(d) Which drug was ordered on April 22, 2007?

_____

(e) Which drug is to be given every 8 hours?

_____

(f) Identify the drug(s) that are to be administered before breakfast?

_____

8. Use the package insert shown in ●**Figure 2.30** to answer the following questions.
   (a) What is the generic name of the drug?

_____

(b) What is the form of the drug?

_____

(c) On what type of diet should the patient, who is receiving Lipitor, be placed?

_____

(d) What is the maximum daily dose of Lipitor recommended for heterozygous familial hypercholesterolemia in pediatric patients (10–17 years of age)?

_____

Lipitor®
(Atorvastatin Calcium)
Tablets

DESCRIPTION

LIPITOR® (atorvastatin calcium) is a synthetic lipid-lowering agent. Atorvastatin is an inhibitor of 3-hydroxy-3-methylglutaryl-coenzyme A (HMG-CoA) reductase. This enzyme catalyzes the conversion of HMG-CoA to mevalonate, an early and rate-limiting step in cholesterol biosynthesis.

DOSAGE AND ADMINISTRATION

The patient should be placed on a standard cholesterol-lowering diet before receiving LIPITOR and should continue on this diet during treatment with LIPITOR.

Hypercholesterolemia (Heterozygous Familial and Nonfamilial) and Mixed Dyslipidemia (_Fredrickson_ Types IIa and IIb)

The recommended starting dose of LIPITOR is 10 or 20 mg once daily. Patients who require a large reduction in LDL-C (more than 45%) may be started at 40 mg once daily. The dosage range of LIPITOR is 10 to 80 mg once daily. LIPITOR can be administered as a single dose at any time of the day, with or without food. The starting dose and maintenance doses of LIPITOR should be individualized according to patient characteristics such as goal of therapy and response (see _NCEP Guidelines,_ summarized in Table 5). After initiation and/or upon titration of LIPITOR, lipid levels should be analyzed within 2 to 4 weeks and dosage adjusted accordingly.

Since the goal of treatment is to lower LDL-C, the NCEP recommends that LDL-C levels be used to initiate and assess treatment response. Only if LDL-C levels are not available, should total-C be used to monitor therapy.

Heterozygous Familial Hypercholesterolemia in Pediatric Patients (10-17 years of age)

The recommended starting dose of LIPITOR is 10 mg/day; the maximum recommended dose is 20 mg/day (doses greater than 20 mg have not been studied in this patient population). Doses should be individualized according to the recommended goal of therapy (see NCEP Pediatric Panel Guidelines[1], CLINICAL PHARMACOLOGY, and...

[1] National Cholesterol Education Program (NCEP): Highlights of the Report of the Expert Panel on Blood Cholesterol Levels in Children Adolescents, _Pediatrics._ 89(3):495-501. 1992.

● **Figure 2.30**
Excerpts from package insert for Lipitor.

(Reg. Trademark of Pfizer Inc. Reproduced with permission.)

MediaLink
www.prenhall.com/olsen

Animated examples, interactive practice questions with animated solutions, and challenge tests for this chapter can be found on the Prentice Hall Dosage Calculation Tutor that accompanies this text. Additional, unique, interactive resources and activities can be found on the Companion Website.

Workspace

Chapter

3

Dimensional Analysis

Learning Outcomes

After completing this chapter, you will be able to

1. Solve simple problems by using Dimensional Analysis.
2. Identify some common units of measurement and their abbreviations.
3. Construct unit fractions from equivalences.
4. Convert a quantity expressed with a single unit of measurement to an equivalent quantity with another single unit of measurement.
5. Convert a quantity expressed as a rate to another rate.
6. Solve complex problems using Dimensional Analysis.

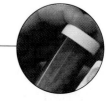

In this chapter, you will learn to use *Dimensional Analysis.* Dimensional Analysis is a simple approach to drug calculations that largely frees you from the need to memorize formulas. It is the method most commonly employed in the physical sciences. Once this technique is mastered, you will be able to calculate drug dosages quickly and safely.

Introduction to Dimensional Analysis

In courses such as chemistry and physics, students learn to routinely change a quantity in one unit of measurement to an equivalent quantity in a different unit of measurement by cancelling matching units of measurement. When the authors of this book first introduced this method into medical dosage calculation texts in 1973, we called this method Dimensional Analysis. We chose this name because the units of measure (for example, feet and inches) are called *dimensions*, and these dimensions have to be *analyzed* in order to see how to do the problems. Dimensional Analysis is rapidly making other dosage computation methods obsolete.

The Mathematical Foundation for Dimensional Analysis

Dimensional Analysis relies on two simple mathematical concepts.

Concept 1   **When a nonzero quantity is divided by the same amount, the result is 1.**

For example: $7 \div 7 = 1$

Because you can also write a division problem in fractional form, you get

$$\frac{7}{7} = 1$$

Since $\frac{7}{7}$ is a fraction equal to 1, and the word "unit" means one, the fraction $\frac{7}{7}$ is called a unit fraction.

In the preceding unit fraction, you may *cancel* the 7s on the top and bottom. That is, you can divide both numerator and denominator by 7.

$$\frac{\cancel{7}}{\cancel{7}} = \frac{1}{1} = 1$$

Units of measurement are the "labels," such as *inches, feet, minutes,* and *hours,* which are sometimes written after a number. They are also referred to as **dimensions**, or simply **units**. For example, in the quantity 7 *days, days* is the unit of measurement.

The equivalent quantities you divide may contain **units of measurement**.

For example: 7 days $\div$ 7 days $= 1$

Or in fractional form: $\dfrac{7 \text{ days}}{7 \text{ days}} = 1$

In the preceding unit fraction, you may cancel the number 7 and the unit of measurement *days* on the top and bottom and obtain the following:

$$\frac{\cancel{7 \text{ days}}}{\cancel{7 \text{ days}}} = \frac{1}{1} = 1$$

Going one step further, now consider this *equivalence:* **7 days = 1 week**.

Because 7 *days* is the same quantity of time as 1 *week,* when you divide these quantities, you must get 1.

So, both 7 days $\div$ 1 week $= 1$ **and**   1 week $\div$ 7 days $= 1$

Or in unit fractional form: $\dfrac{7 \text{ days}}{1 \text{ week}} = 1$ **and** $\dfrac{1 \text{ week}}{7 \text{ days}} = 1$

Other unit fractions can be obtained from the equivalences found in Table 3.1

Table 3.1	**Equivalents for Common Units**
12 inches (in)	= 1 foot (ft)
2 pints (pt)	= 1 quart (qt)
16 ounces (oz)	= 1 pound (lb)
60 seconds (sec)	= 1 minute (min)
60 minutes (min)	= 1 hour (h or hr)
24 hours (h or hr)	= 1 day (d)
12 months (mon)	= 1 year (yr)

Concept 2   When a quantity is multiplied by 1, the quantity is unchanged.

In the following examples, the quantity *2 weeks* will be multiplied by the number 1 and also by the unit fractions $\dfrac{7}{7}, \dfrac{7 \text{ days}}{7 \text{ days}},$ and $\dfrac{7 \text{ days}}{1 \text{ week}}$

$$2 \text{ weeks} \times 1 = \qquad\qquad 2 \text{ weeks}$$

$$2 \text{ weeks} \times \frac{7}{7} = 2 \text{ weeks} \times 1 = 2 \text{ weeks}$$

$$2 \text{ weeks} \times \frac{7 \text{ days}}{7 \text{ days}} = 2 \text{ weeks} \times 1 = 2 \text{ weeks}$$

$$2 \text{ weeks} \times \frac{7 \text{ days}}{1 \text{ week}} = 2 \text{ weeks} \times 1 = 2 \text{ weeks}$$

Consider the previous line again. This time you cancel the *week(s)!*

$$2 \text{ weeks} \times \frac{7 \text{ days}}{1 \text{ week}} = 2 \text{ weeks} \times \frac{7 \text{ days}}{1 \text{ week}} = (2 \times 7) \text{ days} = 14 \text{ days}$$

So, 2 weeks = 14 days.

This shows how to convert a quantity measured in weeks (2 *weeks*) to an equivalent quantity measured in days (14 *days*). With the Dimensional Analysis method, you will be multiplying quantities by unit fractions in order to convert the units of measure. This procedure demonstrates the basic technique of Dimensional Analysis.

Many of the problems in dosage calculation require changing a quantity with a *single unit of measurement* into an equivalent quantity with a different *single unit of measurement*; for example, changing 2 *weeks* to 14 *days* as was done above. Other problems may involve changing *rates of flow* to equivalent *rates of flow*. Both of these types of problems will be addressed in this chapter.

Changing a Single Unit of Measurement to Another Single Unit of Measurement

Simple Problems With Single Units of Measurement

Suppose you want to express 18 *months* in *years*. That is, you want to convert 18 *months* to an equivalent amount of time in *years*.

This is a **simple** problem. Simple problems have only three elements. The elements in this problem are

The given quantity:	18 months
The quantity you want to find:	? years
An equivalence between them:	1 year = 12 months

To begin the Dimensional Analysis process in a logical way, write the quantity you are given (18 *months*) on the left of an equal sign and the unit you want to change it to (*years*) on the right side, as follows:

$$18 \text{ months} = ? \text{ years}$$

It may help to write 18 *months* as the fraction $\dfrac{18 \text{ months}}{1}$

Thus, you now have

$$\frac{18 \text{ months}}{1} = ? \text{ years}$$

Formulate the Appropriate Unit Fraction To change *months* to *years*, you need an equivalence between *months* and *years*. That equivalence is

$$12 \text{ months} = 1 \text{ year}$$

From this equivalence, you can get two possible unit fractions:

$$\frac{12 \text{ months}}{1 \text{ year}} \quad \text{and} \quad \frac{1 \text{ year}}{12 \text{ months}}$$

But which of these fractions shall you choose? If you multiply $\dfrac{18 \text{ months}}{1}$ by the first of these fractions, you get

$$\frac{18 \text{ months}}{1} \times \frac{12 \text{ months}}{1 \text{ year}}$$

Notice that both the *months* units are in the numerators of the fractions.

Because no cancellation of the units is possible in this case, do not select this unit fraction.

If instead you multiply by the second of the unit fractions, you get the following:

$$\frac{18 \text{ months}}{1} \times \frac{1 \text{ year}}{12 \text{ months}} = ? \text{ years}$$

Notice that now *one of the months is in the numerator (top), and the other months is in the denominator (bottom) of a fraction.* Because cancellation of the *months* is now possible, this is the appropriate unit fraction to choose.

Cancel the Units of Measurement $\dfrac{18\,\cancel{months}}{1} \times \dfrac{1\ year}{12\,\cancel{months}} = ?\ years$

After you cancel the *months*, notice that *year* (the unit of measurement that you want to find) is the only remaining unit on the left side.

$$\frac{18\,\cancel{months}}{1} \times \frac{1\,\cancel{year}}{12\,\cancel{months}} = ?\ years$$

Cancel the Numbers and Finish the Multiplication After you are sure that you have *only the unit of measurement that you want (years) remaining on the left side and that it is on the top of a fraction,* you can complete the cancellation and multiplication of the numbers as follows:

$$\frac{\overset{3}{\cancel{18}}\,\cancel{months}}{1} \times \frac{1\ year}{\underset{2}{\cancel{12}}\,\cancel{months}} = \frac{3\ years}{2} \quad or \quad 1\frac{1}{2}\,years$$

So, 18 *months* is equivalent to $1\frac{1}{2}$ *years*.

Example 3.1

Change $2\frac{1}{4}$ *hours* to an equivalent amount of time in *minutes.*
The elements in this problem are

The given quantity:	$2\frac{1}{4}$ hours
The quantity you want to find:	? minutes
An equivalence between them:	1 hour = 60 minutes

$$2\frac{1}{4}\,hours = ?\ minutes$$

Avoid doing multiplication with mixed numbers; change them to improper fractions or decimal numbers. In this case, you can write $2\frac{1}{4}$ *hours* as the improper fraction $\frac{9}{4}$ *hours*. It is better to write the quantity $\frac{9}{4}$ *hours* as $\dfrac{9\ hours}{4}$ in order to make it clear that the unit of measurement (*hours*) is in the numerator of the fraction, not in the denominator.

So, the problem becomes $\dfrac{9\ hours}{4} = ?\ minutes.$

> **NOTE**
>
> The unit you want to find must always appear in the numerator (top) of the fraction.

Formulate the Appropriate Unit Fraction You want to change *hours* to *minutes*, so you need an equivalence between *hours* and *minutes*. That equivalence is

$$1 \text{ hour} = 60 \text{ minutes}$$

From this equivalence, you get two possible fractions, which are both equal to 1:

$$\frac{1 \text{ hour}}{60 \text{ minutes}} \quad \text{and} \quad \frac{60 \text{ minutes}}{1 \text{ hour}}$$

But which of these fractions will lead to cancellation? Because you want to eliminate (cancel) the *hours*, and because *hours* are on the top, as follows:

$$\frac{9 \text{ hours}}{4} = ? \text{ minutes}$$

you need to multiply by the unit fraction with *hour* on the bottom, as follows:

$$\frac{9 \text{ hours}}{4} \times \frac{60 \text{ minutes}}{1 \text{ hour}} = ? \text{ minutes}$$

This is what you want because cancellation of the *hour(s)* is now possible.

Cancel the Units $\dfrac{9 \cancel{\text{ hours}}}{4} \times \dfrac{60 \text{ minutes}}{1 \cancel{\text{ hour}}} = ? \text{ minutes}$

After you cancel the *hour(s)*, make sure that *minutes* (the unit you want) is the only remaining unit of measurement and that it is in a numerator (top) of a fraction.

$$\frac{9 \cancel{\text{ hours}}}{4} \times \frac{60 \cancel{\text{minutes}}}{1 \cancel{\text{ hour}}} = ? \text{ minutes}$$

Cancel the Numbers and Finish the Multiplication

$$\frac{9 \cancel{\text{ hours}}}{\underset{1}{\cancel{4}}} \times \frac{\overset{15}{\cancel{60}} \text{ minutes}}{1 \cancel{\text{ hour}}} = 135 \text{ minutes}$$

So, $2\frac{1}{4}$ hours = 135 minutes.

NOTE

To eliminate a particular unit of measurement in the numerator, use a unit fraction with that same unit of measurement in the denominator.

NOTE

When a unit of measure follows a numeric fraction, write the unit of measure in the numerator (top) of the fraction. For example, write $\frac{1}{2}$ hour as $\dfrac{1 \text{ hour}}{2}$.

Example 3.2

Change $5\frac{1}{2}$ feet to an equivalent length in inches.

The given quantity: $5\frac{1}{2}$ feet

The quantity you want to find: ? inches

An equivalence between them: 1 foot = 12 inches

$$5\frac{1}{2} \text{ feet} = ? \text{ inches}$$

$$\frac{11 \text{ feet}}{2} = ? \text{ inches}$$

You want to cancel *feet* and get the answer in *inches,* so choose a fraction with *feet (foot)* on the bottom and *inches* on top. You need a fraction that looks like $\dfrac{?\text{ inches}}{?\text{ foot}}$

Since 1 foot = 12 inches, therefore the fraction is $\dfrac{12\text{ inches}}{1\text{ foot}}$

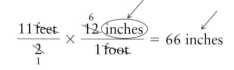

$$\frac{11\;\cancel{\text{feet}}}{\underset{1}{\cancel{2}}} \times \frac{\overset{6}{\cancel{12}}\,\text{inches}}{1\;\cancel{\text{foot}}} = 66\text{ inches}$$

So, $5\frac{1}{2}$ feet = 66 inches.

Example 3.3

An infant weighs 6 pounds 5 ounces. What is the weight of the infant in ounces?

$$6\ pounds\ 5\ ounce \quad \text{means} \quad 6\text{ pounds} + 5\text{ ounces}$$

First, convert 6 *pounds* to *ounces.*

The given quantity: 6 pounds
The quantity you want to find: ? ounces
An equivalence between them: 1 pound = 16 ounces

$$6\text{ pounds} = ?\text{ ounces}$$

$$\frac{6\text{ pounds}}{1} = ?\text{ ounces}$$

You want to cancel *pounds* and get the answer in *ounces.* So, choose a fraction with *pounds* on the bottom and *ounces* on top; that is, a fraction that looks like $\dfrac{?\text{ ounces}}{?\text{ pounds}}$

Since 1 pound = 16 ounces, the fraction is $\dfrac{16\text{ ounces}}{1\text{ pound}}$

$$\frac{6\;\cancel{\text{pounds}}}{1} \times \frac{16\;\text{ounces}}{1\;\cancel{\text{pound}}} = 96\text{ ounces}$$

So, 6 pounds = 96 ounces, and the infant weighs 96 ounces + 5 ounces, or 101 *ounces.*

Dimensional Analysis can be applied to a wide variety of problems, as demonstrated by the next example.

Example 3.4

If the exchange rate in a country is 9 pesos for 1 dollar, how many pesos will be exchanged for $45?

The given quantity: $45
The quantity you want to find: ? pesos

An equivalence between them: 9 pesos = \$1

$$\$45 = ? \text{ pesos}$$

You want to cancel \$ and get the answer in *pesos*. So, multiply \$45 by a fraction that looks like $\dfrac{? \text{ pesos}}{\$?}$

Because 9 pesos = \$1, the fraction you want is $\dfrac{9 \text{ pesos}}{\$1}$

Cancel the \$ signs and do the multiplication to get

$$\frac{\cancel{\$45}}{1} \times \frac{9 \cancel{\text{(pesos)}}}{\cancel{\$1}} = 405 \text{ pesos}$$

So, \$45 will be exchanged for 405 *pesos*.

Complex Problems with Single Units of Measurement

Sometimes you will encounter problems that will require the procedures used previously to be repeated one or more times. We call such problems **complex**. In a complex problem, multiplication by more than one unit fraction is required. The method is very similar to that used with simple problems.

Here is an example: Suppose that you want to change 4 *hours* to an equivalent time in *seconds*.

The given quantity: 4 hours

The quantity you want to find: ? seconds

An equivalence between them: ?

Most people do not know the direct equivalence between hours and seconds. But you do know the following two equivalences related to the units of measurement in this problem: 1 hour = 60 minutes and 1 minute = 60 seconds.

So the problem is

$$4 \text{ hours} = ? \text{ seconds}$$

or

$$\frac{4 \text{ hour}}{1} = ? \text{ hours}$$

First, you want to cancel *hours*. To do this, you must use an equivalence containing *hours* and a unit fraction with *hours* on the bottom. Because 1 hour = 60 minutes, this fraction will be $\dfrac{60 \text{ minutes}}{1 \text{ hour}}$

$$\frac{4 \cancel{\text{hours}}}{1} \times \frac{60 \text{ minutes}}{1 \cancel{\text{hour}}} = ? \text{ seconds}$$

After the *hours* are cancelled, as shown previously, only *minutes* remain on the left side. So, what you have done at this point is changed 4 *hours* to (4 × 60 = 240) *minutes*, but you want to obtain the answer in *seconds*. Therefore, the *minutes* must now be cancelled. Because *minutes* is in the numerator, a fraction with *minutes* in the denominator is required.

Because 1 *minute* = 60 *seconds*, the fraction is $\dfrac{60\ \text{seconds}}{1\ \text{minute}}$

Now multiplying by this unit fraction, you get

$$\frac{4\ \cancel{\text{hours}}}{1} \times \frac{60\ \text{minutes}}{1\ \cancel{\text{hour}}} \times \frac{60\ \text{seconds}}{1\ \text{minute}} = ?\ \text{seconds}$$

Cancel the *minutes* and notice that the only unit of measurement remaining on the left side is *seconds,* the unit that you want to find!

$$\frac{4\ \cancel{\text{hours}}}{1} \times \frac{60\ \cancel{\text{minutes}}}{1\ \cancel{\text{hour}}} \times \frac{60\ \cancelled{\text{seconds}}}{1\ \cancel{\text{minute}}} = ?\ \text{seconds}$$

Now that you have the unit of measurement that you want (seconds) on the left side, cancel the numbers (not possible in this example) and finish the multiplication:

$$\frac{4\ \cancel{\text{hours}}}{1} \times \frac{60\ \cancel{\text{minutes}}}{1\ \cancel{\text{hour}}} \times \frac{60\ \text{seconds}}{1\ \cancel{\text{minute}}} = 14{,}400\ \text{seconds}$$

So, 4 *hours* is equivalent to 14,400 *seconds.*

Example 3.5

Convert 50,400 *minutes* to an equivalent time in *days*

The given quantity: 50,400 minutes

The quantity you want to find: ? days

Equivalences between them: ?

You might not know the direct equivalence between minutes and days. But you do know the following two equivalences related to the units in this problem: 60 minutes = 1 hour and 24 hours = 1 day.

$$50{,}400\ \text{minutes} = ?\ \text{days}$$

You want to cancel *minutes.* To do this, you must use an equivalence containing *minutes* and make a unit fraction with *minutes* on the bottom. Since 60 minutes = 1 hour, this fraction will be $\dfrac{1\ \text{hour}}{60\ \text{minutes}}$.

$$50{,}400\ \cancel{\text{minutes}} \times \frac{1\ \text{hour}}{60\ \cancel{\text{minutes}}} = ?\ \text{days}$$

After the *minutes* are cancelled as shown above, only *hour* remains on the left side, but you want to obtain the answer in *days.* Therefore, the *hour* must now be cancelled. This will require a unit fraction with *hours* in the denominator. Because 1 day = 24 hours, this fraction is $\dfrac{1 \text{ day}}{24 \text{ hours}}$.

After cancelling the *hours*, you now have

$$50{,}400 \ \text{minutes} \times \frac{1 \ \text{hour}}{60 \ \text{minutes}} \times \frac{1 \ \text{day}}{24 \ \text{hours}} = ? \ \text{days}$$

Because only *day* (in the numerator) is on the left side, the numbers can be cancelled.

$$\overset{840}{50{,}400} \ \text{minutes} \times \frac{1 \ \text{hour}}{\underset{1}{60} \ \text{minutes}} \times \frac{1 \ \text{day}}{24 \ \text{hours}} = \frac{840}{24} \text{days} = 35 \ \text{days}$$

So, 50,400 minutes = 35 days

Example 3.6

Kim is having a party for 24 people and is serving hot dogs. Each person will eat 2 hot dogs. How much will the hot dogs for the party cost if a package of 8 hot dogs costs $2.50?

The given single unit of measurement: 24 people or 24 persons

The single unit of measurement
you want to find: ? Cost ($)

You might not know the direct equivalence between people and cost. But you do know the following equivalences supplied in this problem:

2 hot dogs per person   2 hot dogs = 1 person
1 package of hot dogs is $2.50   1 package = $2.50
1 package has 8 hot dogs   1 package = 8 hot dogs

But where do you start?

In this problem, there are two single units of measurement—one that is given (persons) and one you have to find (cost). Cost involves a single unit of measurement, namely dollars ($). *Because you are looking for a quantity measured in a single unit of measurement ($), you should start with the given single unit of measurement (persons).*

$$24 \text{ persons} = ? \ \$$$

You want to cancel *persons*. To do this, you must use an equivalence containing *person(s)* to make a fraction with *person(s)* on the bottom.

NOTE

Don't stop multiplying by unit fractions until the unit of measurement you are looking for is the only remaining unit on the left side. Remember that the unit you are looking for must be in the numerator of a fraction.

From the preceding equivalence, 2 hot dogs = 1 person, this fraction will be $\dfrac{2 \text{ hot dogs}}{\text{person}}$.

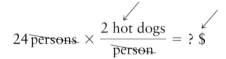

$$24 \,\cancel{\text{persons}} \times \frac{2 \text{ hot dogs}}{\cancel{\text{person}}} = ? \; \$$$

After the *person(s)* are cancelled, only *hot dogs* remains on the left side, and it indicates that 48 *hot dogs* are needed. But you want to obtain the answer in $\$$. Therefore, the *hot dogs* must now be cancelled. This will require a fraction with *hot dogs* in the denominator. From the equivalence 1 package = 8 hot dogs, the unit fraction is $\dfrac{1 \text{ package}}{8 \text{ hot dogs}}$

Thus, you now have

$$24 \,\cancel{\text{persons}} \times \frac{2 \,\cancel{\text{hot dogs}}}{\cancel{\text{person}}} \times \frac{1 \text{ package}}{8 \,\cancel{\text{hot dogs}}} = ? \; \$$$

After the *hot dogs* are cancelled, only *package* remains on the left side, and (if you do the mathematics now) it indicates the number of *packages* (6) that are needed. But you want to obtain the answer in $\$$. Therefore, the *package* must now be cancelled. This will require a fraction with *package* in the denominator. From the equivalence 1 package = $\$2.50$, the unit fraction is $\dfrac{\$2.50}{1 \text{ package}}$.

$$24 \,\cancel{\text{persons}} \times \frac{2 \,\cancel{\text{hot dogs}}}{\cancel{\text{person}}} \times \frac{1 \,\cancel{\text{package}}}{8 \,\cancel{\text{hot dogs}}} \times \frac{\$2.50}{1 \,\cancel{\text{package}}} = ? \; \$$$

Because you now have only $\$$ (in the numerator) on the left side, the numbers can be cancelled and the multiplication finished.

$$\overset{3}{\cancel{24}} \,\cancel{\text{persons}} \times \frac{2 \,\cancel{\text{hot dogs}}}{\cancel{\text{person}}} \times \frac{1 \,\cancel{\text{package}}}{\underset{1}{\cancel{8}} \,\cancel{\text{hot dogs}}} \times \frac{\$2.50}{1 \,\cancel{\text{package}}} = \$15$$

So, the hot dogs for the party will cost $\$15.00$.

Changing One Rate to Another Rate

A *rate* is a fraction with different units of measurement on top and bottom. For example, 50 *miles* per *hour* written as 50 miles/hour and 3 *pounds* per *week* written as 3 pounds/week are rates. In dosage calculation, the bottom unit of measurement is frequently time (for example, *hours* or *minutes*). We sometimes want to change one rate into another rate. These problems are done in a manner similar to the method that was used to do the single-unit-to-single-unit problems.

Simple Problems With Rates

Example 3.7

Convert *5 feet per hour* to an equivalent rate of speed in *inches per hour*.

The given rate: 5 feet per hour

The rate you want to find: ? inches per hour

Because you are looking for a **rate**, you start with the *given* **rate**:

5 feet per hour = ? inches per hour

Write these rates as fractions:

$$\frac{5 \text{ feet}}{\text{hour}} = \frac{? \text{ inches}}{\text{hour}}$$

Notice that you are given a rate with *hour* in the denominator, and the rate you are looking for also has *hour* in the denominator. Therefore, *the denominator does not have to be changed!*

But the given rate has *feet* in the numerator, and the rate you want has a different unit, *inches*, in the numerator. Therefore, *feet* must be changed.

To cancel *feet*, you must use an equivalence containing *feet*, namely, 12 *inches* = 1 *foot*. Because *feet* is in the numerator, you need a unit fraction with *feet* in the denominator. This unit fraction is $\frac{12 \text{ inches}}{1 \text{ foot}}$.

After the *feet* are cancelled, *inches* remain on top, and *hour* remains on the bottom, and those are the units you want. Finally, do the multiplication of the numbers.

$$\frac{5 \text{ feet}}{\text{hour}} \times \frac{12 \text{ inches}}{1 \text{ foot}} = \frac{60 \text{ inches}}{\text{hour}}$$

So, *5 feet per hour* is equivalent to 60 *inches per hour*.

Example 3.8

Convert 90 *feet per hour* to an equivalent rate in *feet per minute*.

The given rate: 90 ft/h

The rate you want to find: ? ft/min

Since you are looking for a rate, you start with the given rate,

90 ft per h = ? ft/min

$$\frac{90 \text{ ft}}{\text{h}} = \frac{? \text{ ft}}{\text{min}}$$

Notice that you are given a rate with *ft* in the numerator, and the answer you are looking for also has *ft* in the numerator. Therefore, the numerator does not have to be changed!

But the given rate has h in the denominator, and the rate you want has a different unit, *min*, in the denominator. Therefore, h must be eliminated. Since h is in the denominator, you need a fraction with h in the numerator.

Use the equivalence 1h $=$ 60 min. This unit fraction is $\dfrac{1\ h}{60\ min}$.

$$\frac{90\,\text{(ft)}}{\text{h}} \times \frac{1\,\text{h}}{60\,\text{(min)}} = \frac{?\ ft}{min}$$

After the h is cancelled, *ft* remains on top and *min* is on the bottom, and those are the units you want. Cancel the numbers and finish the multiplication.

$$\frac{\overset{3}{\cancel{90}}\,\text{ft}}{\text{h}} \times \frac{1\,\text{h}}{\underset{2}{\cancel{60}}\,\text{min}} = \frac{3\ ft}{2\ min} = \frac{1.5\ ft}{min}$$

So, 90 *feet/hour* is equivalent to a rate of 1.5 *feet/minute*.

Complex Problems With Rates

Example 3.9

Convert $10\frac{1}{2}$ *feet/hour* to an equivalent rate in *inches/minute*.

The given rate: $10\frac{1}{2}$ feet/hour
The rate you want to find: ? inches/minute

Since you are looking for a rate, you should start with a rate.

$$10\tfrac{1}{2}\,\text{feet/hour} = ?\ \text{inches/minute}$$

Write $10\frac{1}{2}$ as the improper fraction $\frac{21}{2}$

$$\frac{21\ ft}{2\ h} = \frac{?\ in}{min}$$

You want to cancel *ft*. To do this, you must use an equivalence containing *ft* on the bottom. Because you want to convert to *inches*, use the equivalence 12 *inches* $=$ 1 *foot*, and the unit fraction will be $\dfrac{12\ in}{1\ ft}$.

$$\frac{21\,\cancel{ft}}{2\ h} \times \frac{12\ in}{1\,\cancel{ft}} = \frac{?\ in}{min}$$

After the *ft* are cancelled, *in* is on top, which is what you want. But h is on the bottom and it must be cancelled. This will require a fraction with h in the numerator. From the equivalence 1 hour $=$ 60 minutes, the unit fraction is $\dfrac{1\ h}{60\ min}$.

After cancelling the hours, you now have

$$\frac{21 \cancel{ft}}{2 \cancel{h}} \times \frac{12 \textcircled{in}}{1 \cancel{ft}} \times \frac{1 \cancel{h}}{60 \textcircled{min}} = \frac{? \text{ in}}{\text{min}}$$

You now have *in* on top and *min* on the bottom, so do the cancelling and multiplications of the numbers.

$$\frac{21 \cancel{ft}}{2 \cancel{h}} \times \frac{\overset{1}{\cancel{12}} \text{ in}}{1 \cancel{ft}} \times \frac{1 \cancel{h}}{\underset{5}{\cancel{60}} \text{ min}} = \frac{21 \text{ in}}{10 \text{ min}} \quad \text{or} \quad \frac{2.1 \text{ in}}{\text{min}}$$

So, $10\frac{1}{2}$ feet/hour = 2.1 inches/minute.

Example 3.10

Write 3.2 *inches/second* in *feet/minute*.

The given rate: 3.2 in/sec
The rate you want to find: ? ft/min

Since you are looking for a **rate**, you should start with a **rate**.

$$\frac{3.2 \text{ in}}{\text{sec}} = \frac{? \text{ ft}}{\text{min}}$$

You want to cancel *in*. To do this, you must use an equivalence containing *in* on the bottom. This fraction will be $\dfrac{1 \text{ ft}}{12 \text{ in}}$

$$\frac{3.2 \cancel{in}}{\text{sec}} \times \frac{1 \text{ ft}}{12 \cancel{in}} = \frac{? \text{ ft}}{\text{min}}$$

Now, *ft* is on top, which is what you want. But *sec* is on the bottom and it must be cancelled. This will require a fraction with *sec* in the numerator: $\dfrac{60 \text{ sec}}{1 \text{ min}}$.

Now cancel and multiply the numbers.

$$\frac{3.2 \cancel{in}}{\cancel{sec}} \times \frac{1 \textcircled{ft}}{\underset{1}{\cancel{12}} \cancel{in}} \times \frac{\overset{5}{\cancel{60}} \cancel{sec}}{1 \textcircled{min}} = \frac{16 \text{ ft}}{\text{min}}$$

So, 3.2 inches/second = 16 feet/minute.

Summary

In this chapter, the techniques of Dimensional Analysis were introduced.

Mathematical concepts were reinforced:

- A nonzero number divided by itself equals 1.
- A fraction equal to 1 is called a unit fraction.
- When a quantity is multiplied (or divided) by 1, the quantity is unchanged.
- Cancellation always involves a quantity in a numerator and another quantity in a denominator.

Simple single-unit-to-single-unit problems:

- Start with the **given** single unit of measure on the left side of the = sign.
- Write the single unit of measure you want to **find** on the right side of the = sign.
- Identify an **equivalence** containing the units of measure in the problem.
- Use the equivalence to make a unit fraction with the **given** unit of measure in the **denominator.**
- Multiply by the unit fraction.
- Cancel the units of measure. The only unit of measurement remaining on the left side (in a numerator) will match the unit of measure on the right side.
- Cancel the numbers and finish the multiplication.

Simple rate-to-rate problems:

- Start with the given rate on the left side of the equal sign.
- Write the rate you want to **find** on the right side of the equal sign.
- Identify a unit of measure that must be cancelled.
- Find an **equivalence** containing the unwanted unit of measure you want to cancel.
- Choose a unit fraction that leads to cancellation of the unwanted unit of measurement.
- Cancel the units of measurement. The only units of measurement remaining on the left side (in a numerator) will match the units of measure on the right side.
- Cancel the numbers and finish the multiplication.
- In medical dosage calculations involving rates of flow, time (in minutes or hours) will always be in the denominator

Complex problems:

- Repeat the preceding steps until the only unit of measurement(s) remaining on the left side is the same as the unit of measurement(s) on the right side.

Workspace

Practice Sets

The answers to *Try These for Practice* and *Exercises* appear in Appendix A at the end of the book. Ask your instructor for the answers to the *Additional Exercises*.

Try These for Practice

Test your comprehension after reading the chapter.

1. How many minutes are in 4.5 hours? _____

2. An infant weighs 7 lb 3 oz. What is this weight in ounces? _____

3. How many hours are in $1\frac{1}{2}$ weeks? _____

4. Water is flowing from a hose at 0.1 quarts per minute. Find this rate of flow in quarts per hour. _____

5. A certain animal eats 2.5 ounces of food per day. At this rate, find the number of *pounds of food per week* the animal eats. _____

Exercises

Reinforce your understanding in class or at home.

1. 1.5 min = _____ sec   2. $5\frac{1}{2}$ years = _____ months

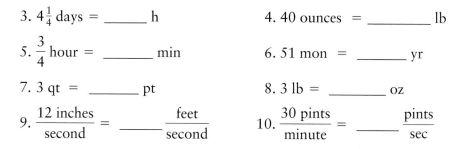

3. $4\frac{1}{4}$ days = _____ h

4. 40 ounces = _____ lb

5. $\frac{3}{4}$ hour = _____ min

6. 51 mon = _____ yr

7. 3 qt = _____ pt

8. 3 lb = _____ oz

9. $\dfrac{12 \text{ inches}}{\text{second}}$ = _____ $\dfrac{\text{feet}}{\text{second}}$

10. $\dfrac{30 \text{ pints}}{\text{minute}}$ = _____ $\dfrac{\text{pints}}{\text{sec}}$

11. An infant weighs 8 pounds 10 ounces at birth. What is the weight in ounces?_____

12. What is the height in inches of a person who is 6 feet 4 inches tall?

    _____

13. If 3 feet = 1 yard, convert 4 yards to an equivalent distance in inches.

    _____

14. If a person measures 42 inches in height, what does the patient measure in feet?_____

15. What fraction of an hour is 2,700 seconds? _____

16. Change $6 \dfrac{\text{pints}}{\text{h}}$ to an equivalent rate in $\dfrac{\text{quarts}}{\text{day}}$. _____

17. Change $6 \dfrac{\text{quarts}}{\text{day}}$ to an equivalent rate in $\dfrac{\text{pints}}{\text{hour}}$. _____

18. Change 1,680 hours to weeks. _____

19. Write 1,209,600 seconds as an equivalent amount of time in weeks.

    _____

20. There are 24 cans of soda in a case. Each can contains 12 ounces of soda. Every 60 ounces of soda contains 1 cup of sugar. How many cups of sugar are in 5 cases of soda? _____

Additional Exercises

Now, test yourself!

1. 540 sec = _____ min

2. 1.25 yr = _____ mon

3. 4 d = _____ h

4. 4 lb = _____ oz

5. $\frac{3}{4}$ min = _____ sec

6. $1\frac{2}{3}$ yr = _____ mon

7. 480 in = _____ ft

8. 12 oz = _____ lb

9. $\dfrac{0.25 \text{ feet}}{\text{sec}}$ = _____ $\dfrac{\text{in}}{\text{sec}}$

10. $\dfrac{120 \text{ qt}}{\text{min}}$ = _____ $\dfrac{\text{qt}}{\text{sec}}$

Workspace

11. An infant weighs 8 pounds at birth. What is the weight in ounces?
_____

12. Convert $1\frac{1}{2}$ yards to feet if 3 feet equal 1 yard. _____

13. How many yards are in 90 inches? _____

14. What part of an hour is 50 minutes? _____

15. How many years are there in 30 months? _____

16. Change 2.25 hours to seconds. _____

17. An IV solution has been infusing for 55 minutes. How many seconds is that? _____

18. $12 \dfrac{qt}{day} =$ _____ $\dfrac{pt}{h}$

19. $0.24 \dfrac{in}{sec} =$ _____ $\dfrac{ft}{min}$

20. If $0.25 is equivalent to 1 Yuan, how many Yuan are equivalent to $500?
_____

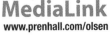

MediaLink
www.prenhall.com/olsen

Animated examples, interactive practice questions with animated solutions, and challenge tests for this chapter can be found on the Prentice Hall Dosage Calculation Tutor that accompanies this text. Additional, unique, interactive resources and activities can be found on the Companion Website.

Unit

2

Systems of Measurement

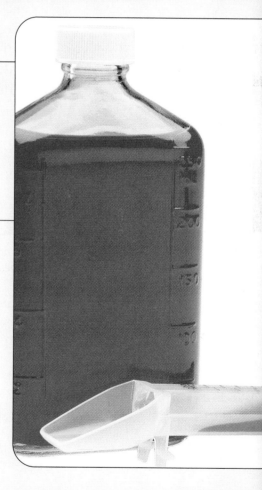

Chapter 4

The Metric, Household, and Apothecary Systems

Chapter 5

Converting From One System of Measurement to Another

The Metric, Household, and Apothecary Systems

Learning Outcomes

After completing this chapter, you will be able to

1. Identify the units of measurement in the metric, household, and apothecary systems.
2. Recognize the abbreviations for the units of measurement in the three systems.
3. State the equivalents for the units of volume for liquids.
4. State the equivalents for the units of weight for solids.
5. Convert from one unit to another within each of the three systems.

At present, there are three systems used to measure drugs: the *International System (SI), the household system, and the apothecary system.* The SI, commonly known as the *metric system*, is replacing the other systems of measurement. However, the other systems are still in use, so you must understand all three systems and learn how to convert from one to another. In this chapter, you will be introduced to the three systems. The metric system uses decimal numbers (i.e., 3.5), the apothecary system uses fractions $\left(i.e., 3\frac{1}{2}\right)$ and the household system, uses both.

The Metric System

The metric system is the most widely used, general system of measurement in the world today, with the United States being the only exception among developed countries. However, in all countries, the metric system is the preferred system for prescribing medications.

The fundamental units of measurement in the metric system are the *liter* (for liquid volume), the *gram* (for weight), and the *meter* (for length). Other units are formed by placing prefixes onto these fundamental units. The prefixes commonly used in medical doses are *kilo, centi, milli,* and *micro.* The equivalences illustrated in this section need to be understood in order to work within the metric system.

Liquid Volume in the Metric System

Drugs in liquid form are measured by volume. The volume of a liquid is the amount of space it occupies. In dosage calculations, *liters* and *milliliters* are used to measure liquid volume (see Table 4.1).

NOTE

The abbreviation mL should be used instead of the abbreviation cc because "c" may be confused with "u" (units) or "cc" with "00" (double zero).

Table 4.1 **Metric Equivalents of Liquid Volume**
1 cubic centimeter (cc or cm³) = 1 milliliter (mL)
1,000 milliliters (mL) = 1 liter (L)

Milliliters are used for smaller amounts of fluids. The prefix milli means $\frac{1}{1,000}$, so

$$1 \text{ liter (L)} = 1,000 \text{ milliliters (mL)}$$

Milliliters are equivalent to *cubic centimeters* (cm^3 or cc), so

$$1 \text{ mL} = 1 \text{ cm}^3 = 1 \text{ cc}$$

You can use dimensional analysis to convert from one unit of measurement to an equivalent unit of measurement within the metric system (the same way you converted units of measurement in Chapter 3). You multiply the given measurement by a unit fraction that is equal to 1; the unit fraction has the **given units of measurement on the bottom** (the denominator) and the **desired units of measurement on top** (the numerator), as the following examples show.

Example 4.1

If the prescriber ordered 0.5 L of 5% dextrose in water, how many milliliters were ordered?

$$0.5 \text{ L} = ? \text{ mL}$$

Cancel the liters and obtain the equivalent amount in milliliters.

$$0.5 \text{ L} \times \frac{? \text{ mL}}{? \text{ L}} = ? \text{ mL}$$

Because 1,000 mL = 1 L, the fraction you want is $\dfrac{1,000 \text{ mL}}{1 \text{ L}}$

$$0.5 \cancel{\text{L}} \times \frac{1,000 \text{ (mL)}}{1 \cancel{\text{L}}} = 500 \text{ mL}$$

So the prescriber ordered 500 mL of 5% dextrose in water.

Example 4.2

Your patient is to receive 1,750 mL of 0.9% NaCl IV q12h. What is the same amount in liters?

$$1,750 \text{ mL} = ? \text{ L}$$

Cancel the milliliters and obtain the equivalent amount in liters.

$$1,750 \text{ mL} \times \frac{? \text{ L}}{? \text{ mL}} = ? \text{ L}$$

Because 1,000 mL = 1 L, the fraction you want is $\dfrac{1 \text{ L}}{1,000 \text{ mL}}$

$$1,750 \cancel{\text{mL}} \times \frac{1 \text{ (L)}}{1,000 \cancel{\text{mL}}} = \frac{1,750 \text{ L}}{1,000} = 1.75 \text{ L}$$

So, 1,750 mL of 0.9% NaCl is the same amount as 1.75 L of 0.9% NaCl.

ALERT

Write 0.5 L instead of $\frac{5}{10}$ or $\frac{1}{2}$ L because in the metric system, quantities are written as decimal numbers instead of fractions.

ALERT

The abbreviation for microgram, mcg, is preferred over the abbreviation μg because μg may be mistaken for the abbreviation for milligram, mg. This error would result in a dose that would be 1,000 times greater than the prescribed dose.

Weight in the Metric System

Drugs in dry form are measured by weight in the metric system. In dosage calculations, *kilograms, grams, milligrams,* and *micrograms* (written in order of size) are used to measure weight. *Kilograms* are the largest of these units of measurement, and *micrograms* are the smallest (see Table 4.2).

Kilograms are used for heavier weights. The prefix kilo means 1,000, so

$$1 \textbf{ kilogram (kg)} = 1,000 \textit{ grams} \text{ (g)}$$

Milligrams are used for lighter weights, and *micrograms* are used for even lighter weights.

The prefix milli means $\dfrac{1}{1,000}$, and micro means $\dfrac{1}{1,000,000}$, so

$$1 \text{ gram (g)} = 1,000 \textbf{ milligrams (mg)}$$

$$1 \text{ milligram (mg)} = 1,000 \textbf{ micrograms (mcg or } \mu g)$$

Table 4.2	**Metric Equivalents of Weight**	
1 kilogram (kg)	=	1,000 grams (g)
1 gram (g)	=	1,000 milligrams (mg)
1 milligram (mg)	=	1,000 micrograms (mcg)

Using dimensional analysis and the information in Table 4.2, you can convert a quantity written in one unit of metric weight to an equivalent quantity in another unit of metric weight. The following examples show you how to do this.

Example 4.3

The order reads 125 mcg of Lanoxin (digoxin) PO daily. How many milligrams of this cardiac medication would you administer to the patient?

$$125 \text{ mcg} = \text{? mg}$$

Cancel the micrograms and obtain the equivalent amount in milligrams.

$$125 \text{ mcg} \times \frac{\text{? mg}}{\text{? mcg}} = \text{? mg}$$

Because 1,000 mcg = 1 mg, you have

$$125 \text{ mcg} \times \frac{1 \text{ (mg)}}{1,000 \text{ mcg}} = 0.125 \text{ mg}$$

So, 125 mcg is the same amount as 0.125 mg, and you would administer 0.125 mg of digoxin.

Example 4.4

The order reads Glucotrol (glipizide) 15 mg PO daily ac breakfast. How many grams of this hypoglycemic agent would you administer?

$$15 \text{ mg} = \text{? g}$$

Cancel the milligrams and obtain the equivalent amount in grams.

$$15 \text{ mg} \times \frac{\text{? g}}{\text{? mg}} = \text{? g}$$

$$15 \text{ mg} \times \frac{1 \text{ (g)}}{1,000 \text{ mg}} = \frac{15}{1,000} \text{ g} = 0.015 \text{ g}$$

So, 15 mg is the same amount as 0.015 g, and you would administer 0.015 g.

Length in the Metric System

Centimeters (cm) are used to measure lengths or heights, and centimeter is the only metric unit of length used in medical dosage calculations. Therefore, no conversions of metric units of length are necessary in medical dosage calculations.

Shortcut for Converting Units in the Metric System

The following chart is useful for a quick method of converting units of measurement within the metric system.

	Kilo-	Fundamental Unit	Milli-	Micro-
Weight	kilogram (kg)	gram (g)	milligram (mg)	microgram (mcg)
Volume		liter (L)	milliliter (mL)	

The metric system, like our number system, is a decimal system because it is **based on the number 10**. Therefore, measurements given in one metric unit can be converted to another metric unit by *merely moving the decimal place*. Using the preceding chart, to change a quantity measured in units from one column to units in the column to its right, move the decimal point **three places** to the right. To change a quantity measured in units from one column to units in the column to its left, move the decimal point **three places** to the left. Therefore, Examples 4.1 through 4.4 could also have been done as shown in the following examples.

Example 4.5

(Shortcut Method) 0.5 L = ? mL

In this problem, you convert from L to mL. The movement from L to mL in the following chart is a movement of one column to the right. Therefore, the conversion is accomplished by moving the decimal point three places to the right.

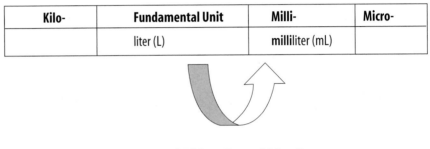

Kilo-	Fundamental Unit	Milli-	Micro-
	liter (L)	milliliter (mL)	

So, 0.5 L = 0. 5 0 0 mL = 0500. mL = 500 mL

Example 4.6

(Shortcut Method) 1750 mL = ? L

In this problem, you convert from mL to L. The movement from mL to L in the following chart is a movement of one column to the left. Therefore, the conversion is accomplished by moving the decimal point three places to the left.

Kilo-	Fundamental Unit	Milli-	Micro-
	liter (L)	milliliter (mL)	

So, 1,750 mL = 1 7 5 0. L = 1.750 L = 1.75 L

Example 4.7

(Shortcut Method) 125 mcg = ? mg

In this problem, you convert from mcg to mg. The movement from mcg to mg in the following chart is a movement of one column to the left.

Therefore, the conversion is accomplished by moving the decimal point three places to the left.

Kilo-	Fundamental Unit	Milli-	Micro-
kilogram (kg)	gram (g)	milligram (mg)	microgram (mcg)

So, 125 mcg = 1 2 5. mg = .125 mg = 0.125 mg

Example 4.8

(Shortcut Method) 15 mg = ? g

In this problem, you convert from mg to g. The movement from mg to g in the following chart is a movement of one column to the left. Therefore, the conversion is accomplished by moving the decimal point three places to the left.

Kilo-	Fundamental Unit	Milli-	Micro-
kilogram (kg)	gram (g)	milligram (mg)	microgram (mcg)

So, 15 mg = 0 1 5. g = .015 g = 0.015 g

ALERT

Because the volume of ordinary household spoons, cups, and glasses may vary, the equivalences in Table 4.3 are only *approximate*. Medications should not be administered using ordinary household utensils.

The Household System

Liquid Volume in the Household System

Occasionally, household measurements are used when prescribing liquid medication. Table 4.3 lists equivalent values, with their abbreviations, for units of liquid measurement in the household system.

Table 4.3 Household Equivalents of Liquid Volume

1 quart (qt)	=	2 pints (pt)
1 pint (pt)	=	16 ounces (oz)
1 glass (usually)	=	8 ounces (oz)
1 measuring cup	=	8 ounces (oz)
1 ounce (oz)	=	2 tablespoons (T)
1 tablespoon (T)	=	3 teaspoons (t)
1 teaspoon (t)	=	60 drops (gtt)

NOTE

The unit *ounce*, which is used to measure liquid volumes, is sometimes referred to as *fluid ounce*.

Example 4.9

How many teaspoons are equivalent to 15 gtt?

$$15 \text{ gtt} = ? \text{ t}$$

Cancel drops and obtain the equivalent amount in teaspoons.

$$15 \text{ gtt} \times \frac{? \text{ t}}{? \text{ gtt}} = ? \text{ t}$$

Because 60 gtt = 1 t, the fraction is $\dfrac{1 \text{ t}}{60 \text{ gtt}}$.

$$\overset{1}{\cancel{15 \text{ gtt}}} \times \frac{\boxed{1 \text{ t}}}{\underset{4}{\cancel{60 \text{ gtt}}}} = \frac{1}{4} \text{ t}$$

So, 15 gtt is approximately the same as $\frac{1}{4}$ t.

Example 4.10

A patient takes 24 oz of the laxative agent, COLYTE. How many glasses did the patient take?

$$24 \text{ oz} = ? \text{ glasses}$$

Cancel the ounces and obtain the equivalent amount in glasses.

$$24 \text{ oz} \times \frac{? \text{ glasses}}{? \text{ oz}} = ? \text{ glasses}$$

Because 1 glass = 8 ounces, the fraction is $\dfrac{1 \text{ glass}}{8 \text{ oz}}$.

$$\overset{3}{\cancel{24 \text{ oz}}} \times \frac{1 \boxed{\text{glass}}}{\underset{1}{\cancel{8 \text{ oz}}}} = 3 \text{ glasses}$$

24 oz is approximately the same as 3 glasses, so the patient took 3 glasses of COLYTE.

NOTE

Ounces used for weight should not be confused with ounces used for volume.

Weight in the Household System

The only units of weight used in the household system are ounces (oz) and pounds (lb), as shown in Table 4.4.

Table 4.4   **Weight in the Household System**
16 ounces (oz) = 1 pound (lb)

Example 4.11

An infant weighs 5 lb 8 oz. What is the weight of the infant in ounces? First change the 5 lb to ounces.

$$5 \text{ lb} = ? \text{ oz}$$

Cancel the pounds and obtain the equivalent amount in ounces.

$$5 \text{ lb} = \frac{? \text{ oz}}{? \text{ lb}} = ? \text{ oz}$$

Because 16 oz = 1 lb, the fraction is $\dfrac{16 \text{ oz}}{1 \text{ lb}}$

$$5 \cancel{\text{lb}} \times \frac{16 \text{ (oz)}}{1 \cancel{\text{lb}}} = 80 \text{ oz}$$

Now add the extra 8 oz.

$$80 \text{ oz} + 8 \text{ oz} = 88 \text{ oz}$$

So, the 5 lb, 8 oz infant weighs 88 oz.

The Apothecary System

The apothecary system is one of the oldest systems of drug measurement. Although the apothecary system was used in the past to write prescriptions, it has largely been replaced by the metric system. Apothecary units are rarely used on drug labels, but when they are, the metric equivalents are also provided.

Liquid Volume in the Apothecary System

The equivalents for the units of measurement for liquid volume in the apothecary system are shown in Table 4.5 along with their abbreviations.

Table 4.5	Common Equivalents for Apothecary Liquid Volume Units
ounce (oz)1	= drams (dr)8
dram (dr)1	= minims 60

> **NOTE**
>
> In the apothecary system, the abbreviation or symbol for the unit is placed before the quantity (as in drams 8). Ounces are used for liquid volume in both the household and apothecary systems. To avoid errors, the abbreviations dr and oz are preferred over ℨ and ℥.

Example 4.12

How many minims would be equivalent to dr $\dfrac{1}{6}$?

$$\text{dr} \frac{1}{6} = \text{minims ?}$$

Cancel the drams and obtain the equivalent amount in minims.

$$\frac{\text{dr } 1}{6} \times \frac{\text{minims ?}}{\text{dr ?}} = \text{minims ?}$$

Because minims 60 = dr 1, the fraction you want is $\dfrac{\text{minims } 60}{\text{dr } 1}$

$$\frac{\cancel{\text{dr}} 1}{6} \times \frac{\text{minims } \overset{10}{\cancel{60}}}{\cancel{\text{dr}} 1} = \text{minims } 10$$

So, dr $\dfrac{1}{6}$ is the same as minims 10.

Example 4.13

How many ounces would be equivalent to dr 4?

$$dr\ 4 = oz\ ?$$

Cancel the drams and get the answer in ounces.

$$dr\ 4 \times \frac{oz\ ?}{dr\ ?} = oz\ ?$$

Because dr 8 = oz 1, the fraction you want is $\dfrac{oz\ 1}{dr\ 8}$

$$\overset{1}{\cancel{dr\ 4}} \times \frac{\boxed{oz\ 1}}{\underset{2}{\cancel{dr\ 8}}} = oz\ \frac{1}{2}$$

So, dr 4 is the same as oz $\frac{1}{2}$.

Weight in the Apothecary System

The grain (gr) is the only unit of weight in the apothecary system that is used in administering medications.

Roman Numerals

Dosages in the apothecary system are sometimes written using Roman numerals. Table 4.6 shows Roman numerals.

Table 4.6 Roman Numerals

Roman Numerals	Symbols	Roman Numerals	Symbols	Roman Numerals	Symbols
1	I	7	VII	$\frac{1}{2}$	ss
2	II	8	VIII	$1\frac{1}{2}$	iss
3	III	9	IX	$7\frac{1}{2}$	viiss
4	IV	10	X		
5	V	15	XV		
6	VI	20	XX		

Summary

In this chapter, the three systems of measurement used in medication administration were introduced, and dimensional analysis was used to perform conversions within these systems.

- The metric, household, and apothecary systems are used in medication administration.

- The metric system is the dominant system.
- Memorize all the abbreviations for the units in the metric and household systems.
- Avoid the use of the abbreviations cc and μg.
- The metric system uses decimal numbers, not fractions.

- Learn the shortcut method of conversion within the metric system by moving the decimal point.
- The apothecary systems uses fractions, not decimal numbers.
- The apothecary system sometimes uses Roman numerals.

- The apothecary system is being phased out.
- Memorize all the equivalences within each of the systems.
- Dimensional analysis can be used to perform conversions within each of the three systems.

Practice Sets

Workspace

The answers to *Try These for Practice, Exercises,* and *Cumulative Review Exercises* appear in Appendix A at the end of the book. Ask your instructor for the answers to the *Additional Exercises.*

Try These for Practice

Test your comprehension after reading the chapter.

1. You need to memorize all the metric, household, and apothecary equivalents. To test yourself, fill in the missing numbers in the following chart.

Metric System

(a) 1 L   = _____ mL

(b) 1 mL   = _____ cc

(c) 1 L   = _____ cc

(d) 1 kg   = _____ g

(e) 1 g   = _____ mg

(f) 1 mg   = _____ mcg

(g) 1 mg   = _____ mcg

Household System

(h) 1 qt   = _____ pt

(i) 1 pt   = _____ oz

(j) 1 glass   = _____ oz

(k) 1 measuring cup   = _____ oz

(l) 1 oz   = _____ T

(m) 1 T   = _____ t

(n) 1 t   = _____ gtt

(o) 1 lb   = _____ oz

Apothecary System

(p) oz 1   = dr _____

(q) dr 1   = minim _____

2. Use the label in ● **Figure 4.1** to determine the number of grams of Oxy-Contin in 1 tablet of the drug.

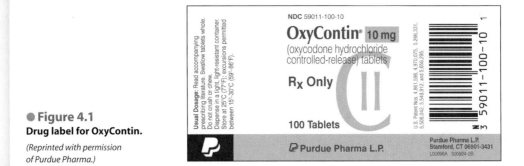

● **Figure 4.1**
Drug label for OxyContin.

(Reprinted with permission of Purdue Pharma.)

3. The prescriber ordered methorexate 2.5 mg PO q12h, for a patient with psoriasis. How many micrograms of this drug are administered in a day?

4. The urinary output of a patient with an indwelling Foley catheter is 1,800 mL. How many liters of urine are in the bag?

5. If a patient drank $1\frac{1}{2}$ quarts of water, how many pints of water did the patient drink?

Exercises

Reinforce your understanding in class or at home.

1. 400 mg = _____ g

2. 0.003 g = _____ mg

3. 0.07 g = _____ mg

4. 3 L = _____ mL

5. 2,500 mL = _____ L

6. 600 mcg = _____ mg

7. 1.7 L = _____ mL

8. $4\frac{1}{2}$ qt = _____ pt

9. 2.5 kg = _____ g

10. 4 T = _____ t

11. 5 T = _____ oz

12. 32 oz = _____ pt

13. Using the drug label in ● **Figure 4.2**, determine the number of micrograms of Diovan in one tablet.

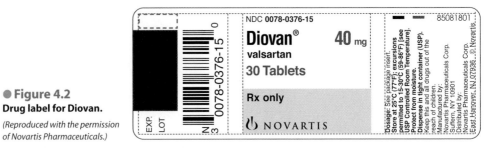

● **Figure 4.2**
Drug label for Diovan.

(Reproduced with the permission of Novartis Pharmaceuticals.)

14. The physician ordered a loading dose of digoxin 520 mcg PO stat. How many milligrams are in this dose?

15. According to the physician's order sheet in ● **Figure 4.3**, what is the dose in grams of the chlorpromazine?

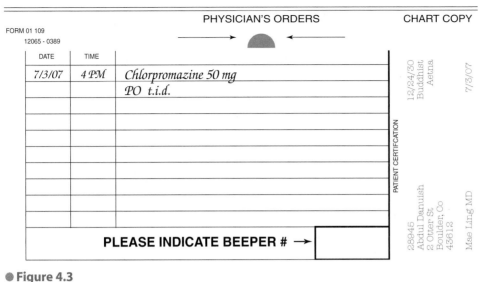

PHYSICIAN'S ORDERS   CHART COPY

FORM 01 109
12065 - 0389

DATE	TIME		
7/3/07	4 PM	Chlorpromazine 50 mg	
		PO t.i.d.	

PLEASE INDICATE BEEPER # →

12/24/30 Buddhist Aetna   7/3/07

PATIENT CERTIFCATION

28945 Abdul Damush 2 Otter St. Boulder, Co 43612   Mae Ling MD

● **Figure 4.3**
Physician's order sheet.

16. A patient is drinking $\frac{1}{2}$ pint of orange juice every two hours. At this rate, how many quarts of orange juice will the patient drink in eight hours?

17. Use the label in ● **Figure 4.4** to determine the number of grams in one capsule of Zonegran.

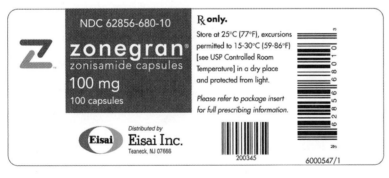

● **Figure 4.4**
Drug label for Zonegran.
(Reproduced with the permission of Eisai Inc.)

18. An infant weighs 3,400 grams. How much does the infant weigh in kilograms?

19. drams 12 = ounces _____

20. drams $1\frac{1}{2}$ = minims _____

Additional Exercises

Now, test yourself!

1. 6.5 mg = _____ mcg

2. 0.05 g = _____ mg

3. 0.04 g = _____ mg

4. 4.75 L = _____ mL

5. drams 3 = minims _____

6. oz 64 = dr _____

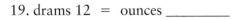

7. 120 mL = _____ cc   10. 6 T = _____ t

8. 100,000 mcg = _____ mg   11. 8 pt = _____ qt

9. 2 qt = _____ pt   12. 0.26 kg = _____ g

13. The label in ● **Figure 4.5** indicates the quantity of Wellbutrin in one tablet. Change milligrams to grams.

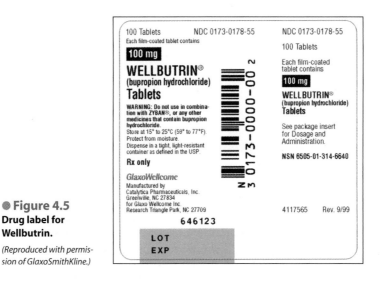

● **Figure 4.5**
Drug label for Wellbutrin.

(Reproduced with permission of GlaxoSmithKline.)

14. The physician ordered ProBanthine 30 mg PO ac hs. What is this dose in PO grams?

15. According to the physician's order sheet in ● **Figure 4.6**, what is the dose of Timentin in milligrams?

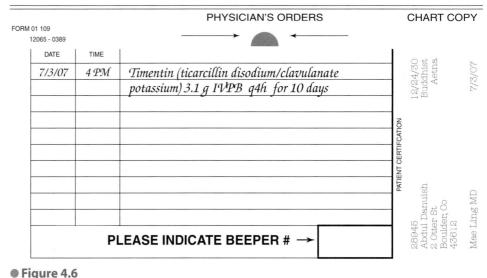

● **Figure 4.6**
Physician's order sheet.

16. The prescriber ordered the following:

Orange juice $\frac{1}{2}$ pint PO q2h

How many ounces of orange juice should be given q2h?

17. A patient is receiving 1 tablet of Xanax. Read the label in ● **Figure 4.7**. How many grams of Xanax is the patient receiving?

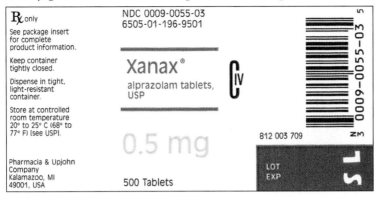

● **Figure 4.7**
Drug label for Xanax.

18. The label in ● **Figure 4.8** indicates the amount of Zantac in each tablet. Convert milligrams to grams.

● **Figure 4.8**
Drug label for Zantac.

(Reproduced with permission of GlaxoSmithKline.)

19. An infant weighs 2.8 kg. How much does the infant weigh in grams?

20. Read the order on the physician's order sheet in ● **Figure 4.9**. Convert the dose to grams.

PHYSICIAN'S ORDERS   CHART COPY

FORM 01 109
12065 - 0389

DATE	TIME	
8/4/07	8AM	Cimetidine 400 mg PO b.i.d.

PLEASE INDICATE BEEPER # →

12/24/16
R.C.
Medicare

PATIENT CERTIFICATION

612408
Frank Kiernan
3 Elm St.
Bethpage, NY
11720

● **Figure 4.9**
Physician's order sheet.

Cumulative Review Exercises

Review your mastery of earlier chapters.

1. 7.8 g = _____ mg   4. oz 28 = dr _____

2. 0.25 mg = _____ mcg   5. 1,200 mL = _____ L

3. 4.5 L = _____ mL   6. 7.6 kg = _____ g

7. Convert 750 mL to liters.

8. How many teaspoons are contained in 5 T?

9. The order reads Carafate 1 g PO q.i.d. Convert this dose to milligrams.

10. The patient must receive 250 mg of Cloxacillin PO q6h. Change to grams.

11. Change 0.65 mg to micrograms.

12. The physician ordered 2 T of Mylanta PO q2h. How many teaspoons of this antacid would you prepare?

13. The order is Colace 150 mg PO t.i.d. the label reads 150 mg/15 mL. How many milliliters would you prepare?

14. Change 250 mL to liters.

15. Change 0.032 g to milligrams.

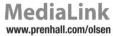 **MediaLink**   Animated examples, interactive practice questions with animated solutions, and challenge tests for this
www.prenhall.com/olsen   chapter can be found on the Prentice Hall Dosage Calculation Tutor that accompanies this text. Addi-
tional, unique, interactive resources and activities can be found on the Companion Website.

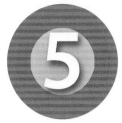
Converting From One System of Measurement to Another

Learning Outcomes

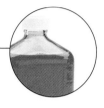

After completing this chapter, you will be able to

1. State the equivalent units of weight among the metric, household, and apothecary systems.
2. State the equivalent units of volume among the metric, household, and apothecary systems.
3. State the equivalent units of length between the metric and household systems.
4. Convert a quantity from one system of measurement to its equivalent in another system of measurement.

When calculating drug dosages, you will sometimes need to convert a quantity expressed in one system of measurement to an equivalent quantity expressed in a different system of measurement. For example, you might need to convert a quantity measured in ounces to the same quantity measured in milliliters. This chapter will show you how to use dimensional analysis to accomplish such conversions.

Equivalents of Common Units of Measurement

NOTE

Here are some useful equivalents:

1 t = 5 mL = dr 1

2 T = 30 mL = oz 1 = dr 8

Equivalent values for units of weight, volume, and length can also be found on the inside front cover of this text.

To get started, you will need to learn some basic equivalent values of the various units in the different systems. Tables 5.1 through Table 5.3 list some common equivalent values for weight, volume, and length in the metric, household, and apothecary systems of measurement. Although these equivalents are considered standards, many of them are approximations.

Table 5.1   Equivalent Values for Units of Weight

Metric		Apothecary		Household
60 milligrams (mg)	=	grain (gr) 1		
1 gram (g)	=	grains (gr) 15		
1 kilogram (kg)			=	2.2 pounds (lb)

Table 5.2   Equivalent Values for Units of Volume

Metric		Apothecary		Household
1 milliliter (mL)	=	minims 15		
5 milliliters (mL)	=	dram (dr) 1	=	1 teaspoon (t)
15 milliliters (mL)	=	ounce (oz) $\frac{1}{2}$	=	1 tablespoon (T)
30 milliliters (mL)	=	ounce (oz) 1	=	2 tablespoons (T)
500 milliliters	=	ounces (oz) 16	=	1 pint (pt)
1,000 milliliters	=	ounces (oz) 32	=	1 quart (qt)

Table 5.3   Equivalent Values for Units of Length

Metric		Household
2.5 centimeters (cm)	=	1 inch (in)

You can use dimensional analysis to convert from one system to another in exactly the same way you converted from one unit to another within the same system. ● **Figure 5.1** depicts some useful equivalents of volume measurements among the three systems.

●**Figure 5.1**
Measuring cups showing equivalent units.

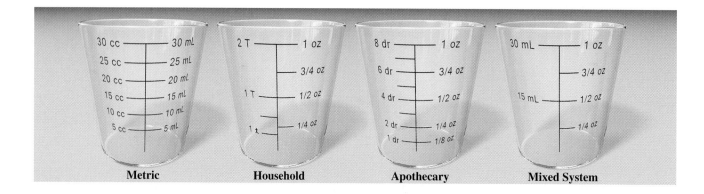

| Metric | Household | Apothecary | Mixed System |

The surface of a liquid, called the meniscus, in a medication cup is not flat (● **Figure 5.2**). It is curved. We read the amount of liquid at the level of the bottom of the meniscus.

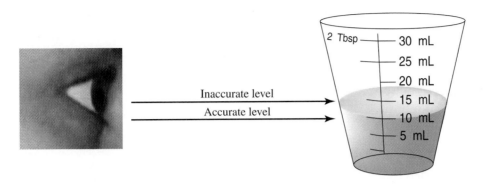

●**Figure 5.2**
Medication cup.

Metric–Household Conversions

Example 5.1

Convert 8 teaspoons to milliliters.

$$8 \text{ t} = ? \text{ mL}$$

You want to cancel the teaspoons and obtain the equivalent in milliliters.

$$8 \text{ t} \times \frac{? \text{ mL}}{? \text{ t}} = ? \text{ mL}$$

You use the equivalence 5 mL = 1 t.
So, the unit fraction is $\dfrac{5 \text{ mL}}{1\text{t}}$.

$$8\cancel{\text{t}} \times \frac{5 \text{ mL}}{1 \cancel{\text{t}}} = 40 \text{ mL}$$

So, 8 teaspoons are equivalent to 40 milliliters.

Example 5.2

Change $1\frac{1}{2}$ pints to milliliters.

$$1\tfrac{1}{2} \text{ pt} = ? \text{ mL}$$

You want to cancel the pints and obtain the equivalent amount in milliliters.

$$\frac{3 \text{ pt}}{2} \times \frac{? \text{ mL}}{? \text{ pt}} = ? \text{ mL}$$

Because 500 mL = 1 pt, the fraction is $\dfrac{500 \text{ mL}}{1 \text{ pt}}$.

$$\frac{3 \cancel{\text{pt}}}{\underset{1}{\cancel{2}}} \times \frac{\overset{250}{\cancel{500}} \text{ mL}}{1 \cancel{\text{pt}}} = 750 \text{ mL}$$

So, $1\frac{1}{2}$ pints is equivalent to 750 milliliters.

Example 5.3

Adam is 6 feet 3 inches tall. What is his height in centimeters?

$$6 \text{ ft } 3 \text{ in} \quad \text{means} \quad 6 \text{ ft} + 3 \text{ in}$$

First determine Adam's height in inches. To do this, convert 6 feet to inches.

$$6 \text{ ft} = ? \text{ in}$$

You want to cancel feet and obtain the equivalent height in inches.

$$6 \text{ ft} \times \frac{? \text{ in}}{? \text{ ft}} = ? \text{ in}$$

Because 1 ft = 12 in, the fraction is $\dfrac{12 \text{ in}}{1 \text{ ft}}$

$$6 \cancel{\text{ft}} \times \frac{12 \text{ in}}{1 \cancel{\text{ft}}} = 72 \text{ in}$$

Now, add the extra 3 inches.

$$72 \text{ in} + 3 \text{ in} = 75 \text{ in}$$

Now convert 75 inches to centimeters.

$$75 \text{ in} = ? \text{ cm}$$

You want to cancel inches and obtain the equivalent length in centimeters.

$$75 \text{ in} \times \frac{? \text{ cm}}{? \text{ in}} = ? \text{ cm}$$

Because 1 in = 2.5 cm, the fraction is $\dfrac{2.5 \text{ cm}}{1 \text{ in}}$

$$75 \cancel{\text{in}} \times \frac{2.5 \text{ cm}}{1 \cancel{\text{in}}} = 187.5 \text{ cm}$$

So, Adam is 187.5 centimeters tall.

Example 5.4

Jennifer weighs 115 pounds 8 ounces. What is her weight in kilograms?

$$115 \text{ lb } 8 \text{ oz} \quad \text{means} \quad 115 \text{ lb} + 8 \text{ oz}$$

First determine Jennifer's weight in pounds. To do this, convert 8 ounces to pounds.

$$8 \text{ oz} = ? \text{ lb}$$

You want to cancel ounces and obtain the equivalent amount in pounds.

$$8 \text{ oz} \times \frac{? \text{ lb}}{? \text{ oz}} = ? \text{ lb}$$

Because 1 lb = 16 oz, the fraction is $\dfrac{1 \text{ lb}}{16 \text{ oz}}$

$$\overset{1}{\cancel{8 \text{ oz}}} \times \frac{1 \text{ lb}}{\underset{2}{\cancel{16 \text{ oz}}}} = \frac{1}{2} \text{ lb}$$

So, Jennifer weighs 115 lb + $\frac{1}{2}$ lb or 115.5 pounds.

Now, convert 115.5 pounds to kilograms.

$$115.5 \text{ lb} = ? \text{ kg}$$

You want to cancel pounds and obtain the equivalent amount in kilograms.

$$115.5 \text{ lb} \times \frac{? \text{ kg}}{? \text{ lb}} = ? \text{ kg}$$

Because 1 kg = 2.2 lb, the fraction is $\dfrac{1 \text{ kg}}{2.2 \text{ lb}}$

$$115.5 \cancel{\text{ lb}} \times \frac{1 \text{ kg}}{2.2 \cancel{\text{ lb}}} = 52.5 \text{ kg}$$

So, Jennifer weighs 52.5 kilograms.

Metric–Apothecary Conversions

Example 5.5

Convert 40 milligrams to grains.

$$40 \text{ mg} = \text{gr } ?$$

Cancel the milligrams and obtain the equivalent amount in grains.

$$40 \text{ mg} \times \frac{\text{gr } ?}{? \text{ mg}} = \text{gr } ?$$

Because 60 mg = gr 1, the fraction is $\dfrac{\text{gr } 1}{60 \text{ mg}}$

$$\overset{2}{\cancel{40 \text{ mg}}} \times \frac{\text{gr } 1}{\underset{3}{\cancel{60 \text{ mg}}}} = \text{gr } \frac{2}{3}$$

So, 40 milligrams are equivalent to grain $\dfrac{2}{3}$.

Example 5.6

Convert 0.12 milligrams to grains.

$$0.12 \text{ mg} = \text{gr } ?$$

You want to cancel the milligrams and get the equivalent amount in grains.

$$0.12 \text{ mg} \times \frac{\text{gr } ?}{? \text{ mg}} = \text{gr } ?$$

Because 60 mg = gr 1, the fraction is $\dfrac{\text{gr } 1}{60 \text{ mg}}$.

$$0.12 \text{ mg} \times \frac{\text{gr } 1}{60 \text{ mg}} = \text{gr } \frac{0.12}{60} \times \frac{100}{100} = \text{gr } \frac{12}{6{,}000} = \text{gr } \frac{1}{500}$$

So, 0.12 mg is equivalent to grains $\frac{1}{500}$.

Example 5.7

Read the information on the label in ● **Figure 5.3** and convert the quantity of drug in the vial to grains.

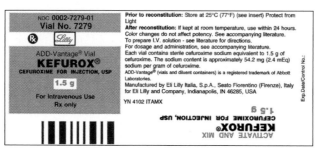

●**Figure 5.3**
Drug label for Kefurox.

(Copyright Eli Lilly and Company. Used with permission.)

$$1.5 \text{ g} = \text{gr ?}$$

You want to cancel the grams and obtain the equivalent amount in grains.

$$1.5 \text{ g} \times \frac{\text{gr ?}}{\text{? g}} = \text{gr ?}$$

Because 1 g = gr 15, the fraction is $\dfrac{\text{gr } 15}{1 \text{ g}}$

$$1.5 \text{ g} \times \frac{\text{gr } 15}{1 \text{ g}} = \text{gr } 22.5 \quad \text{or} \quad \text{gr } 22\frac{1}{2}$$

So, 1.5 grams is equivalent to grains $22\frac{1}{2}$.

> **NOTE**
>
> Grains are apothecary units and are therefore expressed as fractions or whole numbers. Therefore, grains 22.5 should be expressed as grains $22\frac{1}{2}$.

Example 5.8

Convert grain $\frac{1}{300}$ to milligrams.

$$\text{gr } \frac{1}{300} = \text{? mg}$$

You want to cancel the grain and obtain the equivalent amount in milligrams.

$$\text{gr } \frac{1}{300} \times \frac{\text{? mg}}{\text{gr ?}} = \text{? mg}$$

Because 60 mg = gr 1, the fraction is $\dfrac{60 \text{ mg}}{\text{gr } 1}$

$$\text{gr } \frac{1}{\underset{5}{\cancel{300}}} \times \frac{\overset{1}{\cancel{60}} \text{ mg}}{\cancel{\text{gr }} 1} = \frac{1}{5} \text{ mg} \quad \text{or} \quad 0.2 \text{ mg}$$

So, grain $\frac{1}{300}$ is equivalent to 0.2 mg.

Example 5.9

Convert grains $7\frac{1}{2}$ to grams.

$$\text{gr } 7\frac{1}{2} = ? \text{ g}$$

You want to cancel the grains and obtain the equivalent amount in grams.

$$\text{gr } \frac{15}{2} \times \frac{? \text{ g}}{\text{gr } ?} = ? \text{ g}$$

Since 1 g = gr 15, the fraction is $\dfrac{1 \text{ g}}{\text{gr } 15}$

$$\cancel{\text{gr}} \frac{\overset{1}{\cancel{15}}}{2} \times \frac{1 \text{ g}}{\underset{1}{\cancel{\text{gr } 15}}} = \frac{1}{2} \text{ g} = 0.5 \text{ g}$$

So, grains $7\frac{1}{2}$ are equivalent to 0.5 gram.

NOTE

Grams are metric units so they are expressed as decimals or whole numbers. Therefore, $\frac{1}{2}$ gram is expressed as 0.5 gram.

Household–Apothecary Conversions

Example 5.10

Convert ounces 2 to tablespoons.

$$\text{ounces 2} = ? \text{ tablespoons}$$

You want to cancel the ounces and obtain the equivalent amount in tablespoons.

$$\text{oz 2} \times \frac{? \text{ T}}{\text{oz } ?} = ? \text{ T}$$

Because 1 tablespoon = ounce $\frac{1}{2}$, the fraction is $\dfrac{1 \text{ T}}{\text{oz } \frac{1}{2}}$

$$\cancel{\text{oz}} \, 2 \times \frac{1 \text{ T}}{\cancel{\text{oz}} \, \frac{1}{2}} = \frac{2}{\frac{1}{2}} \text{T} = 4 \text{ T}$$

So, ounces 2 is equivalent to 4 tablespoons.

Summary

In this chapter, quantities measured in one system of measurement were converted to equivalent quantities measured in a different system of measurement.

- It is important to memorize all the equivalences for volume, weight, and length between the various systems of measurement.

- Dimensional analysis can be used to perform conversions between any two of the three systems.

- The equivalences between systems are not exact equivalences; they are approximate equivalences.

- When performing conversions between two systems, your answers are not exact; they are approximate.

- When performing conversions between two systems, answers may differ somewhat, depending on which approximate equivalences are used.

Workspace

Practice Sets

The answers to *Try These for Practice, Exercises,* and *Cumulative Review Exercises* appear in Appendix A at the end of the book. Ask your instructor for the answers to the *Additional Exercises*.

Try These for Practice

Test your comprehension after reading the chapter.

1. In order to do the exercises at the end of this chapter, you need to memorize all the equivalents presented so far. To test yourself, fill in the missing numbers in the following chart.

Metric System

(a) 1 mL = _____ cc

(b) 1 L = _____ mL

(c) 1 kg = _____ g

(d) 1,000 mg = _____ g

(e) 1,000 mcg = _____ mg

Household System

(f) 1 glass = _____ oz

(g) 1 oz = _____ T

(h) 1 T = _____ t

(i) 1 lb = _____ oz

(j) 1 ft = _____ in

(k) 1 qt = _____ pt

(l) 1 pt = _____ oz

Apothecary System

(m) oz 1 = dr _____

(n) dr 1 = minims _____

Mixed Systems

(o) dr 1 = _____ t = minims _____ = _____ mL

(p) oz 1 = _____ T = dr _____ = _____ mL

(q) 1 measuring cup = _____ glass = oz _____ = _____ pt

(r) gr 1 = _____ mg

(s) 1 g = gr _____

(t) 1 kg = _____ lb

(u) 1 in = _____ cm

2. A patient is receiving 5 mL of Indocin. Read the label in ● **Figure 5.4** to determine the number of grams the patient is receiving.

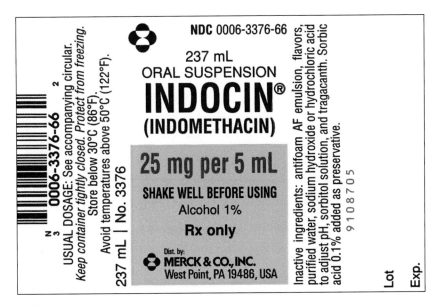

● **Figure 5.4**
Drug label for Indocin.

(The labels for the products Indocin 25mg per 5mL are reproduced with permission of Merck & Co., Inc., copyright owner.)

3. How many pounds is a person who weighs 50 kilograms?

4. Read the label in ● **Figure 5.5** and determine how many teaspoons of this antiviral drug would contain 50 milligrams of Retrovir.

5. How many milligrams of aspirin are contained in a grains 5 aspirin tablet?

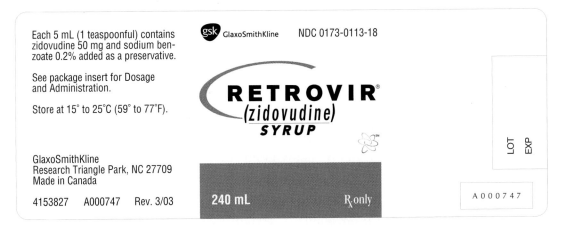

● **Figure 5.5**
Drug label for Retrovir.

(Reproduced with permission of GlaxoSmithKline.)

Exercises

Reinforce your understanding in class or at home.

1. 4,500 mcg = _____ mg

2. 1.5 L = _____ mL

3. 4 t = _____ mL

4. 15 mL = _____ t

5. 45 kg = _____ lb

6. 110 lb = _____ kg

7. 48 oz = _____ pt

8. 3 oz = _____ T

9. 10 cm = _____ in

10. 6 in = _____ cm

11. A patient is 6 feet 2 inches tall. Find the height of the patient in centimeters.

12. Using the label in ●**Figure 5.6,** determine the number of ounces of the solution that would contain 10 mg of the antifungal drug fluconazole.

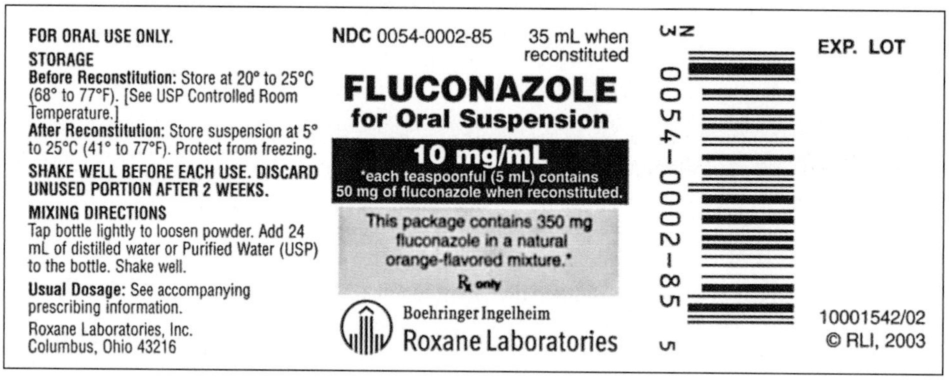

●**Figure 5.6**
Drug label for fluconazole.

(Courtesy of Roxane Laboratories Inc.)

13. A woman weighs 165 pounds. What is her weight in kilograms?

14. A patient takes 2 teaspoons of Robitussin (guaifenesin). How many milliliters of this cough suppressant did the patient take?

15. The prescriber ordered methotrexate 25 mg IM daily for 5 days. The label reads 25 mg/mL. How many grains of this antineoplastic drug are contained in one dose?

16. Read the information in ●**Figure 5.7** and determine the number of teaspoons of the bronchodilator metaproterenol you will administer if the label reads "10 mg/5 mL."

17. A patient drank 12 ounces of orange juice. How many milliliters did the patient drink?

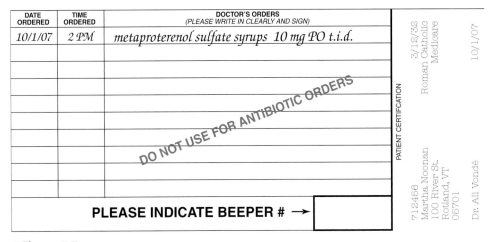

UNIVERSITY HOSPITAL

AUTHORIZATION IS HEPEBY GIVEN TO DISPENSE THE GENERIC OR CHEMICAL EQUIVALENT UNLESS OTHERWISE INDICATED BY THE WORDS — **NO SUBSTITUTE**

DATE ORDERED	TIME ORDERED	DOCTOR'S ORDERS *(PLEASE WRITE IN CLEARLY AND SIGN)*	
10/1/07	2 PM	metaproterenol sulfate syrups 10 mg PO t.i.d.	

DO NOT USE FOR ANTIBIOTIC ORDERS

PATIENT CERTIFICATION

3/12/32
Roman Catholic
Medicare

10/1/07

712456
Martha Noonan
100 River St.
Rotland, VT
05701

Dr. Ali Vordé

PLEASE INDICATE BEEPER # →

●**Figure 5.7**
Physician's order sheet.

18. Use the label in ●**Figure 5.8** to determine the number of milligrams of Rhinocort in one metered spray.

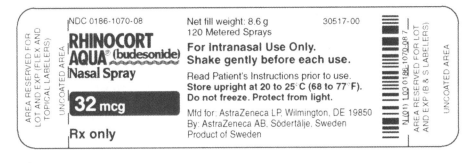

● **Figure 5.8**
Drug label for Rhinocort.

(Courtesy of AstraZeneca Pharmaceuticals LP.)

19. The label in Figure 5.8 indicates that in the container there are 120 metered sprays, each of which contains 32 mcg of Rhinocort. Use this information to determine the total number of milligrams of this corticosteroid inhalant that are in the container.

20. Read the label in ●**Figure 5.9** and determine the number of grains in 3 tablets of this antihypertensive drug.

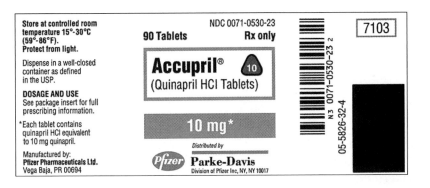

● **Figure 5.9**
Drug label for Accupril.

(Reg. Trademark of Pfizer Inc. Reproduced with permission.)

Additional Exercises

Now, test yourself!

1. Convert 3,200 micrograms to milligrams.

2. How many milligrams are contained in 250 grams?

3. 0.005 g = _____ mg

4. 0.004 mg = _____ mcg

5. 8 oz = _____ mL

6. 0.006 mg = gr _____

7. 0.7 mg = _____ g

8. 8.25 L = _____ mL

9. 10,700 mL = _____ L

10. gr $3\frac{3}{4}$ = _____ mg

11. Read the label in ●**Figure 5.10**. How many grams of codeine are contained in 5 milliliters?

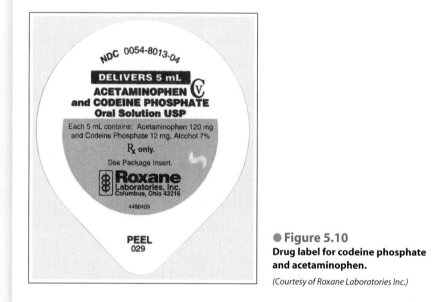

●**Figure 5.10**
Drug label for codeine phosphate and acetaminophen.
(Courtesy of Roxane Laboratories Inc.)

12. A capsule of acetaminophen (Tylenol), an antipyretic drug, contains 0.5 gram. One capsule contains how many milligrams?

13. A prescriber ordered

Chlorpromazine 30 mg PO q4h stat

Using the label in ●**Figure 5.11,** determine the number of milliliters of this antianxiety drug you would give your patient.

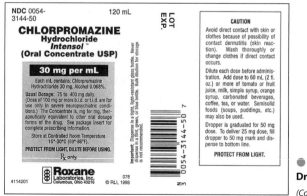

●**Figure 5.11**
Drug label for Chlorpromazine.
(Courtesy of Roxane Laboratories Inc.)

14. How many teaspoons of the drug in ●**Figure 5.12** will contain 100 mg of the antibiotic Zyvox?

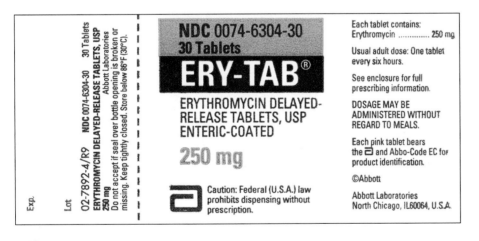

NDC 0009-5136-01

ZYVOX™

linezolid for
oral suspension

100 mg /5 mL

150 mL
(when constituted)   *PHARMACIA*

℞ only
See package insert for dosage and
complete product information.
Warning: Not for injection.
Store at 25°C (77°F) (see insert).
Gently invert the bottle 3 to 5 times before
using. **DO NOT SHAKE.** Keep container
tightly closed. Protect from light and
moisture. Constituted product may be
used for 21 days. Store constituted
suspension at room temperature. Discard
unused portion after 21 days.
Mixing Directions: Gently tap bottle to
loosen powder. Add a total of 123 mL
distilled water in two portions. After
adding the first half, shake vigorously to
wet all of the powder. Then add the
second half of the water and shake
vigorously to obtain a uniform suspension.
Each 5 mL of suspension contains 100 mg
linezolid.

U.S. Patent No. 5,688,792
Pharmacia &
Upjohn Company   ● 818070002
A subsidiary of
Pharmacia   LOT
Corporation
Kalamazoo, MI   EXP   **S L**
49001, USA

● **Figure 5.12**
Drug label for Zyvox.

15. Read the label in ●**Figure 5.13** to determine the number of grains in 1 tablet of the antibiotic ERY-TAB.

NDC 0074-6304-30
30 Tablets

ERY-TAB®

ERYTHROMYCIN DELAYED-
RELEASE TABLETS, USP
ENTERIC-COATED

250 mg

Caution: Federal (U.S.A.) law
prohibits dispensing without
prescription.

Each tablet contains:
Erythromycin .... 250 mg

Usual adult dose: One tablet
every six hours.

See enclosure for full
prescribing information.

DOSAGE MAY BE
ADMINISTERED WITHOUT
REGARD TO MEALS.

Each pink tablet bears
the ⼕ and Abbo-Code EC for
product identification.

©Abbott

Abbott Laboratories
North Chicago, IL60064, U.S.A.

● **Figure 5.13**
Drug label for Ery-Tab.

(Reproduced with permission of Abbott Laboratories.)

16. The order is *Benadryl syrup (diphenhydramine HCl) 12.5 mg PO q6h.* The label reads 12.5 mg/5 mL. How many teaspoons of this antihistamine will you administer to your patient?

17. Read the label in ●**Figure 5.14** and determine the number of milligrams of this cardiac medication in one milliliter of this elixir.

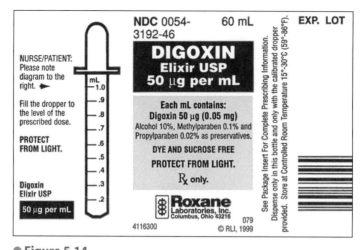

● **Figure 5.14**
Drug label for digoxin.

(Courtesy of Roxane Laboratories Inc.)

18. Read the information on the physician's order sheet in ● **Figure 5.15**. How many grains of this antihypertensive drug will the patient receive in a day?

UNIVERSITY HOSPITAL

AUTHORIZATION IS HEPEBY GIVEN TO DISPENSE THE GENERIC OR CHEMICAL EQUIVALENT UNLESS OTHERWISE INDICATED BY THE WORDS — **NO SUBSTITUTE**

DATE ORDERED	TIME ORDERED	DOCTOR'S ORDERS (PLEASE WRITE IN CLEARLY AND SIGN)		
10/1/07	2 PM	*clonidine 0.3 mg PO b.i.d.*		
			DO NOT USE FOR ANTIBIOTIC ORDERS	
		PLEASE INDICATE BEEPER # →		

PATIENT CERTIFCATION 3/12/32 Roman Catholic Medicare 10/1/07

712456 Martha Noonan 100 River St. Rotland, VT 05701 Dr. Ali Vondé

● **Figure 5.15**
Physician's order sheet.

19. Read the label in ● **Figure 5.16** and determine the number of grams in 1 tablet of this oral hypoglycemic drug.

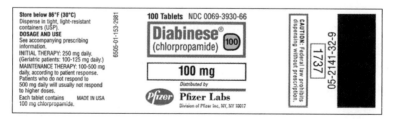

● **Figure 5.16**
Drug label for Diabinese.

(Reg. Trademark of Pfizer Inc. Reproduced with permission.)

20. Convert grains 45 to grams.

Cumulative Review Exercises

Review your mastery of earlier chapters.

1. Convert 0.125 milligrams to micrograms.

2. 0.009 g = _____ mg

3. How many grams are contained in 5.65 kilograms?

4. 0.1 mg = _____ mcg

5. 0.06 g = _____ mg

6. gr 75 = _____ mg

7. 7.75 L = _____ mL

8. 0.6 mg = _____ mcg

9. 1,250 mL = _____ L

10. 30 mg = gr _____

11. Read the label in ●Figure 5.17. How many grains of Agenerase are contained in 3 capsules?

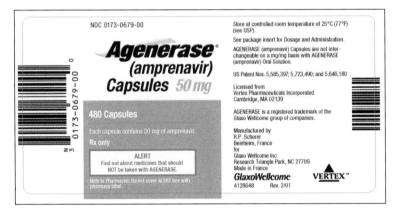

●**Figure 5.17**
Drug label for Agenerase.
(Reproduced with permission of GlaxoSmithKline.)

12. Read the label in Figure 5.17. How many grams of the antiretroviral drug Agenerase are contained in 3 capsules?

13. Read the label in ●Figure 5.18. Calculate the number of grams in 1 tablet of this antihistamine.

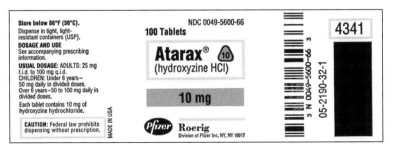

●**Figure 5.18**
Drug label for Atarax.
(Reg. Trademark of Pfizer Inc. Reproduced with permission.)

14. Read the label in ● **Figure 5.19** and determine the total number of tablets in the container.

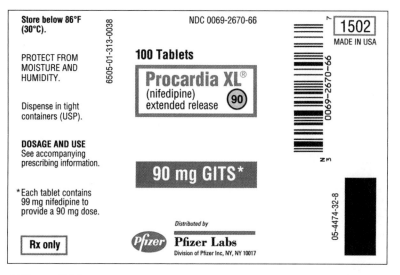

Store below 86°F (30°C).

6505-01-313-0038

PROTECT FROM MOISTURE AND HUMIDITY.

Dispense in tight containers (USP).

DOSAGE AND USE
See accompanying prescribing information.

*Each tablet contains 99 mg nifedipine to provide a 90 mg dose.

Rx only

NDC 0069-2670-66

100 Tablets

Procardia XL®
(nifedipine)
extended release (90)

90 mg GITS*

Distributed by

Pfizer **Pfizer Labs**
Division of Pfizer Inc, NY, NY 10017

1502
MADE IN USA

0069-2670-66

05-4474-32-8

● **Figure 5.19**
Drug label for Procardia XL.

(Reg. Trademark of Pfizer Inc. Reproduced with permission.)

15. Read the label in Figure 5.19 and determine the number of grams in 1 tablet of this antianginal drug.

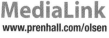

MediaLink
www.prenhall.com/olsen

Animated examples, interactive practice questions with animated solutions, and challenge tests for this chapter can be found on the Prentice Hall Dosage Calculation Tutor that accompanies this text. Additional, unique, interactive resources and activities can be found on the Companion Website.

Unit

Oral and Parenteral Medications

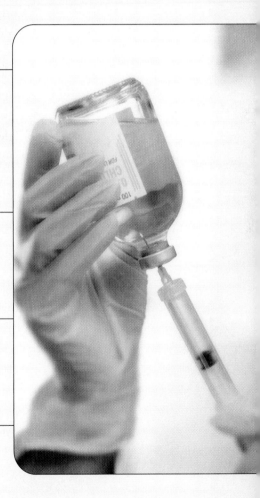

Calculating Oral Medication Doses

Learning Outcomes

After completing this chapter, you will be able to

1. Calculate simple problems for oral medications in solid and liquid form.
2. Calculate complex problems for oral medications in solid and liquid form.
3. Calculate doses for medications measured in milliequivalents.
4. Interpret drug labels in order to calculate doses for oral medication.
5. Calculate doses based on body weight.
6. Calculate doses based on body surface area (BSA) using a formula or a nomogram.

In this chapter you will learn how to calculate doses of oral medications in solid or liquid form. You will also be introduced to problems that utilize body weight or body surface area (BSA) to calculate dosages.

Simple Problems

In the calculations you have done in previous chapters, all the equivalents have come from standard tables, for example, 60 mg = gr 1. In this chapter, the equivalent used will depend on the strength of the drug that is available; for example 1 tab = 15 mg. In the following examples, the equivalent is found on the label of the drug container.

Medication in Solid Form

Example 6.1

The order reads Cymbalta (duloxetine HCl) 120 mg PO daily.

Read the drug label shown in ● **Figure 6.1**. How many capsules of this antidepressant drug will you administer to the patient?

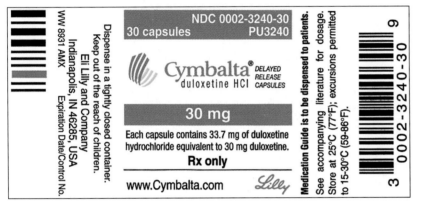

● **Figure 6.1**
Drug label for Cymbalta.

(Copyright Eli Lilly and Company. Used with permission).

Convert 120 mg to capsules.

$$120 \text{ mg} = ? \text{ cap}$$

Cancel the milligrams and calculate the equivalent amount in capsules.

$$120 \text{ mg} \times \frac{? \text{ cap}}{? \text{ mg}} = ? \text{ cap}$$

Because the label indicates that each capsule contains 30 mg, you use the unit fraction $\frac{1 \text{ cap}}{30 \text{ mg}}$

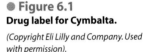

$$\overset{4}{\cancel{120}} \text{ mg} \times \frac{\boxed{1 \text{ cap}}}{\underset{1}{\cancel{30}} \text{ mg}} = 4 \text{ cap}$$

So, you would give 4 capsules by mouth once a day to the patient.

Example 6.2

The prescriber orders Diovan (valsartan) 120 mg PO once daily for a patient with hypertension. Read the drug label shown in ● **Figure 6.2** and determine how many tablets you would give to the patient.

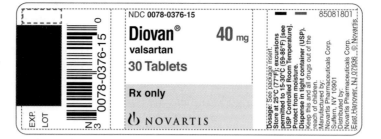

● **Figure 6.2**
Drug label for Diovan.

(Reproduced with the permission of Novartis Pharmaceuticals.)

Convert 120 mg to tablets.

$$120 \text{ mg} = ? \text{ tab}$$

Cancel the milligrams and obtain the equivalent amount in tablets.

$$120 \text{ mg} \times \frac{? \text{ tab}}{? \text{ mg}} = ? \text{ tab}$$

Because 1 tab = 40 mg, the unit fraction is $\dfrac{1 \text{ tab}}{40 \text{ mg}}$

$$\overset{3}{\cancel{120}} \text{ mg} \times \frac{\boxed{1 \text{ tab}}}{\underset{1}{\cancel{40} \text{ mg}}} = 3 \text{ tab}$$

So, you would give 3 tablets by mouth daily to the patient.

Example 6.3

Read the label in ● **Figure 6.3**. The physician's order is Lotrel 5 mg/20 mg PO daily. How many capsules of this antihypertensive drug should be administered per day?

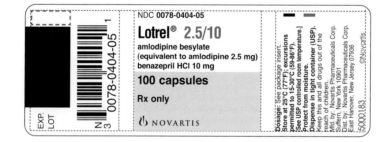

● **Figure 6.3**
Drug label for Lotrel.

(Reproduced with the permission of Novartis Pharmaceuticals.)

Lotrel is a combination drug (see Figures 2.16 and 2.17 in Chapter 2) composed of amlodipine and benazepril; therefore, for computational purposes we need only address the first listed drug (amlodipine).

Since the order requires 5 mg of amlodipine, convert the 5 mg to capsules.

$$5 \text{ mg} = ? \text{ cap}$$

Cancel the milligrams and obtain the equivalent amount in capsules.

$$5 \text{ mg} \times \frac{? \text{ cap}}{? \text{ mg}} = ? \text{ cap}$$

The label indicates that 1 capsule contains 2.5 mg of amlodipine.

Therefore, the fraction is $\dfrac{1 \text{ cap}}{2.5 \text{ mg}}$

$$\overset{2}{\cancel{5}} \text{ mg} \times \dfrac{\boxed{1 \text{ cap}}}{\underset{1}{\cancel{2.5} \text{ mg}}} = 2 \text{ cap}$$

So, you would give 2 capsules by mouth daily to the patient.

Example 6.4

The order is codeine sulfate grain $\frac{1}{2}$ PO q4h prn pain. The label reads gr$\frac{1}{4}$ per tablet. How many tablets should you give a patient?
In this problem you want to convert the grain $\frac{1}{2}$ to tablets.

$$\text{gr } \dfrac{1}{2} = ? \text{ tab}$$

Cancel the grain and determine the equivalent amount in tablets.
Because 1 tab = gr$\frac{1}{4}$, the fraction is $\dfrac{1 \text{ tab}}{\text{gr}\frac{1}{4}}$

$$\cancel{\text{gr}} \dfrac{1}{2} \times \dfrac{\boxed{1 \text{ tab}}}{\cancel{\text{gr}}\dfrac{1}{4}} = \dfrac{1 \text{ tab}}{\dfrac{2}{4}} = 1 \text{ tab} \div \dfrac{2}{4} = 1 \text{ tab} \times \dfrac{4}{2} = 2 \text{ tab}$$

Since 2 tablets contain grain $\frac{1}{2}$ of codeine sulfate, you would give 2 tablets by mouth every 4 hours as necessary for pain.

Medication in Liquid Form

Since pediatric and geriatric patients, as well as patients with neurological conditions, may be unable to swallow medication in tablet form, sometimes oral medications are ordered in liquid form. The label states how much drug is contained in a given amount of liquid.

> **NOTE**
>
> Some liquid oral medications are supplied with special calibrated droppers or oral syringes that are used *only* for these medications (e.g., digoxin and Lasix).

Example 6.5

The physician orders Lexapro (escitalopram oxalate) 10 mg PO once daily. Read the label in ●**Figure 6.4** and determine the number of milliliters you would administer to the patient.

Convert 10 milligrams to milliliters.

$$10 \text{ mg} = ? \text{ mL}$$

Cancel the milligrams and calculate the equivalent amount in mL.

$$10 \text{ mg} \times \dfrac{? \text{ mL}}{? \text{ mg}} = ? \text{ mL}$$

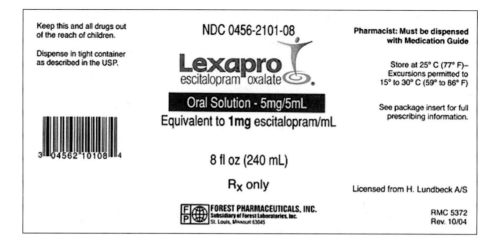

● **Figure 6.4**
Drug label for Lexapro.
(Courtesy of Forest Pharmaceuticals, Inc.)

Because the label indicates that every 5 mL of the solution contains 5 mg of Lexapro, use the unit fraction $\dfrac{5 \text{ mL}}{5 \text{ mg}}$

$$10 \text{ mg} \times \frac{5 \text{ mL}}{5 \text{ mg}} = 10 \text{ mL}$$

So, you would give 10 mL by mouth once a day to the patient.

Example 6.6

The physician orders Omnicef (cefdinir) 500 mg PO q12h. Read the label in ●**Figure 6.5**. Determine the number of mL you would administer to the patient.

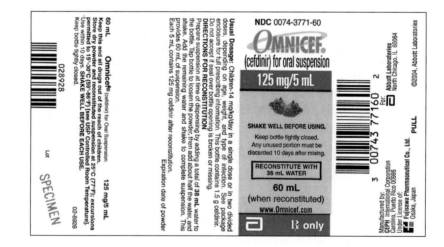

● **Figure 6.5**
Drug label for Omnicef.
(Reproduced with permission of Abbott Laboratories.)

Convert 500 mL to mg.

$$500 \text{ mg} = ? \text{ mL}$$

Cancel the milligrams and calculate the equivalent amount in milliliters.

$$500 \text{ mg} \times \frac{? \text{ mL}}{? \text{ mg}} = ? \text{ mL}$$

Because the label indicates that every 5 mL of the solution contains 123 mg of Omnicef, use the unit fraction $\dfrac{5 \text{ mL}}{125 \text{ mg}}$

$$\overset{4}{\cancel{500}} \text{ mg} \times \frac{5 \text{ \textcircled{mL}}}{\underset{1}{\cancel{125}} \text{ mg}} = 20 \text{ mL}$$

So, you would give 20 mL by mouth every 12 hours to the patient.

Medications Measured in Milliequivalents

Some drugs are measured in milliequivalents, which are abbreviated as mEq. Pharmaceutical companies label electrolytes in milligrams as well as milliequivalents.

Example 6.7

The physician orders K-Tab (potassium chloride) 30 mEq PO daily.

Read the label in ●**Figure 6.6** and determine how many tablets of this electrolyte supplement you should administer.

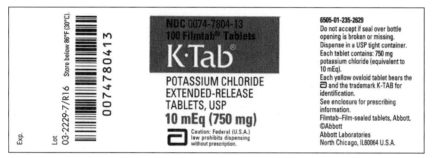

●**Figure 6.6**
Drug label for K-Tab.

(Reproduced with permission of Abbott Laboratories.)

In this problem you want to change 30 mEq to tablets.

$$30 \text{ mEq} \longrightarrow ? \text{ tab}$$

You can do this on one line as follows:

$$30 \text{ mEq} \times \frac{? \text{ tab}}{? \text{ mEq}} = ? \text{ tab}$$

Because the label indicates that each tablet contains 10 mEq, the unit fraction is $\dfrac{1 \text{ tab}}{10 \text{ mEq}}$

$$\overset{3}{\cancel{30}} \text{ \cancel{mEq}} \times \frac{\text{\textcircled{1 tab}}}{\cancel{10} \text{ \cancel{mEq}}} = 3 \text{ tab}$$

So, you would administer 3 tablets of K-Tab by mouth once daily.

Complex Problems

Sometimes dosage calculations will require that multiplication by unit fractions be repeated one or more times. Recall that we examined complex problems in Chapter 3.

For example, if each tablet of a drug contains 2.5 mg, how many tablets would contain 0.0025 gram?

It helps to organize the information you will need for the computation as follows:

Given quantity:	0.0025 mg
Strength:	1 tab = 2.5 mg
Quantity you want to find:	? tab

You do not know the direct equivalence between grams and tablets.

This is a **complex** problem because you need to convert 0.0025 g to milligrams and then convert milligrams to tablets.

$$0.0025 \text{ g} \longrightarrow \text{? mg} \longrightarrow \text{? tab}$$

So the problem is 0.0025 g = ? tab

First, you want to cancel *grams (g)*. To do this you must use an equivalence containing *grams* to make a unit fraction with *grams* in the denominator.

From the equivalence 1 g = 1,000 mg, the unit fraction is $\dfrac{1,000 \text{ mg}}{1 \text{ g}}$

$$0.0025 \text{ \cancel{g}} \times \frac{1,000 \text{ \textcircled{mg}}}{1 \text{ \cancel{g}}} = \text{? tab}$$

After the *grams* are cancelled, only *milligrams* remain on the left side. Now you need to change the *milligrams* to *tablets*. From the strength 2.5 mg = 1 tab, the unit fraction is $\dfrac{1 \text{ tab}}{2.5 \text{ mg}}$

$$0.0025 \text{ \cancel{g}} \times \frac{1,000 \text{ \cancel{mg}}}{1 \text{ \cancel{g}}} \times \frac{1 \text{ \textcircled{tab}}}{2.5 \text{ \cancel{mg}}} = \text{? tab}$$

After cancelling the milligrams, only tablets remain on the left side. Now complete your calculation by multiplying the numbers.

$$0.0025 \text{ \cancel{g}} \times \frac{1,000 \text{ \cancel{mg}}}{1 \text{ \cancel{g}}} \times \frac{1 \text{ \textcircled{tab}}}{2.5 \text{ \cancel{mg}}} = \frac{2.5 \text{ tab}}{2.5} = 1 \text{ tab}$$

So, 1 tablet contains 0.0025 g.

Example 6.8

The physician's order is aspirin (acetylsalicylic acid) 600 mg PO stat. The label reads *gr 5 per caplet*. How many caplets of this antipyretic drug should be given to the patient?

Given quantity: 600 mg
Strength: 1 cap = gr 5
Quantity you want to find: ? cap

There is no direct equivalence between milligrams and caplets.
This is a **complex** problem because you need to convert 600 mg to grains
and then convert grains to caplets.

$$600 \text{ mg} \longrightarrow \text{gr?} \longrightarrow \text{? cap}$$

First change milligrams to grains. To do this, you must use an equivalence containing *milligrams* to make a unit fraction with *milligrams* in
the denominator. From the equivalence gr 1 = 60 mg, the
unit fraction is $\dfrac{\text{gr } 1}{60 \text{ mg}}$.

$$600 \ \cancel{\text{mg}} \times \frac{\textcircled{\text{gr}}\, 1}{60 \ \cancel{\text{mg}}} = \text{? cap}$$

After the milligrams are cancelled, only grains remain on the left
side. Now you need to change the grains to caplets. From the strength
gr 5 = 1 cap, the unit fraction is $\dfrac{1 \text{ cap}}{\text{gr } 5}$.

$$600 \ \cancel{\text{mg}} \times \frac{\cancel{\text{gr}}\, 1}{60 \ \cancel{\text{mg}}} \times \frac{1 \ \textcircled{\text{cap}}}{\cancel{\text{gr}}\, 5} = \text{? cap}$$

Now complete your calculation.

$$\overset{10}{\cancel{600}} \ \cancel{\text{mg}} \times \frac{\cancel{\text{gr}}\, 1}{\underset{1}{\cancel{60}} \ \cancel{\text{mg}}} \times \frac{1 \text{ cap}}{\cancel{\text{gr}}\, 5} = \frac{10 \text{ cap}}{5} = 2 \text{ caplets}$$

So, you should give 2 caplets by mouth immediately to the patient.

Example 6.9

The order is Diflucan (fluconazole) 0.4 gram PO daily. Read the label
shown in ●**Figure 6.7** and calculate the number of tablets of this antifungal drug that should be given to the patient.

Given quantity: 0.4 g
Strength: 1 tab = 100 mg
Quantity you want to find: ? tab

In this problem you want to convert 0.4 gram to milligrams and then
convert milligrams to tablets.

$$0.4 \text{ g} \longrightarrow \text{? mg} \longrightarrow \text{? tab}$$

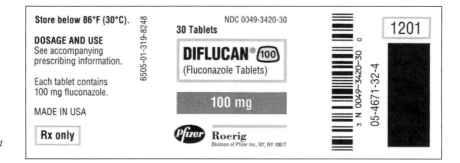

● Figure 6.7
Drug label for Diflucan.

(Reg. Trademark of Pfizer Inc. Reproduced with permission.)

You can do this on one line as follows:

$$0.4 \text{ g} \times \frac{? \text{ mg}}{? \text{ g}} \times \frac{? \text{ tab}}{? \text{ mg}} = ? \text{ tab}$$

Because 1,000 mg = 1 g, the first unit fraction is $\dfrac{1,000 \text{ mg}}{1 \text{ g}}$

Because 100 mg = 1 tab, the second unit fraction is $\dfrac{1 \text{ tab}}{100 \text{ mg}}$

$$0.4 \text{ g} \times \frac{\overset{10}{\cancel{1,000} \text{ mg}}}{1 \text{ g}} \times \frac{1 \text{ tab}}{\underset{1}{\cancel{100} \text{ mg}}} = 4 \text{ tab}$$

So, you should give 4 tablets by mouth once a day to the patient.

NOTE

Although Example 6.10 would be simpler using the milligrams, we will do the calculation using micrograms in order to practice complex problems. For safety purposes, drug manufacturers often place both microgram and milligram concentrations on drug labels.

Example 6.10

The order is Tikosyn (dofetilide) 0.5 mg PO b.i.d. Read the label shown in ● **Figure 6.8**. Calculate how many capsules of this antifungal drug should be given to the patient. Although there are two strengths on the label (mcg and mg), calculate the problem using microgram strength.

Given quantity:	0.5 mg
Strength:	1 tab = 125 mcg
Quantity you want to find:	? cap

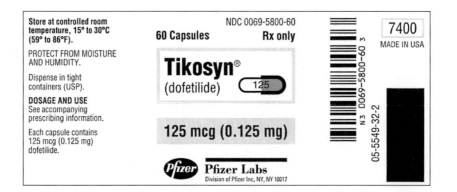

● Figure 6.8
Drug label for Tikosyn.

(Reg. Trademark of Pfizer Inc. Reproduced with permission.)

In this problem you want to convert 0.5 milligrams to micrograms and then convert micrograms to capsules.

$$0.5 \text{ mg} \longrightarrow \text{? mcg} \longrightarrow \text{? cap}$$

You can do this on one line as follows:

$$0.5 \text{ mg} \times \frac{\text{? mcg}}{\text{? mg}} \times \frac{1 \text{ cap}}{\text{? mcg}} = \text{? cap}$$

Because 1,000 mcg = 1 mg, the first unit fraction is $\dfrac{1{,}000 \text{ mcg}}{1 \text{ mg}}$

Because 1 cap = 125 mcg, the second unit fraction is $\dfrac{1 \text{ cap}}{125 \text{ mcg}}$

$$0.5 \text{ mg} \times \frac{\overset{8}{\cancel{1{,}000} \text{ mcg}}}{1 \text{ mg}} \times \frac{1 \text{ cap}}{\underset{1}{\cancel{125} \text{ mcg}}} = 4 \text{ cap}$$

So, you should give 4 capsules by mouth twice a day to the patient.

Example 6.11

The order is Daypro (oxaprozin) 1.8 g PO once daily each morning. The drug is supplied as 600 mg per caplet. How many caplets of this anti-arthritic drug should be given the patient?

Given quantity:	1.8 g
Strength:	1 cap = 600 mg
Quantity you want to find:	? cap

In this problem you want to convert 1.8 grams to milligrams and then convert milligrams to caplets.

$$1.8 \text{ g} \longrightarrow \text{? mg} \longrightarrow \text{? cap}$$

You can do this on one line as follows:

$$1.8 \text{ g} \times \frac{\text{? mg}}{\text{? g}} \times \frac{\text{? cap}}{\text{? mg}} = \text{? cap}$$

Because 1,000 mg = 1 g, the first unit fraction is $\dfrac{1{,}000 \text{ mg}}{1 \text{ g}}$

Because 1 cap = 600 mg, the second unit fraction is $\dfrac{1 \text{ cap}}{600 \text{ mg}}$

$$1.8 \text{ g} \times \frac{1{,}000 \text{ mg}}{1 \text{ g}} \times \frac{1 \text{ cap}}{600 \text{ mg}} = \frac{18 \text{ cap}}{6} = 3 \text{ cap}$$

So, you should give 3 caplets by mouth to the patient once a day in the morning.

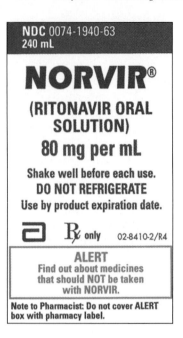

● Figure 6.9
Drug label for Norvir.

(Reproduced with permission of Abbott Laboratories.)

Example 6.12

The physician orders Norvir (ritonavir) 0.6 g PO q12 hours. Read the label in ● **Figure 6.9** and determine the number of mL of this protease inhibitor your patient would receive.

Given quantity:	0.6 g
Strength:	80 mg/mL
The quantity you want to find:	? mL

In this problem you want to convert 0.6 grams to milligrams and then convert milligrams to milliliters.

$$0.6 \text{ g} \longrightarrow ? \text{ mg} \longrightarrow ? \text{ mL}$$

You can do this on one line as follows:

$$0.6 \text{ g} \times \frac{? \text{ mg}}{? \text{ g}} \times \frac{? \text{ mL}}{? \text{ mg}} = ? \text{ mL}$$

Because 1,000 mg = 1 g, the first unit fraction is $\dfrac{1,000 \text{ mg}}{1 \text{ g}}$

Because 1 mL = 80 mg, the second unit fraction is $\dfrac{1 \text{ mL}}{80 \text{ mg}}$

$$0.6 \text{ g} \times \frac{1,000 \text{ mg}}{1 \text{ g}} \times \frac{1 \text{ mL}}{80 \text{ mg}} = \frac{60}{8} \text{ mL} = 7.5 \text{ mL}$$

So, you would give 7.5 mL by mouth to the patient every 12 hours.

Example 6.13

The order is Indocin (indomethacin) 75 mg PO daily in 3 divided doses. Read the label in ● **Figure 6.10** and determine the number of teaspoons of this antiinflammatory drug you should administer.

● Figure 6.10
Drug label for Indocin.

(The labels for the products Indocin 25mg per 5mL are reproduced with permission of Merck & Co., Inc., copyright owner.)

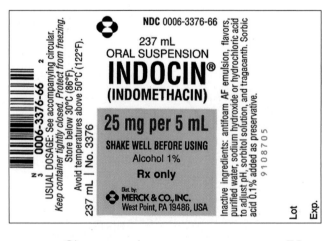

Given quantity:	75 mg
Strength:	25 mg per 5 mL
The quantity you want to find:	? t

In this problem you want to convert 75 milligrams to milliliters and then convert mL to teaspoons.

$$75 \text{ mg} \longrightarrow ? \text{ mL} \longrightarrow ? \text{ t}$$

You can do this on one line as follows:

$$75 \text{ mg} \times \frac{? \text{ mL}}{? \text{ mg}} \times \frac{? \text{ t}}{? \text{ mL}} = ? \text{ t}$$

Because 25 mg = 5 mL, the first unit fraction is $\dfrac{5 \text{ mL}}{25 \text{ mg}}$

Because 5 mL = 1 t, the second unit fraction is $\dfrac{1 \text{ t}}{5 \text{ mL}}$

$$75 \text{ mg} \times \frac{5 \text{ mL}}{25 \text{ mg}} \times \frac{1 \text{ t}}{5 \text{ mL}} = \frac{75}{25} \text{ t} \quad \text{or} \quad 3 \text{ t}$$

Because the order specifies "3 divided doses", the 3 t must be divided into 3 equal amounts over 24 hours. Therefore, each dose would be 1 teaspoon (25 mg), and you would give 1 teaspoon of Indocin by mouth to the patient every 8 hours.

NOTE

In Example 6.13, the order states "in three divided doses." This instructs the practitioner to separate the total daily dose into 3 equal parts over a 24-hour period. To ensure even distribution of the medication, the frequency of the doses should also be regular and consistent, so the drug is administered every 8 hours.

Calculating Dosage by Body Weight

Sometimes the amount of medication is prescribed based on the patient's body weight. A patient who weighs more will receive a larger dose of the drug, and a patient who weighs less will receive a smaller dose of the drug.

Example 6.14

The prescriber orders 15 milligrams per kilogram of a drug for a patient who weighs 80 kilograms. How many milligrams of this drug should the patient receive?

Body weight:	80 kg
Order:	15 mg/kg
Find:	? mg

Convert body weight to dosage.

$$80 \text{ kg (of body weight)} \longrightarrow ? \text{ mg (of drug)}$$

$$80 \text{ kg (of body weight)} \times \frac{? \text{ mg (of drug)}}{? \text{ kg (of body weight)}} = ? \text{ mg (of drug)}$$

Since the order is 15mg/kg, you use the unit fraction $\dfrac{15 \text{ mg}}{1 \text{ kg}}$

$$80 \text{ kg} \times \frac{15 \text{ mg}}{1 \text{ kg}} = 1{,}200 \text{ mg}$$

Therefore, the patient should receive 1,200 mg of the drug.

NOTE

The expression 15 mg/kg means that the patient is to receive 15 milligrams of the drug for each kilogram of body weight. Therefore, you will use the equivalent 15 mg (of drug) = 1 kg (of body weight).

Example 6.15

The prescriber orders Klonopin (clonazepam) 0.05 mg/kg PO daily in three divided doses for a patient who weighs 60 kilograms. If each tablet contains 1 mg, how many tablets of this anticonvulsant drug should the patient receive per day? How many tablets would the patient receive per dose?

Body weight:	60 kg
Order:	0.05 mg/kg
Strength:	1 tab = 1 mg
Find:	? tab

When drugs are prescribed based on body weight, you generally start the problem with the weight of the patient. You first change the single unit of measurement, kilograms (kg of body weight), to another single unit of measurement, milligrams (mg of drug), and then convert the milligrams to tablets.

$$60 \text{ kg (of body weight)} \longrightarrow \text{ ? mg (of drug)} \longrightarrow \text{ ? tab}$$

$$\frac{60 \text{ kg}}{\text{(of body weight)}} \times \frac{\text{? mg (of drug)}}{\text{? kg (of body weight)}} \times \frac{\text{? tab}}{\text{? mg (of drug)}} = \text{ ? tab}$$

Because the order is for 0.05 mg per kg, the first unit fraction is $\dfrac{0.05 \text{ mg}}{1 \text{ kg}}$.

Since each tablet contains 1 mg, the second unit fraction is $\dfrac{1 \text{ tab}}{1 \text{ mg}}$

$$60 \text{ kg} \times \frac{0.05 \text{ mg}}{1 \text{ kg}} \times \frac{1 \text{ tab}}{1 \text{ mg}} = 3 \text{ tabs}$$

The patient should receive 3 tablets of Klonopin by mouth per day in 3 divided doses, and therefore the patient should receive 1 tablet every 8 hours.

Example 6.16

The physician orders Biaxin (clarithromycin) 7.5 milligrams per kilogram PO b.i.d. If the drug strength is 250 milligrams per 5 mL, how many mL of this antibiotic drug should be administered to a patient who weighs 70 kilograms?

Body weight:	70 kg
Order:	7.5 mg/kg
Strength:	250 mg/5 mL
Find:	? ml

Convert body weight to dosage.

$$70 \text{ kg} \longrightarrow \text{ ? mg} \longrightarrow \text{ ? mL}$$

$$70 \text{ kg} \times \frac{\text{? mg}}{\text{? kg}} \times \frac{\text{? mL}}{\text{? mg}} = \text{ ? mL}$$

Since the order specifies 7.5 mg per kg, the first fraction is $\dfrac{7.5 \text{ mL}}{\text{kg}}$

Since the strength is 250 mg per 5 mL, the second fraction is $\dfrac{5 \text{ mL}}{250 \text{ mg}}$

$$70 \text{ kg} \times \frac{7.5 \text{ mg}}{\text{kg}} \times \frac{5 \text{ mL}}{250 \text{ mg}} = 10.5 \text{ mL}$$

The patient should receive 10.5 mL of Biaxin by mouth 2 times per day.

Calculating Dosage by Body Surface Area

In some cases, **body surface area (BSA)** may be used rather than **weight** in determining appropriate drug dosages. This is particularly true when calculating dosages for children, those receiving cancer therapy, burn patients, and patients requiring critical care. A patient's BSA can be estimated by using formulas or nomograms.

BSA Formulas

Body surface area can be approximated by formula using either a hand-held calculator or an online website. BSA, which is measured in square meters (m^2), can be determined by using either of the following two mathematical formulas:

Formula for metric units:

$$BSA = \sqrt{\frac{\text{weight in kilograms} \times \text{height in centimeters}}{3{,}600}}$$

Formula for household units:

$$BSA = \sqrt{\frac{\text{weight in pounds} \times \text{height in inches}}{3{,}131}}$$

Example 6.17

Find the BSA of an adult who is 183 cm tall and weighs 92 kg.

Because this example has metric units (kilograms and centimeters), we use the following formula:

$$BSA = \sqrt{\frac{\text{weight in kilograms} \times \text{height in centimeters}}{3{,}600}}$$

$$= \sqrt{\frac{92 \times 183}{3{,}600}}$$

At this point we need a calculator with a square root key.

$$= \sqrt{4.6767}$$

$$= 2.16256$$

Therefore, the BSA of this adult is 2.16 m^2.

> **NOTE**
>
> In Example 6.17, the metric formula for BSA was used, and in Example 6.18, the household formula for BSA was used. However, each formula provided the BSA measured is square meters (m^2). In this book, we will round off BSA to *two* decimal places.

Example 6.18

What is the BSA of a man who is 4 feet 10 inches tall and weighs 142 pounds?

First you convert 4 feet 10 inches to 58 inches.

Because the example has household units (pounds and inches), we use the following formula:

$$\text{BSA} = \sqrt{\frac{\text{weight in pounds} \times \text{height in inches}}{3{,}131}}$$

$$= \sqrt{\frac{142 \times 58}{3{,}131}}$$

$$= \sqrt{26{,}305}$$

$$= 1.62187$$

Therefore, the BSA of this adult is 1.62 m².

Nomograms

BSA can also be approximated by using a chart called a nomogram (●**Figure 6.11**). The nomogram includes height, weight, and body surface area. If a straight line is drawn on the nomogram from the patient's height (left column) to the patient's weight (right column), the line will cross the center column at the approximate BSA of the patient. Before handheld calculators were used, the nomogram was the best tool available for determining BSA. Since electronic technology has been incorporated into most healthcare settings to ensure more accurate measurements, nomograms are becoming obsolete.

In Example 6.17 we used the formula to calculate the BSA of an 183 cm, 92 kg patient to be 2.16 m². Now let's use the adult nomogram to do the same problem. In ●**Figure 6.12**, you can see that the line from 183 cm to 92 kg intersects the BSA column at about 2.20 m².

In Example 6.18, by using the formula we calculated the BSA of a 4 ft 10 in, 142 lb patient to be 1.62 m². If we use the adult nomogram to determine the BSA (●**Figure 6.13**), we get 1.59 m².

Example 6.19

The physician orders 40 mg/m² of a drug PO once daily. How many milligrams of the drug would you administer to an adult patient weighing 88 kg with a height of 150 cm?

The first step is to determine the BSA of the patient. This can be done by formula or nomogram.

Using the formula, you get

$$\text{BSA} = \sqrt{\frac{88 \times 150}{3{,}600}}$$

$$= \sqrt{3.6667}$$

$$= 1.91 \text{ m}^2$$

Using the adult nomogram, you get 1.81 m². So, you can use either 1.91 m² or 1.81 m² as the BSA. If you choose to use 1.81 m², you want to convert BSA to dosage in mg.

BSA:	1.81 m²
Order:	40 mg/m²
Find:	? mg

$$1.81 \text{ m}^2 = \text{? mg}$$

$$1.81 \text{ m}^2 \times \frac{\text{? mg}}{\text{m}^2} = \text{? mg}$$

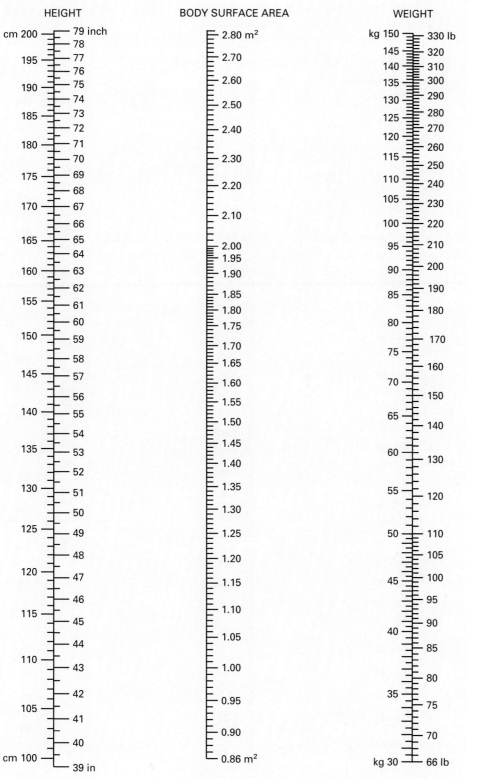

● **Figure 6.11**
Adult nomogram.

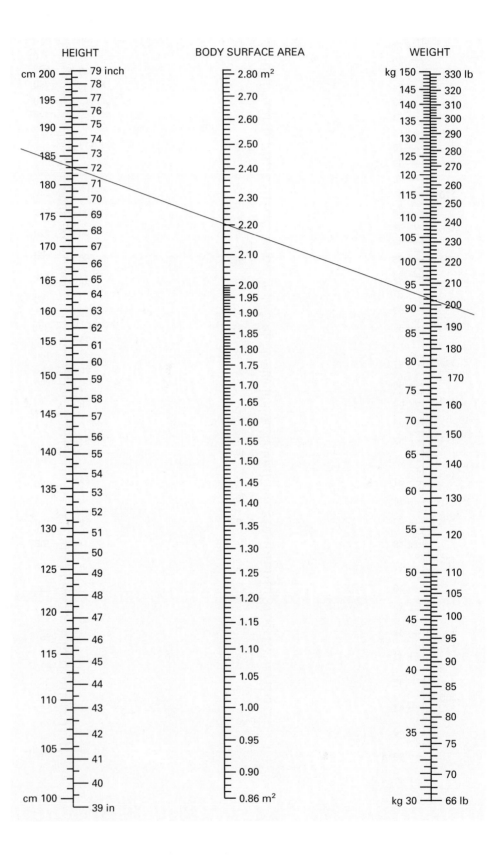

HEIGHT   BODY SURFACE AREA   WEIGHT

● **Figure 6.12**
Nomogram for Example 6.17.

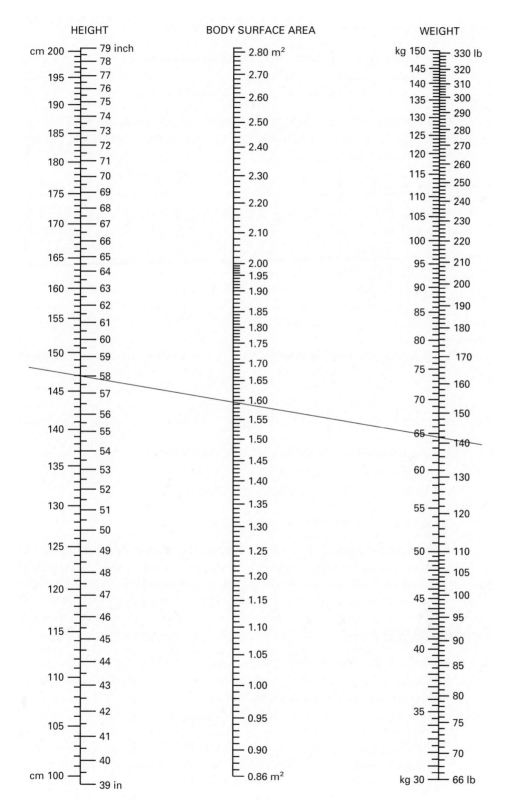

HEIGHT

BODY SURFACE AREA

WEIGHT

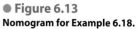

● **Figure 6.13**
Nomogram for Example 6.18.

Since the order is 40 mg/m^2, the unit fraction is $\dfrac{40 \text{ mg}}{\text{m}^2}$

$$1.81 \text{ m}^2 \times \frac{40 \text{ mg}}{\text{m}^2} = 72.4 \text{ mg}$$

If you use the BSA of 1.91 m^2, the calculations are similar.

$$1.91 \text{ m}^2 \times \frac{40 \text{ mg}}{\text{m}^2} = 76.4 \text{ mg}$$

So, if you use 1.81 m^2, you would administer 72.4 mg. However if you use 1.91 m^2, you would administer 76.4 mg of the drug to the patient.

Example 6.20

The prescriber ordered 30 mg/m^2 of a drug PO stat for a patient who has a BSA of 1.65 m^2. The "safe dose range" for this drug is 20 to 40 mg per day. Calculate the prescribed dose in milligrams and determine if it is within the safe range.

BSA:	1.65 m^2
Order:	30 mg/m^2
Find:	? mg

You want to convert the BSA of 1.65 m^2 to the number of milligrams ordered.

$$1.65 \text{ m}^2 = ? \text{ mg}$$

$$1.65 \text{ m}^2 \times \frac{? \text{ mg}}{\text{m}^2} = ? \text{ mg}$$

Because the order is 30 mg per m^2, the unit fraction is $\dfrac{30 \text{ mg}}{\text{m}^2}$

$$1.65 \text{ m}^2 \times \frac{30 \text{ mg}}{\text{m}^2} = 49.5 \text{ mg}$$

The safe dose range is 20–40 mg per day.

So, the dose prescribed, 49.5 mg, is higher than the upper limit (40 mg) of the daily "safe dose range." Therefore, the prescribed dose is not safe, and you would not administer this drug. You would consult with the prescriber.

Example 6.21

The order is Trexall (methotrexate) 3.3 mg/m^2 PO q12h for three doses. How many scored 5 mg tablets of this antineoplastic drug would you administer to patient with a BSA of 2.29 m^2?

BSA:	2.29 m^2
Order:	3.3 mg/m^2
Strength:	1 tab = 5 mg
Find:	? tab

Convert the body surface area to tablets.

$$2.29 \text{ m}^2 \longrightarrow ? \text{ mg} \longrightarrow ? \text{ tabs}$$

$$2.29 \text{ m}^2 \times \frac{? \text{ mg}}{\text{m}^2} \times \frac{? \text{ tab}}{? \text{ mg}} = ? \text{ tab}$$

Because the order is 3.3 mg/m^2, the first unit fraction is $\dfrac{3.3 \text{ mg}}{\text{m}^2}$.

Because 1 scored tablet contains 5 mg, the second unit fraction is $\dfrac{1 \text{ tab}}{5 \text{ mg}}$.

$$2.29 \ \cancel{\text{m}^2} \times \frac{3.3 \ \cancel{\text{mg}}}{\cancel{\text{m}^2}} \times \frac{1 \ \text{tab}}{5 \ \cancel{\text{mg}}} = 1.51 \text{ tabs}$$

The patient should receive $1\frac{1}{2}$ scored tablets of Trexall by mouth every 12 hours for 3 doses.

Summary

In this chapter, you learned the computations necessary to calculate dosages of oral medications in liquid and solid form.

Calculating doses for oral medications in solid and liquid form

- The label states the strength of the drug (e.g., 10 mg/tab, 15 mg/mL).
- Sometimes oral medications are ordered in liquid form for special populations such as pediatrics, geriatrics, and patients with neurological conditions.
- Special calibrated droppers or oral syringes that are supplied with some liquid oral medications may be used to administer *only those medications.*
- Some drugs, such as electrolytes, are measured in milliequivalents (mEq).

Calculating doses by body weight

- Dosages based on body weight are generally measured in milligrams per kilogram (mg/kg).
- Start calculations with the weight of the patient.
- Medications may be prescribed by body weight in special populations such as pediatrics and geriatrics.
- It is crucial to ensure that every medication administered is within the recommended safe dosage range.

Calculating doses by body surface area

- Body surface area (BSA) is measured in square meters (m^2).
- Start calculations with the BSA of the patient.
- BSA is determined by using either a formula or a nomogram.
- BSA may be utilized to determine dosages for special patient populations such as those receiving cancer therapy, burn therapy, and for patients requiring critical care.

Case Study 6.1

Mr. M. is a 68-year-old male patient with a past medical history of diabetes mellitus Type II and severe ischemic cardiomyopathy. He reported that for 6 weeks he had been experiencing shortness of breath and fatigue with moderate activity, difficulty sleeping at night, and has a weight gain of 5 lbs, even though he described his appetite as poor. There is no evidence of smoking or illegal drug use. Upon examination, the practitioner noted periorbital edema and bi-lateral 4+ pitting edema in both lower extremities. His present weight is 154 lb and his vital signs are BP 160/100, T 98.4, P 104, and R 28. Mr. M. was admitted for intravenous support and aggressive diuresis.

His orders are as follows:

- Complete CBC and SMA18
- Coronary angiogram; ECG; stress perfusion scan; chest X-ray.

- Low-salt diet (2 g/day)
- Lasix (furosemide) 80 mg PO stat
- Lasix (furosemide) 60 mg PO q12h to begin 12 hours after the stat dose
- Digoxin 0.25 mg PO once daily
- Micro-K 10 Extencaps (potassium chloride) 20 mEq PO daily
- Diabinese (chlorpropamide) 125 mg PO each morning with breakfast
- Colace (docusate sodium) 100 mg PO t.i.d.
- Ativan (lorazepam) 3 mg PO HS
- Fluid restriction 1,500 mL/24 h
- Strict intake and output
- Foley catheter to bedside drainage

1. The patient drank 650 mL of H_2O, 150 mL of cranberry juice, and 200 mL of ginger ale during the 7 A.M. to 7 P.M. shift. How many mL of fluid may the patient can be given over the next 12 hours?

2. At 8 P.M., Mr. M.'s wife fed him $1\frac{1}{2}$ cups of an organic brand of chicken broth, which contains 390 mg salt in each 1 cup serving.
   (a) How many mL of chicken broth did the patient receive?
   (b) How many grams of salt did he consume?
   (c) How much more salt should Mr. M. consume for the remainder of the day?

3. The diuretic drug Lasix (furosemide) is available in 20 mg tablets.
   (a) How many tablets will you administer for the stat dose?
   (b) How many tablets will the patient have received within the first 20 hours?

4. How many milliequivalents of the electrolyte supplement micro-K will the patient have received after 5 days of therapy?

5. Colace (docusate sodium), a stool-softening drug, is supplied as an oral liquid, 20 mg/5 mL.
   (a) How many times a day does the patient receive this medication?
   (b) How many mL would the patient receive in two days?

6. The available strength of Ativan (lorazepam) is 1 mg/tab. How many tablets of this sedative contain the prescribed dose?

7. The cardiac drug digoxin is supplied in the following strengths: 50 mcg, 100 mcg, and 200 mcg tablets. Which combination of tablets would yield the least number of tablets that would deliver the prescribed dose?

8. Mr. M. remains hospitalized for one week.
   (a) How many milligrams of Diabinese (chlorpropamide) would he have received by the end of the first seven days?
   (b) The Diabinese is available in 250 mg scored tablets. How many tablets would Mr. M. have received by the end of the seven days?

Practice Reading Labels

Calculate the following doses using the labels shown. You will find the answers in Appendix A in the back of the book.

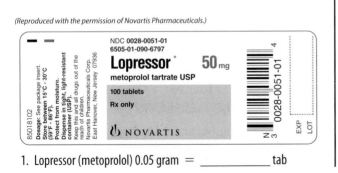

(Reproduced with the permission of Novartis Pharmaceuticals.)

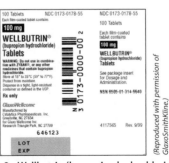

1. Lopressor (metoprolol) 0.05 gram = _____ tab

2. Wellbutrin (bupropion hydrochloride) 200 mg = _____ tab

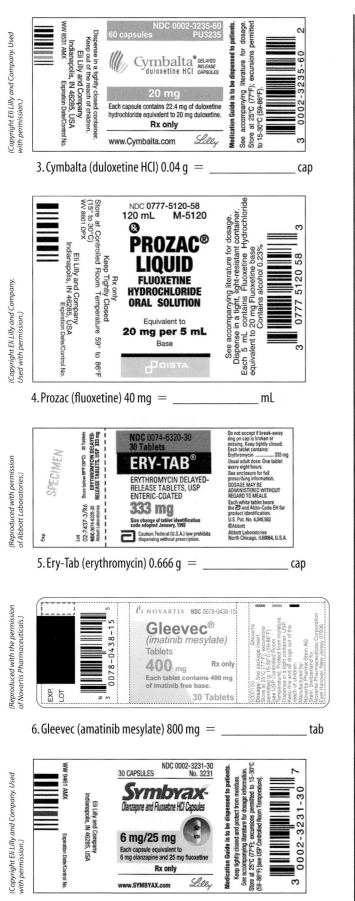

3. Cymbalta (duloxetine HCl) 0.04 g = _____ cap

4. Prozac (fluoxetine) 40 mg = _____ mL

5. Ery-Tab (erythromycin) 0.666 g = _____ cap

6. Gleevec (amatinib mesylate) 800 mg = _____ tab

7. Symbyax (olanzapine / fluoxetine) 12mg / 50mg = _____ cap

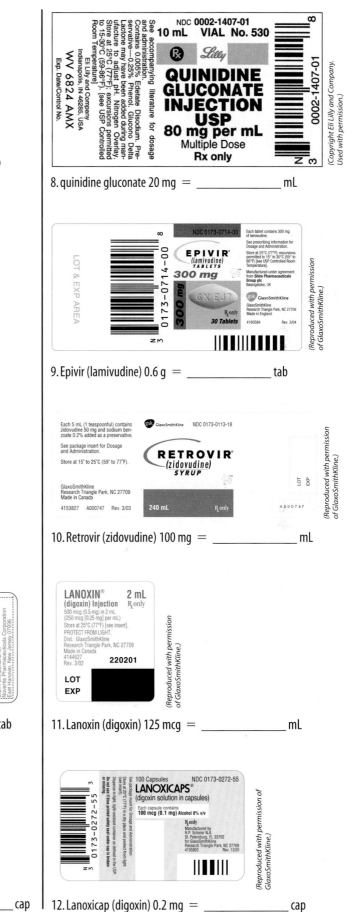

8. quinidine gluconate 20 mg = _____ mL

9. Epivir (lamivudine) 0.6 g = _____ tab

10. Retrovir (zidovudine) 100 mg = _____ mL

11. Lanoxin (digoxin) 125 mcg = _____ mL

12. Lanoxicap (digoxin) 0.2 mg = _____ cap

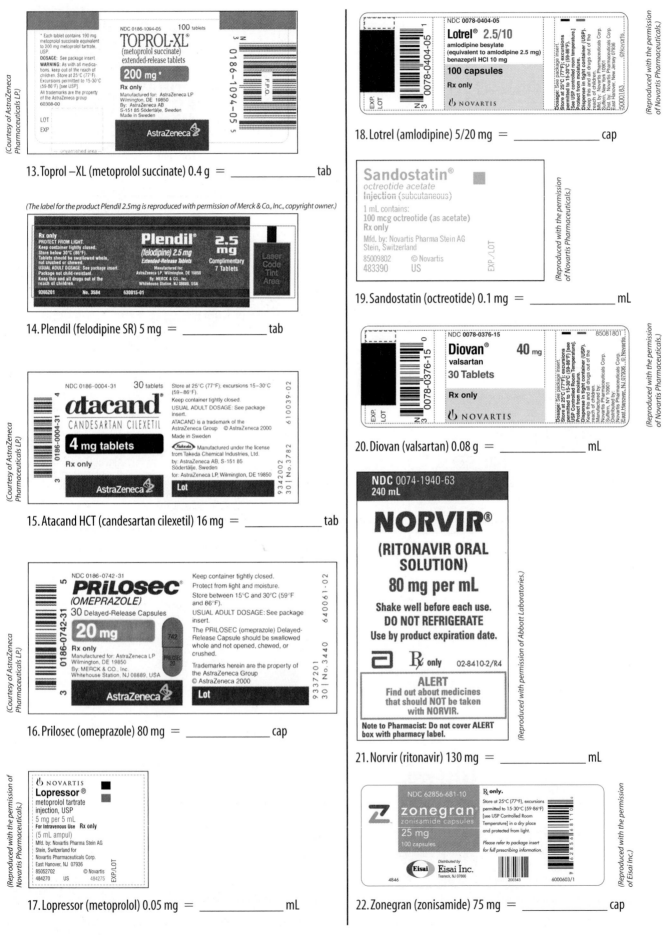

NDC 0186-1094-05   100 tablets

TOPROL-XL®
(metoprolol succinate)
extended-release tablets

200 mg*

Rx only

* Each tablet contains 190 mg metoprolol succinate equivalent to 200 mg metoprolol tartrate, USP.

DOSAGE: See package insert
WARNING: As with all medications, keep out of the reach of children. Store at 25°C (77°F). Excursions permitted to 15–30°C (59–86°F) [see USP]
All trademarks are the property of the AstraZeneca group
60308-00

LOT
EXP

Manufactured by: AstraZeneca LP
Wilmington, DE 19850
By: AstraZeneca AB
S-151 85 Södertälje, Sweden
Made in Sweden

AstraZeneca

13. Toprol –XL (metoprolol succinate) 0.4 g = _____ tab

Rx only
PROTECT FROM LIGHT.
Keep container tightly closed.
Store below 30°C (86°F).
Tablets should be swallowed whole, not crushed or chewed.
USUAL ADULT DOSAGE: See package insert.
Package not child-resistant.
Keep this and all drugs out of the reach of children.

Plendil®
(felodipine) 2.5 mg
Extended-Release Tablets

Manufactured for:
AstraZeneca LP, Wilmington, DE 19850
By: MERCK & CO., Inc.
Whitehouse Station, NJ 08889, USA

2.5 mg
Complimentary
7 Tablets

Laser Code Tint Area

14. Plendil (felodipine SR) 5 mg = _____ tab

NDC 0186-0004-31   30 tablets

atacand®
CANDESARTAN CILEXETIL

4 mg tablets

Rx only

AstraZeneca

Store at 25°C (77°F); excursions 15–30°C (59–86°F).
Keep container tightly closed.
USUAL ADULT DOSAGE: See package insert.
ATACAND is a trademark of the AstraZeneca Group © AstraZeneca 2000
Made in Sweden
Takeda Manufactured under the license from Takeda Chemical Industries, Ltd.
by: AstraZeneca AB, S-151 85 Södertälje, Sweden
for: AstraZeneca LP, Wilmington, DE 19850

Lot

15. Atacand HCT (candesartan cilexetil) 16 mg = _____ tab

NDC 0186-0742-31

PRiLOSEC®
(OMEPRAZOLE)

30 Delayed-Release Capsules

20 mg

Rx only

Manufactured for: AstraZeneca LP
Wilmington, DE 19850
By: MERCK & CO., Inc.
Whitehouse Station, NJ 08889, USA

AstraZeneca

Keep container tightly closed.
Protect from light and moisture.
Store between 15°C and 30°C (59°F and 86°F).
USUAL ADULT DOSAGE: See package insert.
The PRILOSEC (omeprazole) Delayed-Release Capsule should be swallowed whole and not opened, chewed, or crushed.
Trademarks herein are the property of the AstraZeneca Group
© AstraZeneca 2000

Lot

16. Prilosec (omeprazole) 80 mg = _____ cap

NOVARTIS
Lopressor®
metoprolol tartrate
injection, USP
5 mg per 5 mL
For Intravenous Use Rx only
(5 mL ampul)
Mfd. by: Novartis Pharma Stein AG
Stein, Switzerland for
Novartis Pharmaceuticals Corp.
East Hanover, NJ 07936
85052702   © Novartis
484270   US   484275

17. Lopressor (metoprolol) 0.05 mg = _____ mL

NDC 0078-0404-05

Lotrel® 2.5/10
amlodipine besylate
(equivalent to amlodipine 2.5 mg)
benazepril HCl 10 mg

100 capsules

Rx only

NOVARTIS

Dosage: See package insert.
Store at 25°C (77°F); excursions permitted to 15–30°C (59–86°F)
See USP Controlled room temperature.
Protect from moisture.
Dispense in tight container (USP).
Keep this and all drugs out of the reach of children.
Mfd. by: Novartis Pharmaceuticals Corp.
Suffern, New York 10901
Dist. by: Novartis Pharmaceuticals Corp.
East Hanover, New Jersey 07936
5000183

18. Lotrel (amlodipine) 5/20 mg = _____ cap

Sandostatin®
octreotide acetate
Injection (subcutaneous)

1 mL contains:
100 mcg octreotide (as acetate)
Rx only
Mfd. by: Novartis Pharma Stein AG
Stein, Switzerland
85009802   © Novartis
483390   US

19. Sandostatin (octreotide) 0.1 mg = _____ mL

NDC 0078-0376-15

Diovan®   **40** mg
valsartan

30 Tablets

Rx only

NOVARTIS

Dosage: See package insert.
Store at 25°C (77°F); excursions permitted to 15–30°C (59–86°F) [see USP Controlled Room Temperature].
Protect from moisture.
Keep this and all drugs out of the reach of children.
Manufactured by: Novartis Pharmaceuticals Corp.
Suffern, NY 10901
Distributed by: Novartis Pharmaceuticals Corp.
East Hanover, NJ 07936. © Novartis.

20. Diovan (valsartan) 0.08 g = _____ mL

NDC 0074-1940-63
240 mL

NORVIR®

(RITONAVIR ORAL SOLUTION)

80 mg per mL

Shake well before each use.
DO NOT REFRIGERATE
Use by product expiration date.

℞ only   02-8410-2/R4

ALERT
Find out about medicines that should NOT be taken with NORVIR.

Note to Pharmacist: Do not cover ALERT box with pharmacy label.

21. Norvir (ritonavir) 130 mg = _____ mL

NDC 62856-681-10

zonegran®
zonisamide capsules
25 mg
100 capsules

Distributed by
Eisai Inc.
Teaneck, NJ 07666
4846

℞ only.
Store at 25°C (77°F), excursions permitted to 15-30°C (59-86°F) [see USP Controlled Room Temperature] in a dry place and protected from light.
Please refer to package insert for full prescribing information.

6000603/1

22. Zonegran (zonisamide) 75 mg = _____ cap

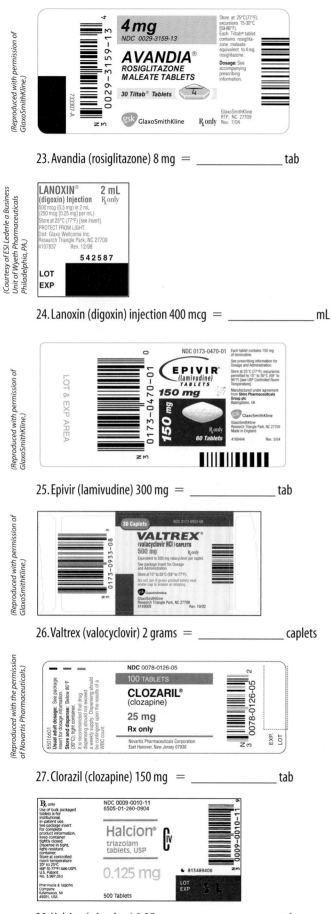

(Reproduced with permission of GlaxoSmithKline.)

4 mg
NDC 0029-3159-13

Store at 25°C (77°F); excursions 15-30°C (59-86°F). Each Tiltab® tablet contains rosiglitazone maleate equivalent to 4 mg rosiglitazone.

Dosage: See accompanying prescribing information.

AVANDIA®
ROSIGLITAZONE
MALEATE TABLETS

30 Tiltab® Tablets

GlaxoSmithKline
RTP, NC 27709
Rev. 7/04

gsk GlaxoSmithKline   Rx only

23. Avandia (rosiglitazone) 8 mg = _____ tab

(Courtesy of ESI Lederle a Business Unit of Wyeth Pharmaceuticals Philadelphia, PA.)

LANOXIN®   2 mL
(digoxin) Injection   Rx only
500 mcg (0.5 mg) in 2 mL
(250 mcg [0.25 mg] per mL)
Store at 25°C (77°F) [see insert].
PROTECT FROM LIGHT.
Dist: Glaxo Wellcome Inc.
Research Triangle Park, NC 27709
4107837   Rev. 12/98

542587

LOT
EXP

24. Lanoxin (digoxin) injection 400 mcg = _____ mL

(Reproduced with permission of GlaxoSmithKline.)

LOT & EXP AREA

NDC 0173-0470-01

Each tablet contains 150 mg of lamivudine.

See prescribing information for Dosage and Administration.

Store at 25°C (77°F); excursions permitted to 15° to 30°C (59° to 86°F) [see USP Controlled Room Temperature.]

Manufactured under agreement from Shire Pharmaceuticals Group plc
Basingstoke, UK

EPIVIR®
(lamivudine)
TABLETS

150 mg

gsk GlaxoSmithKline
Research Triangle Park, NC 27709
Made in England

Rx only
60 Tablets
4160444   Rev. 3/04

25. Epivir (lamivudine) 300 mg = _____ tab

(Reproduced with permission of GlaxoSmithKline.)

30 Caplets   NDC 0173-0933-08

VALTREX®
(valacyclovir HCl) CAPLETS
500 mg   Rx only
Equivalent to 500 mg valacyclovir per caplet.
See package insert for Dosage and Administration.
Store at 15° to 25°C (59° to 77°F).
Do not use if green printed safety seal under cap is broken or missing.

gsk GlaxoSmithKline
Research Triangle Park, NC 27709
4149009   Rev. 10/02

26. Valtrex (valocyclovir) 2 grams = _____ caplets

(Reproduced with the permission of Novartis Pharmaceuticals.)

8501 6601
Usual adult dosage: See package insert for dosage information.
Store and dispense: Below 86°F (30°C); tight container.
It is recommended that drug dispensing should not exceed a weekly supply. Dispensing should be contingent upon the results of a WBC count.

NDC 0078-0126-05

100 TABLETS

CLOZARIL®
(clozapine)

25 mg

Rx only

Novartis Pharmaceuticals Corporation
East Hanover, New Jersey 07936

0078-0126-05

EXP.
LOT

27. Clorazil (clozapine) 150 mg = _____ tab

Rx only
Use of bulk packaged tablets is for institutional, in-patient use.
See package insert for complete product information.
Keep container tightly closed. Dispense in tight, light-resistant container.
Store at controlled room temperature 20° to 25°C
(68° to 77°F [see USP].
U.S. Patent
U.S. 5,907,052

Pharmacia & Upjohn Company
Kalamazoo, MI 49001, USA

NDC 0009-0010-11
6505-01-260-0904

Halcion® C IV
triazolam
tablets, USP

0.125 mg

815489406

0009-0010-11

500 Tablets

LOT
EXP

28. Halcion (triazolam) 0.25 mg = _____ tab

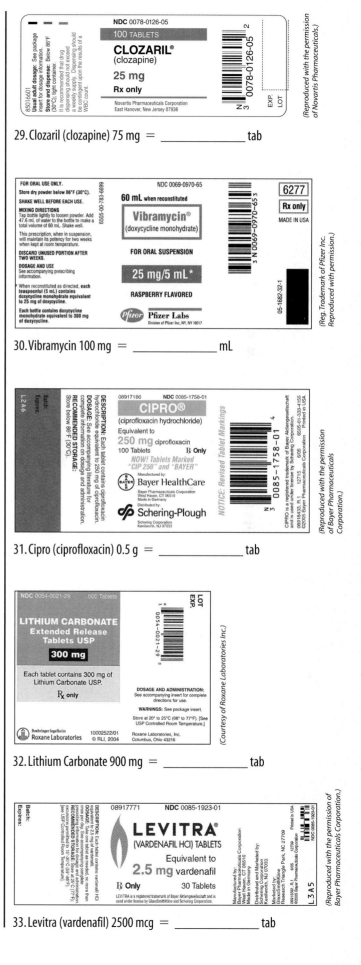

(Reproduced with the permission of Novartis Pharmaceuticals.)

8501 6601
Usual adult dosage: See package insert for dosage information.
Store and dispense: Below 86°F (30°C); tight container.
It is recommended that drug dispensing should not exceed a weekly supply. Dispensing should be contingent upon the results of a WBC count.

NDC 0078-0126-05

100 TABLETS

CLOZARIL®
(clozapine)

25 mg

Rx only

Novartis Pharmaceuticals Corporation
East Hanover, New Jersey 07936

0078-0126-05

EXP.
LOT

29. Clozaril (clozapine) 75 mg = _____ tab

(Reg. Trademark of Pfizer Inc. Reproduced with permission.)

FOR ORAL USE ONLY.
Store dry powder below 86°F (30°C).
SHAKE WELL BEFORE EACH USE.
MIXING DIRECTIONS
Tap bottle lightly to loosen powder. Add 47.6 mL of water to the bottle to make a total volume of 60 mL. Shake well.
This prescription, when in suspension, will maintain its potency for two weeks when kept at room temperature.
DISCARD UNUSED PORTION AFTER TWO WEEKS.
DOSAGE AND USE
See accompanying prescribing information.
* When reconstituted as directed, each teaspoonful (5 mL) contains doxycycline monohydrate equivalent to 25 mg of doxycycline.
Each bottle contains doxycycline monohydrate equivalent to 300 mg of doxycycline.

NDC 0069-0970-65

6277

60 mL when reconstituted

Rx only
MADE IN USA

Vibramycin®
(doxycycline monohydrate)

FOR ORAL SUSPENSION

25 mg/5 mL*

RASPBERRY FLAVORED

Pfizer **Pfizer Labs**
Division of Pfizer Inc, NY, NY 10017

05-1682-32-1

0069-0970-65

30. Vibramycin 100 mg = _____ mL

(Reproduced with the permission of Bayer Pharmaceuticals Corporation.)

Bottle Expires:

08917186   NDC 0085-1758-01

CIPRO®

(ciprofloxacin hydrochloride)
Equivalent to
250 mg ciprofloxacin
100 Tablets   Rx Only

NOW! Tablets Marked "CIP 250" and "BAYER"

DESCRIPTION: Each tablet contains ciprofloxacin hydrochloride equivalent to 250 mg of ciprofloxacin.
DOSAGE: See accompanying literature for complete information on dosage and administration.
RECOMMENDED STORAGE: Store below 86°F (30°C).

Manufactured by:
BAYER **Bayer HealthCare**
Bayer Pharmaceuticals Corporation
West Haven, CT 06516
Made in Germany

Distributed by:
Schering-Plough
Schering Corporation
Kenilworth, NJ 07033

NOTICE: Revised Tablet Markings

CIPRO is a registered trademark of Bayer Aktiengesellschaft and is used under license by Schering Corporation.
©2005 Bayer Pharmaceuticals Corporation   Printed in USA

0085-1758-01

31. Cipro (ciprofloxacin) 0.5 g = _____ tab

(Courtesy of Roxane Laboratories Inc.)

NDC 0054-0021-28   500 Tablets

LITHIUM CARBONATE
Extended Release
Tablets USP
300 mg

Each tablet contains 300 mg of Lithium Carbonate USP.

Rx only

DOSAGE AND ADMINISTRATION:
See accompanying insert for complete directions for use.
WARNINGS: See package insert.
Store at 20° to 25°C (68° to 77°F). [See USP Controlled Room Temperature.]

Boehringer Ingelheim
Roxane Laboratories

10002522/01
© RLI, 2004

Roxane Laboratories, Inc.
Columbus, Ohio 43216

0054-0021-29

LOT
EXP.

32. Lithium Carbonate 900 mg = _____ tab

(Reproduced with the permission of Bayer Pharmaceuticals Corporation.)

Batch:
Expires:

08917771   NDC 0085-1923-01

LEVITRA®
(VARDENAFIL HCl) TABLETS

Equivalent to
2.5 mg vardenafil

Rx Only   30 Tablets

DESCRIPTION: Each tablet contains vardenafil HCl equivalent to 2.5 mg of vardenafil.
DOSAGE: See accompanying prescribing information for dosage and administration.
RECOMMENDED STORAGE: Store at 25°C (77°F); excursions permitted to 15°-30°C (59°-86°F) [see USP Controlled Room Temperature.]

Manufactured by:
Bayer Pharmaceuticals Corporation
West Haven, CT 06516
Made in Germany

Distributed and Marketed by:
Schering Corporation
Kenilworth, NJ 07033

Marketed by:
GlaxoSmithKline
Research Triangle Park, NC 27709

©2005 Bayer Pharmaceuticals Corporation

LEVITRA is a registered trademark of Bayer Aktiengesellschaft and is used under license by GlaxoSmithKline and Schering Corporation.

NDC 0085-1923-01

L 3 A 5

33. Levitra (vardenafil) 2500 mcg = _____ tab

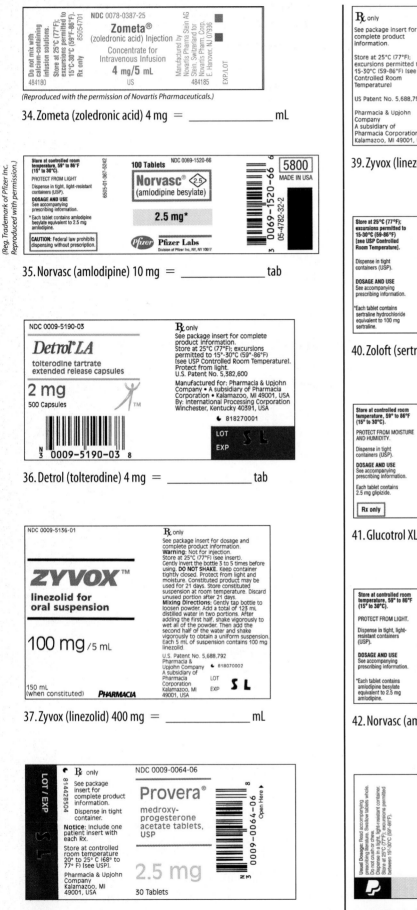

(Reproduced with the permission of Novartis Pharmaceuticals.)

34. Zometa (zoledronic acid) 4 mg = _____ mL

(Reg. Trademark of Pfizer Inc. Reproduced with permission.)

35. Norvasc (amlodipine) 10 mg = _____ tab

36. Detrol (tolterodine) 4 mg = _____ tab

37. Zyvox (linezolid) 400 mg = _____ mL

38. Provera (medroxyprogesterone) 20 mg = _____ tab

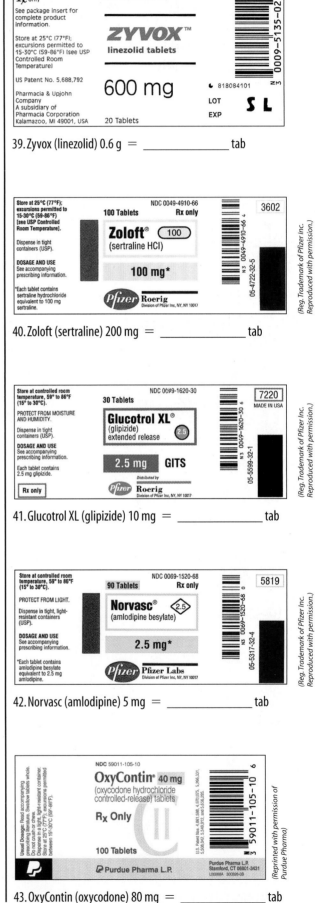

39. Zyvox (linezolid) 0.6 g = _____ tab

40. Zoloft (sertraline) 200 mg = _____ tab

(Reg. Trademark of Pfizer Inc. Reproduced with permission.)

41. Glucotrol XL (glipizide) 10 mg = _____ tab

(Reg. Trademark of Pfizer Inc. Reproduced with permission.)

42. Norvasc (amlodipine) 5 mg = _____ tab

(Reprinted with permission of Purdue Pharma)

43. OxyContin (oxycodone) 80 mg = _____ tab

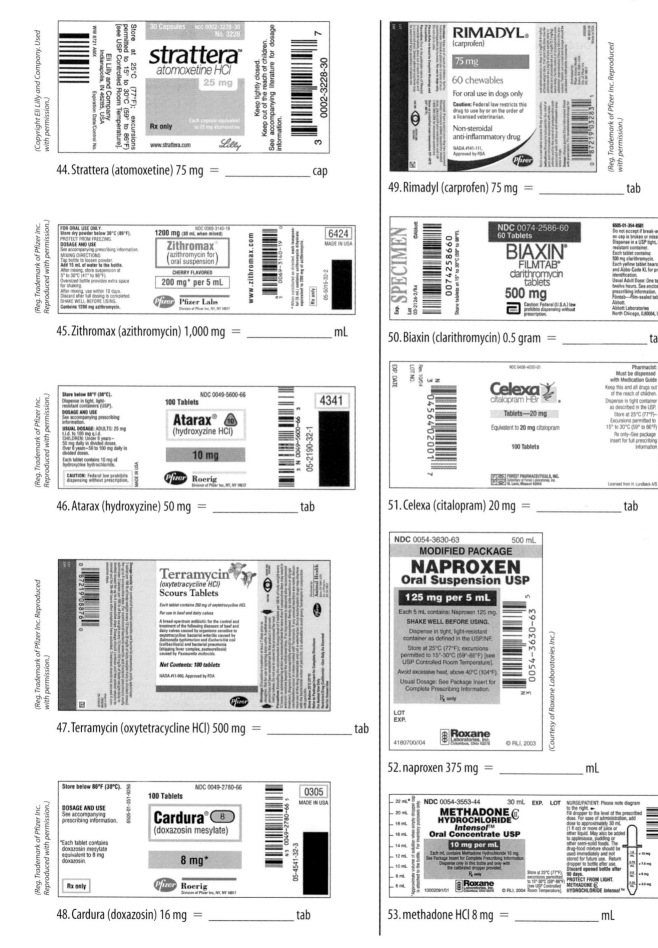

44. Strattera (atomoxetine) 75 mg = _____ cap

45. Zithromax (azithromycin) 1,000 mg = _____ mL

46. Atarax (hydroxyzine) 50 mg = _____ tab

47. Terramycin (oxytetracycline HCl) 500 mg = _____ tab

48. Cardura (doxazosin) 16 mg = _____ tab

49. Rimadyl (carprofen) 75 mg = _____ tab

50. Biaxin (clarithromycin) 0.5 gram = _____ tab

51. Celexa (citalopram) 20 mg = _____ tab

52. naproxen 375 mg = _____ mL

53. methadone HCl 8 mg = _____ mL

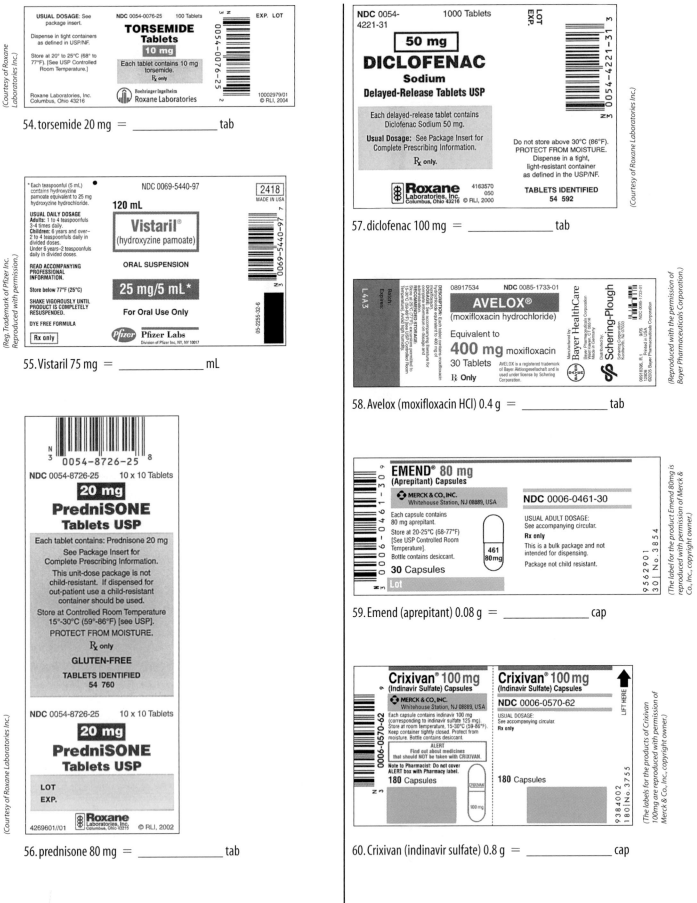

(Courtesy of Roxane Laboratories Inc.)

USUAL DOSAGE: See package insert.

Dispense in tight containers as defined in USP/NF.

Store at 20° to 25°C (68° to 77°F). [See USP Controlled Room Temperature.]

Roxane Laboratories, Inc.
Columbus, Ohio 43216

NDC 0054-0076-25   100 Tablets

TORSEMIDE
Tablets
10 mg

Each tablet contains 10 mg torsemide.
℞ only

Boehringer Ingelheim
Roxane Laboratories

EXP. LOT

10002979/01
© RLI, 2004

54. torsemide 20 mg = _____ tab

(Reg. Trademark of Pfizer Inc. Reproduced with permission.)

* Each teaspoonful (5 mL) contains hydroxyzine pamoate equivalent to 25 mg hydroxyzine hydrochloride.

USUAL DAILY DOSAGE
Adults: 1 to 4 teaspoonfuls 3-4 times daily.
Children: 6 years and over– 2 to 4 teaspoonfuls daily in divided doses.
Under 6 years–2 teaspoonfuls daily in divided doses.

READ ACCOMPANYING PROFESSIONAL INFORMATION.

Store below 77°F (25°C)

SHAKE VIGOROUSLY UNTIL PRODUCT IS COMPLETELY RESUSPENDED.

DYE FREE FORMULA

℞ only

NDC 0069-5440-97

120 mL

Vistaril®
(hydroxyzine pamoate)

ORAL SUSPENSION

25 mg/5 mL*

For Oral Use Only

Pfizer **Pfizer Labs**
Division of Pfizer Inc, NY, NY 10017

2418
MADE IN USA

55. Vistaril 75 mg = _____ mL

(Courtesy of Roxane Laboratories Inc.)

NDC 0054-8726-25   10 x 10 Tablets

20 mg

PredniSONE
Tablets USP

Each tablet contains: Prednisone 20 mg

See Package Insert for Complete Prescribing Information.

This unit-dose package is not child-resistant. If dispensed for out-patient use a child-resistant container should be used.

Store at Controlled Room Temperature 15°-30°C (59°-86°F) [see USP].

PROTECT FROM MOISTURE.

℞ only

GLUTEN-FREE

TABLETS IDENTIFIED
54 760

NDC 0054-8726-25   10 x 10 Tablets

20 mg

PredniSONE
Tablets USP

LOT
EXP.

Roxane
Laboratories, Inc.
Columbus, Ohio 43216

4269601//01   © RLI, 2002

56. prednisone 80 mg = _____ tab

NDC 0054-4221-31   1000 Tablets

LOT
EXP.

50 mg

DICLOFENAC
Sodium
Delayed-Release Tablets USP

Each delayed-release tablet contains Diclofenac Sodium 50 mg.

Usual Dosage: See Package Insert for Complete Prescribing Information.

℞ only.

Roxane
Laboratories, Inc.
Columbus, Ohio 43216 © RLI, 2000

4163570
050

Do not store above 30°C (86°F). PROTECT FROM MOISTURE. Dispense in a tight, light-resistant container as defined in the USP/NF.

TABLETS IDENTIFIED
54 592

(Courtesy of Roxane Laboratories Inc.)

57. diclofenac 100 mg = _____ tab

08917534   NDC 0085-1733-01

AVELOX®
(moxifloxacin hydrochloride)

Equivalent to

400 mg moxifloxacin

30 Tablets

℞ Only

Manufactured by
Bayer HealthCare
Bayer Pharmaceuticals Corporation
West Haven, CT 06516
Made in Germany

Distributed by
Schering-Plough
Schering Corporation
Kenilworth, NJ 07033

AVELOX is a registered trademark of Bayer Aktiengesellschaft and is used under license by Schering Corporation.

(Reproduced with the permission of Bayer Pharmaceuticals Corporation.)

58. Avelox (moxifloxacin HCl) 0.4 g = _____ tab

EMEND® 80 mg
(Aprepitant) Capsules

MERCK & CO., INC.
Whitehouse Station, NJ 08889, USA

Each capsule contains 80 mg aprepitant.

Store at 20-25°C (68-77°F) [See USP Controlled Room Temperature].

Bottle contains desiccant.

30 Capsules

Lot

461
80mg

NDC 0006-0461-30

USUAL ADULT DOSAGE:
See accompanying circular.

Rx only

This is a bulk package and not intended for dispensing.

Package not child resistant.

(The label for the product Emend 80mg is reproduced with permission of Merck & Co., Inc., copyright owner.)

59. Emend (aprepitant) 0.08 g = _____ cap

Crixivan® 100 mg
(Indinavir Sulfate) Capsules

MERCK & CO., INC.
Whitehouse Station, NJ 08889, USA

Each capsule contains indinavir 100 mg (corresponding to indinavir sulfate 125 mg). Store at room temperature, 15-30°C (59-86°F). Keep container tightly closed. Protect from moisture. Bottle contains desiccant.

ALERT
Find out about medicines that should NOT be taken with CRIXIVAN.

Note to Pharmacist: Do not cover ALERT box with Pharmacy label.

180 Capsules

Crixivan® 100 mg
(Indinavir Sulfate) Capsules

NDC 0006-0570-62

USUAL DOSAGE:
See accompanying circular.
Rx only

LIFT HERE

180 Capsules

(The labels for the products of Crixivan 100mg are reproduced with permission of Merck & Co., Inc., copyright owner.)

60. Crixivan (indinavir sulfate) 0.8 g = _____ cap

Practice Sets

The answers to *Try These for Practice, Exercises,* and *Cumulative Review* appear in Appendix A at the end of the book. Ask your instructor for answers to the *Additional Exercises.*

Try These for Practice

Test your comprehension after reading the chapter.

1. The order is Accupril (quinapril HCl) 30 mg PO b.i.d.
   (a) Read the label in ● **Figure 6.14** to determine how many tablets of this antihypertensive drug you will administer.
   (b) Express the daily dose in grams.

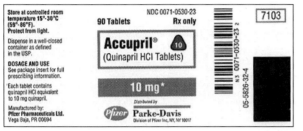

● **Figure 6.14**
Drug label for Accupril.

(Reg. Trademark of Pfizer Inc. Reproduced with permission.)

2. The physician orders Trexall (methotrexate) 25 mg/m^2 PO twice per week to treat leukemia. How many milligrams would you administer in one week if the patient is 150 centimeters tall and weighs 70 kg?

3. The physician ordered E.E.S (erythromycin ethylsuccinate) 300 mg PO q6h. Read the label in ● **Figure 6.15**. How many mL of this antibacterial drug will the patient receive in 24 hours?

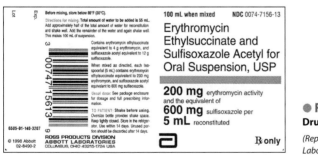

● **Figure 6.15**
Drug label for Erythromycin.

(Reproduced with permission of Abbott Laboratories.)

4. A physician's order reads: Lyrica (pregabalin) 50 mg PO t.i.d. The bottle contains 25-mg capsules. How many capsules of this anticonvulsive medication would you administer in 24 hours?

5. The physician orders Mellaril (thioridazine HCl) 80 mg PO t.i.d. for a patient with schizrenia. If you have 10, 15, and 50 mg nonscored tablets to chose from, which combination of tablets would contain the exact dosage with the smallest number of tablets?

Exercises

Reinforce your understanding in class or at home.

1. Paxil (paroxetine HCl) 40 mg PO daily has been ordered for your patient. Each tablet contains 0.02 gram. How many tablets of this antidepressant will you prepare?

2. The physician prescribes 500 mcg of Baraclude (entecavir) per day via NG (nasogastric tube) for a patient with chronic hepatitis B virus infection. The oral solution contains 0.05 mg of entecavir per milliliter. How many mL of this antiviral medication would you deliver?

3. The order reads Prilosec (omeprazole) 40 mg PO once daily for 4 weeks. Read the drug label in ● **Figure 6.16** and determine the total number of delayed-release capsules of this antacid drug you would administer to the patient over the entire treatment period.

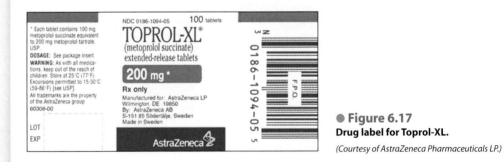

● **Figure 6.16**
Drug label for Prilosec.

(Courtesy of AstraZeneca Pharmaceuticals LP.)

4. The prescriber ordered Precose (acarbose) 75 mg PO t.i.d. with meals. The medication is available in 25 mg tablets. How many tablets of this α glucosidase inhibitor (antidiabetic agent) will you give your patient in 24 hours?

5. Toprol-XL (metoprolol succinate) extended-release tablets 200 mg PO daily has been prescribed for a patient. After reading the label in ● **Figure 6.17,** how many tablets of this antihypertensive drug would the patient have received after 7 days?

● **Figure 6.17**
Drug label for Toprol-XL.

(Courtesy of AstraZeneca Pharmaceuticals LP.)

6. Keftab (cephalexin) is prescribed for an elderly patient who weighs 40 kilograms. The order is 50 milligrams per kilogram PO in two equally divided doses. Each tablet contains 500 mg. How many tablets of this cephalosporin antibiotic will the patient receive per dose?

7. Zyvox (linezolid) 600 mg PO q12h has been prescribed for an elderly patient with pneumonia. Read the label in ● **Figure 6.18** and determine how many milliliters of the antibacterial suspension you would administer.

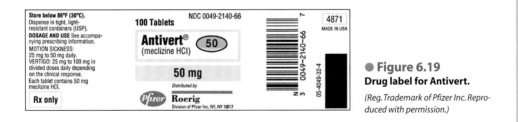

● **Figure 6.18**
Drug label for Zyvox.

8. A patient is scheduled to receive 0.015 g of a drug by mouth every morning. The drug is available as 7.5 mg tablets. How many tablets would you administer?

9. A patient with osteoarthritis is ordered Voltaren (diclofenac sodium) 150 mg PO per day in 3 divided doses. There are 25-milligram tablets available. How many tablets will you give in a single dose?

10. An elderly patient with depression is ordered Aventyl (nortriptyline HCl) 25 mg PO t.i.d. The label reads Aventyl Oral Solution 10 mg/5 mL. How many mL will you administer?

11. Antivert (meclizine HCl) 25 mg PO once daily for three days has been ordered for a patient with a history of motion sickness who is planning extensive traveling. Read the information on the label in ● **Figure 6.19** and calculate the number of scored tablets that the patient will receive when the prescription is completed at the end of the three days.

● **Figure 6.19**
Drug label for Antivert.

(Reg. Trademark of Pfizer Inc. Reproduced with permission.)

12. The physician orders 7.5 mg of Tranxene SD (clorazepate dipotassium) PO t.i.d. for an elderly patient with extreme anxiety. This drug is available in 15 mg scored tablets. How many tablets would the patient receive in 24 hours?

13. A patient develops a mild skin reaction to a transfusion of a unit of packed red blood cells and is given 75 milligrams of Benadryl (diphenhydramine HCl) PO stat. The only drug strength available is 25 mg capsules. How many capsules will you give?

14. The physician orders two Tylenol #3 (codeine 30 mg, acetaminophen 300 mg) PO every 6 hours for a postpartum patient experiencing discom-

fort from afterpains. How many milligrams of acetaminophen will the patient have received by the end of the day?

15. The physician orders Detrol LA (tolterodine tartrate) 4 mg PO daily for a patient with an overactive bladder. Read the label in ● **Figure 6.20** and determine how many tablets you will give this patient.

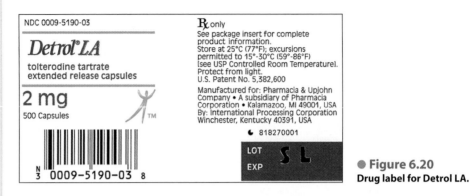

● **Figure 6.20**
Drug label for Detrol LA.

16. A patient with difficulty sleeping is medicated for insomnia with 0.25 g PO at bedtime of a sedative drug. The drug is available as 500 mg per scored tablet. How many tablets will you administer to your patient?

17. The physician orders Coumadin (warfarin sodium) 6.5 mg PO every other day from Monday through Sunday. How many milligrams of Coumadin will your patient receive in that week?

18. A physician is treating a patient for H. influenzae. He writes the following prescription:

   Vantin (cefpodoxime proxetil) 200 mg PO q12h for 14 days

   Read the label in ● **Figure 6.21** and determine how many mL you will give this patient.

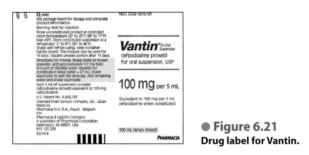

● **Figure 6.21**
Drug label for Vantin.

19. The physician orders Deltasone (prednisone) 60 mg/m^2 PO daily as part of the treatment protocol for a patient with leukemia.
    (a) How many milligrams of this steroid drug would you administer if the patient is 5 feet 6 inches tall and weighs 140 pounds?
    (b) The drug is supplied in 50 mg per tablet. How many tablets will you administer?

20. The antibiotic, Zithromax (azithromycin), is ordered to treat a patient with a bacterial exacerbation of Chronic Obstructive Pulmonary Disease (COPD). The order is:

   Zithromax (azithromycin) 500 mg PO as a single dose on day one, followed by 250 mg once daily on days 2 through 5

   How many milligrams will the patient receive by the completion of the prescription?

Additional Exercises

Now, test yourself!

1. A drug (40 mg PO daily) has been ordered for your client. Each tablet contains 0.02 grams. How many tablets of this drug will you prepare?

2. The physician ordered a drug (0.55 mg/kg PO). The patient weighs 32 kilograms. The drug is supplied with a strength of 30 mg/mL. Calculate the number of milliliters you would administer.

3. Glucophage (metformin) 850 mg PO ac breakfast and dinner has been prescribed for your client. What is the patient's daily dose expressed in grams?

4. Prescriber's order:

   Micronase (glyburide) 5 mg PO with breakfast

   Each tablet contains 2.5 mg. How many tablets will you prepare?

5. Ditropan XL (oxybutynin chloride) 20 mg per day PO for 5 days has been prescribed for a patient. Each tablet contains 5 mg. How many tablets of this anticholinergic medication will the patient receive by the end of the treatment?

6. Norvasc (amlodipine) 5 mg PO once daily for 7 days has been ordered for a patient with angina. Each tablet contains 0.0025 grams. How many tablets will you administer to this patient for the week?

7. Vasotec (enalapril maleate) 7.5 mg PO daily has been prescribed. Tablets available are 2.5 mg, 5 mg, 10 mg, and 20 mg. Which combination of tablets would yeld the least number of tablets that would deliver this ACE-inhibiting antihypertensive drug?

8. Alprazolam 0.5 mg PO t.i.d. has been prescribed for your client. Read the information on the label in ● **Figure 6.22**. How many mL of this antianxiety drug will you administer to your patient?

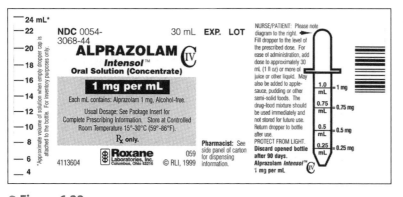

● **Figure 6.22**
Drug label for Alprazolam Intensol.

(Courtesy of Roxane Laboratories Inc.)

9. A patient is to receive 0.01 g PO qhs of a drug. Each tablet contains 0.005 g. How many tablets will you administer to your patient?

10. Order:

    Coumadin (warfarin sodium) 2.5 mg PO Monday, Wednesday, and Friday and 1 mg PO Tuesday, Thursday, Saturday, and Sunday

    How many milligrams of Coumadin will your patient receive in one week?

11. A drug (0.5 g PO stat) has been ordered for your patient. Each tablet contains 0.25 gram. How many tablets of this drug will you give to your patient?

12. Decadron (dexamethasone) 3 mg PO q12 h has been ordered for a patient. The drug is supplied in 1.5 mg tablets. Calculate the number of tablets of this steroid that the patient will receive in 24 hours.

13. Physician's order:

    furosemide 80 mg PO daily

    The drug is supplied in 20 mg tablets. What would the patient's daily dose be if it were expressed in grams?

14. Physician's order:

    Pavabid (papaverine) 300 mg PO q12h

    Each tablet contains 0.15 g. How many tablets would you administer?

15. Prescriber's order:

    Motrin (ibuprofen) 600 mg PO q8h for five days only

    Each caplet contains 200 mg. How many caplets will you give this patient in the 5 days?

16. The antigout medication colchicine 1.2 mg PO q1h for 8 doses has been ordered. Each tablet contains 0.6 mg. How many milligrams of colchicine will the patient receive in eight hours?

17. Physician's order:

    Cytovene (ganciclovir) 500 mg PO q3h while awake

    The drug is available in 250 mg capsules. How many capsules will you administer?

18. The physician ordered Retrovir (zidovudine) PO, an antiviral drug used for the treatment of CMV retinitis. The order is 160 mg/m^2 every 8 hours. The patient weighs 60 kg and is 140 cm in height. How many milligrams of this drug will you give the patient per day? (Use the formula for BSA.)

19. Physician's order: Cytoxan (cyclophosphamide) 3 mg/kg twice weekly. The client weighs 148 lb. The drug is supplied in 50 mg tablets. How many tablets will you prepare?

20. Physician's order: prednisone 40 mg PO q12h for 5 days for a patient with acute asthma. The drug is supplied in 20 mg tablets. How many tablets will you give this patient?

Cumulative Review Exercises

Review your mastery of earlier chapters.

1. Physician's order: *atropine sulfate gr 1/150 PO now*

   Each tablet contains 0.4 mg. How many tablets will you prepare for your patient? _____

2. Lorabid (loracarbef) 400 mg PO q12h. The label reads 200 mg in 5 mL. How many mL will you give your patient? _____

3. Azithromycin 0.2 g PO has been ordered. Convert this dose to grains. _____

4. 0.4 g = _____ mg

5. 2.5 liters = _____ milliliters

6. 7 lb 11 oz = _____ g

7. 1 pint = _____ cups

8. The order reads 267 mg/m^2 of a drug PO. The patient weighs 72 kg and is 70 in tall. The label reads 50 mg/mL. How many mL will you administer to this patient? Use the nomogram to estimate the BSA.

9. A physician orders Tylenol (acetamenophen) 650 mg PO q8h. The label reads as follows: Each capsule contains 325 mg. How many capsules will you give this patient?

10. The order reads Tenormin (atenolol) 100 mg PO daily. Each tablet contains 0.025 g. How many tablets will you prepare?

11. The physician orders Parlodel (bromocriptine mesylate), 7.5 mg PO b.i.d. with meals. Each tablet contains 2.5 mg. How many tablets of this anti-Parkinsonian drug will you prepare?

12. A patient must receive 60 mEq of potassium chloride PO stat. Each tablet is labeled 20 mEq/tab. How many tablets will you prepare?

13. 200 mg = _____ g

14. A patient must receive Videx (didanosine) 2.2 mg/kg PO. The patient weighs 90 kg. How many tablets will the patient receive if each tablet contains 100 mg?

15. 1 t = _____ mL

MediaLink
www.prenhall.com/olsen
Animated examples, interactive practice questions with animated solutions, and challenge tests for this chapter can be found on the Prentice Hall Dosage Calculation Tutor that accompanies this text. Additional, unique, interactive resources and activities can be found on the Companion Website.

Syringes

Learning Outcomes

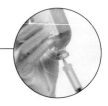

After completing this chapter, you will be able to

1. Identify the parts of a syringe and needle.
2. Identify various types of syringes.
3. Read and measure dosages on syringes.
4. Select the appropriate syringe to administer prescribed doses.
5. Read the calibrations on hypodermic, tuberculin, insulin, and prefilled syringes.
6. Measure single insulin dosages.
7. Measure combined insulin dosages.

I n this chapter, you will learn how to use various types of syringes to measure medication dosages. You will also discuss the difference between the types of insulin and how to measure single insulin dosages and combined insulin dosages.

Syringes are made of plastic or glass, designed for one-time use, and are packaged either separately or together with needles of appropriate sizes. After use, syringes must be discarded in special puncture-resistant containers.

Parts of a Syringe

A syringe consists of a barrel, plunger, and tip.

- **Barrel:** a hollow cylinder that holds the medication. It has calibrations (markings) on the outer surface.

- **Plunger:** fits in the barrel and is moved back and forth. Pulling back on the plunger draws medication or air into the syringe. Pushing in the plunger forces air or medication out of the syringe.

- **Tip:** the end of the syringe that holds the needle. The needle slips onto the tip or can be twisted and locked in place (Leur-Lok).

The inside of the barrel, plunger, and tip (shown in ● **Figure 7.1**) must always be sterile.

Needles

Needles are made of stainless steel and come in various lengths and diameters. They are packaged with a protective cover that keeps them from being contaminated. The parts of a needle are the **hub**, which attaches to the syringe, the **shaft**, the long part of the needle that is embedded in the hub, and the **bevel**, the slanted portion of the tip. The **length** of the needle is the distance

Parts of a 10 mL Leur-Lock Hypodermic Syringe and Needle

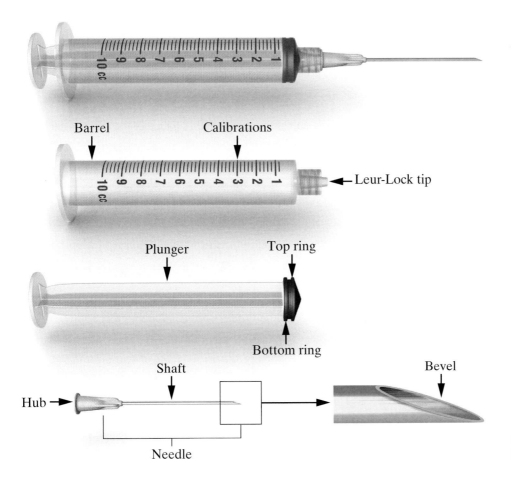

● **Figure 7.1**
Parts of a Syringe and needle.

from the point to the hub. Needles most commonly used in medication administration range from $\frac{3}{8}$ inch to 2 inches. The **gauge** of the needle refers to the thickness of the inside of the needle and varies from 18 to 28 (the larger the gauge, the thinner the needle). The parts of a needle are shown in Figure 7.1.

Types of Syringes

The two major types of syringes are hypodermic and oral. In 1853, Drs. Charles Pravaz and Alexander Wood were the first to develop a syringe with a needle that was fine enough to pierce the skin. This is known as a **hypodermic syringe**. (Use of oral syringes will be discussed in Chapter 12.)

Hypodermic syringes are calibrated (marked) in cubic centimeters (cc), milliliters (mL), or units. Practitioners often refer to syringes by the volume of cubic centimeters they contain, for example, a 3 cc syringe. Although many syringes are still labeled in cubic centimeters, manufacturers are now phasing in syringes labeled in milliliters. In this text, we will generally use mL instead of cc.

The smaller capacity syringes (1, 2, 2 $\frac{1}{2}$, and 3 mL) are used most often for subcutaneous or intramuscular injections of medication. The larger sizes (5, 6, 10, and 12 mL) are commonly used to draw blood or prepare medications for intravenous administration. Syringes 20 mL and larger are used to inject large volumes of sterile solutions. A representative sample of commonly used syringes is shown in ●**Figure 7.2**.

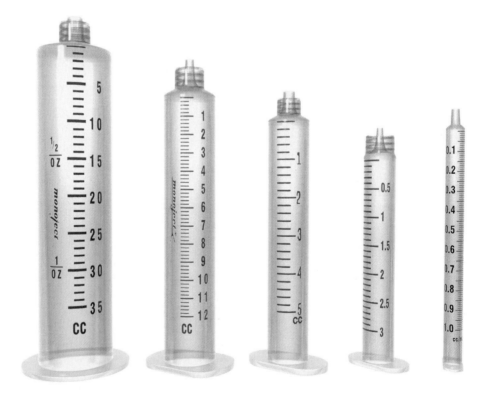

●**Figure 7.2**
A sample of commonly used hypodermic syringes (35 cc, 12 cc, 5 cc, 3 mL, and 1 mL).

A 35 cc syringe is shown in ●**Figure 7.3**. Each line on the barrel represents 1 mL, and the longer lines represent 5 mL.

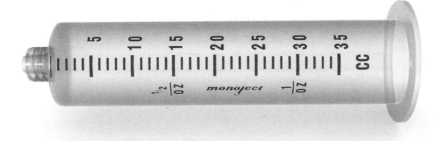

● **Figure 7.3**
35 cc syringe.

A 12 cc syringe is shown in ●**Figure 7.4**. Each line on the barrel represents 0.2 mL, and the longer lines represent 1 mL.

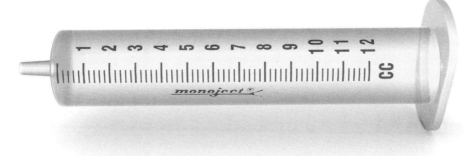

● **Figure 7.4**
12 cc syringe.

A 5 cc syringe is shown in ●**Figure 7.5**. Each line on the barrel represents 0.2 mL, and the longer lines represent 1 mL.

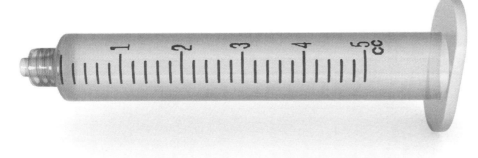

● **Figure 7.5**
5 cc syringe.

In ●**Figure 7.6**, a 3 cc/mL syringe is shown. There are 10 spaces between the largest markings. This indicates that the syringe is measured in tenths of a milliliter. So, each of the lines is 0.1 mL. The longer lines indicate half and full milliliter measures. The liquid volume in a syringe is read from the *top ring*, **not** the bottom ring or the raised section in the middle of the plunger. Therefore, this syringe contains 0.9 mL.

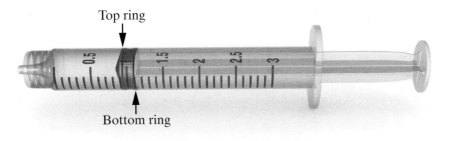

● **Figure 7.6**
Partially filled 3 cc/mL syringe.

NOTE

The syringe in Figure 7.6 is calibrated in both cc and mL. The use of the minim scale (apothecary) found on some 3 mL syringes is being phased out.

Example 7.1

How much liquid is in the 12 cc syringe shown in ● **Figure 7.7**?

The top ring of the plunger is at the second line after the 5 mL line. Because each line measures 0.2 mL, the second line measures 0.4 mL. Therefore, the amount in the syringe is 5.4 mL.

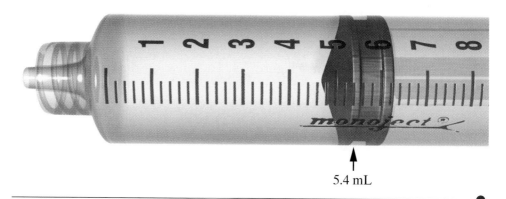

● **Figure 7.7**
A partially filled 12 cc syringe.

5.4 mL

Example 7.2

How much liquid is in the 5 cc syringe shown in ● **Figure 7.8**?

The top ring of the plunger is at the second line after 4 mL. Because each line measures 0.2 mL, the second line measures 0.4 mL. Therefore, the amount of liquid in the syringe is 4.4 mL.

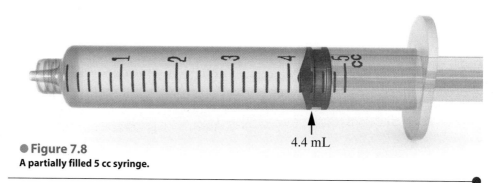

● **Figure 7.8**
A partially filled 5 cc syringe.

4.4 mL

Example 7.3

How much liquid is in the 3 mL syringe in ● **Figure 7.9**?

The top ring of the plunger is at the second line after 1 mL. Because each line measures 0.1 mL, the two lines measure 0.2 mL. Therefore, the amount in the syringe is 1.2 mL.

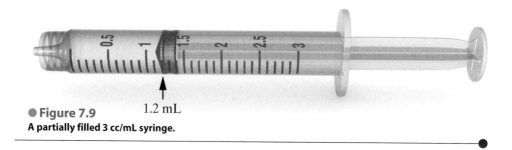

● **Figure 7.9**
A partially filled 3 cc/mL syringe.

1.2 mL

The 1 mL syringe, also called a **tuberculin syringe,** shown in ●Figure 7.10, is calibrated in hundredths of a milliliter. Because there are 100 lines on the syringe, each line represents 0.01 mL. This syringe is used for intradermal injection of very small amounts of substances in tests for tuberculosis and allergies, as well as for intramuscular injection of small quantities of medication. The tuberculin syringe is the preferred syringe for use in measuring medications less than 1 mL.

0.52 mL

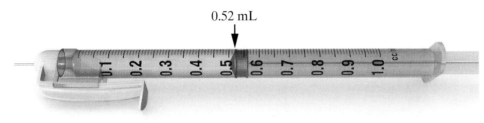

● **Figure 7.10**
A partially filled 1 mL tuberculin syringe.

The top ring of the plunger is at the second line after 0.5 mL. Therefore, the amount in the syringe is 0.52 mL.

Example 7.4

How much liquid is shown in the portion of the 1 mL tuberculin syringe shown in ●Figure 7.11?

The top ring of the plunger is 6 lines after the 0.3 mL calibration. Because each line represents 0.01 mL, the amount of liquid in the syringe is 0.36 mL.

3.6 mL

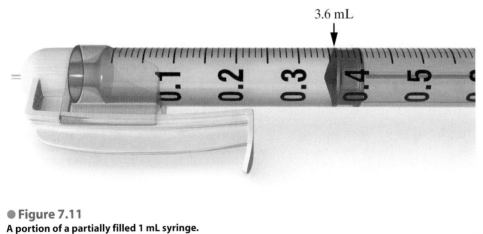

● **Figure 7.11**
A portion of a partially filled 1 mL syringe.

NOTE

Because the 1 mL tuberculin syringe can accurately measure amounts to hundredths of a milliliter, the volume of fluid to be measured in this syringe is rounded off to the nearest hundredth; for example, 0.358 mL is rounded off to 0.36 mL. The 3 mL syringe can accurately measure amounts to tenths of a milliliter. The volume of fluid to be measured in this syringe is rounded off to the nearest tenth of a milliliter; for example, 2.358 mL is rounded off to 2.4 mL.

Insulin syringes are used for the subcutaneous injection of insulin and are calibrated in *units* rather than *milliliters*. Insulin is a hormone used to treat patients who have insulin-dependent diabetes mellitus (IDDM). It is supplied as a premixed liquid measured in standardized units of potency rather than by weight or volume. These standardized units are called **USP** *units*, which are often shortened to *units*. The most commonly prepared concentration of insulin is 100 units per milliliter, which is referred to as *units 100 insulin* and is abbreviated as U-100 on insulin labels. Although a 500 unit concentration of insulin (U-500) is also available, it is used only for the rare patient who is markedly insulin-resistant. U-40 insulin is used in some countries; however in the United States, insulin is standardized to U-100. Exubera, the first inhalable version of insulin, is available as a dry powder and is inhaled through the mouth using the handheld Exubera Inhaler. For the rest of this text, we will refer to U-100 insulin only.

Insulin syringes have three different capacities: the standard 100 unit capacity, and the **Lo-Dose** 50 unit or 30 unit capacities. The plunger of the insulin syringe is flat, and the liquid volume is measured from the top ring.

●**Figure 7.12** shows a *single-scale standard* 100 unit insulin syringe calibrated in 2 unit increments. Any odd number of units (e.g., 23, 35) is measured between the even calibrations. These calibrations and spaces are very small, so this is not the syringe of choice for a person with impaired vision.

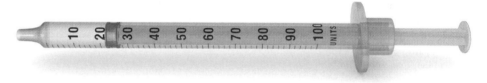

●**Figure 7.12**
A single-scale standard 100 unit insulin syringe with 22 units of insulin.

The dual-scale version of this syringe is easier to read. ●**Figure 7.13** shows a *dual-scale* 100 unit insulin syringe, also calibrated in 2 unit increments. However, it has a scale with *even* numbers on one side and a scale with *odd* numbers on the opposite side. Both the even and odd sides are shown.

Each line on the barrel represents 2 units.

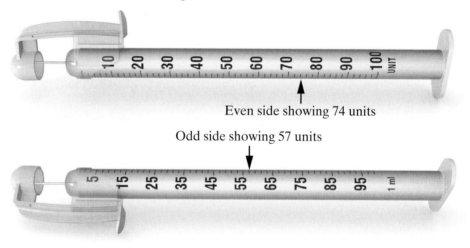

Even side showing 74 units

Odd side showing 57 units

●**Figure 7.13**
Two views of the same dual-scale standard 100 unit insulin syringe.

A 50 unit Lo-Dose insulin syringe, shown in ●**Figure 7.14**, is a single-scale syringe with 50 units. It is calibrated in 1 unit increments.

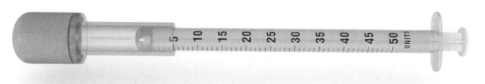

●**Figure 7.14**
A 50 unit Lo-Dose insulin syringe.

A 30 unit Lo-Dose insulin syringe, shown in ● **Figure 7.15**, is a syringe with 30 units. It is calibrated in 1 unit increments and is used when the dose is less than 30 units.

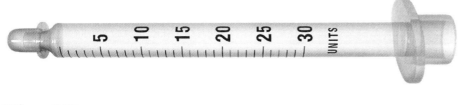

● **Figure 7.15**
A 30 unit Lo-Dose insulin syringe.

Measuring Insulin Doses

Measuring a Single Dose of Insulin in an Insulin Syringe

Insulin is available in 100 units/mL multidose vials. The major route of administration of insulin is by subcutaneous injection. *Insulin is never given intramuscularly.* It can also be administered with an insulin pen that contains a cartridge filled with insulin or with a CSII pump (Continuous Subcutaneous Insulin Infusion). The CSII pump is used to administer a programmed dose of a rapid-acting 100 units insulin at a set rate of units per hour.

The *source* of insulin (animal or human) and *type* (rapid, short, intermediate, or long-acting) are indicated on the label. Today, the most commonly used *source* is human insulin. Insulin from a human source is designated on the label as recombinant DNA (rDNA origin). The *type* of insulin relates to both the *onset and duration of action.* It is indicated by the uppercase bold letter that follows the trade name on the label, for example, Humulin **R (Regular)**, Humulin **L (Lente)**, Humulin **N (NPH)**, and Humulin **U (Ultralente)**. These letters are important visual identifiers when selecting the insulin type. ● **Figure 7.16**.

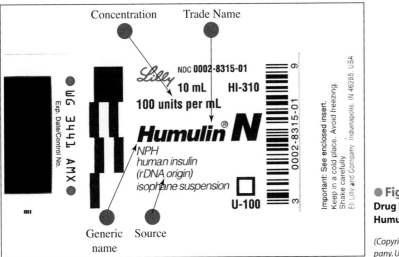

● **Figure 7.16**
Drug label for Humulin N insulin.

(Copyright Eli Lilly and Company. Used with permission.)

Healthcare providers must be familiar with the various **types of insulin,** as summarized in Table 7.1.

Table 7.1 **Type of Insulin**

Type	Name		How It Works
Rapid Acting (generic)	**Humalog (lispro)**	**Novolog (aspart)**	Rapid-acting insulin covers insulin needs for meals eaten at the time of injection. Usually taken 15 minutes before meals or given just after a meal. This type of insulin is also given to cover until longer-acting insulins take effect.
Onset	15–30 minutes	10–20 minutes	
Peak	30 minutes to $2\frac{1}{2}$ hours	1–3 hours	
Duration	3–5 hours	3–5 hours	
Short Acting regular	**Humulin R, Novolin, or Semilente**	**Velosulin** (for use in an insulin pump)	Short-acting insulin covers insulin needs for meals eaten within 30–60 minutes. Usually taken 30 to 40 minutes before meals.
Onset	30 minutes to 1 hour	30 minutes to 1 hour	
Peak	2–5 hours	2–3 hours	
Duration	5–8 hours	2–3 hours	
Intermediate Acting	**NPH (N)**	**Lente (L)**	Intermediate-acting insulin covers insulin needs for about half the day or overnight. Taken up to 1 hour before meals. This type of insulin is often combined with rapid- or short-acting insulin.
Onset	2–4 hours	1–$2\frac{1}{2}$ hours	
Peak	4–10 hours	4–12 hours	
Duration	14–16 hours	12–18 hours	
Long Acting	**Ultralente (U)**	**Lantus (glargine)**	Long-acting insulin covers insulin needs for about 1 full day, not timed to meals. Some are given once or twice daily, and others once a day. Lantus once a day should be given at the same time. This type of insulin is often combined, when needed, with rapid- or short-acting insulin.
Onset	30 minutes–3 hours	1–$1\frac{1}{2}$ hours	
Peak	peakless	No peak time; insulin is delivered at a steady level	
Duration	20–36 hours	20–24 hours	

Premixed Insulin Combinations					How It Works
Premixed	**Humulin 70/30**	**Novolin 70/30**	**Novolog 70/30**	**Humulin 50/50**	**Humalog mix 75/25**	Premixed insulin is a combination of specific proportions of intermediate-acting and short-acting insulin. The numbers after the name indicate the percentage of each insulin.

These products are generally taken twice a day before mealtime, 15–45 minutes before meals. |
Onset	30 minutes	30 minutes	10–20 minutes	30 minutes	15 minutes	
Peak	2–4 hours	2–12 hours	1–4 hours	2–5 hours	30 minutes–$2\frac{1}{2}$ hours	
Duration	14–24 hours	up to 24 hours	up to 24 hours	18 to 24 hours	16–20 hours	

Example 7.5

What is the dose of insulin in the single-scale 100 unit insulin syringe shown in ● **Figure 7.17**?

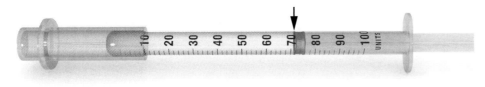

● **Figure 7.17**
A single-scale 100 unit insulin syringe.

The top ring of the plunger is one line after 70. Because each line represents 2 units, the dose is 72 units of insulin.

Example 7.6

What is the dose of insulin in the dual-scale 100 unit insulin syringe shown in ● **Figure 7.18**?

100 Unit Dual-scale Syringe

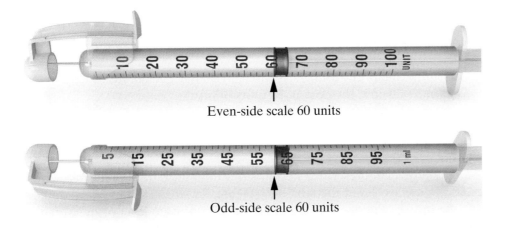

Even-side scale 60 units

Odd-side scale 60 units

● **Figure 7.18**
Three views of a dual-scale insulin syringe.

The top ring of the plunger is slightly more than 2 lines after 55 on the odd side. Notice how difficult it would be to determine where 60 units would measure using the odd side of the syringe. However, on the even side, the plunger falls exactly on the 60.

Example 7.7

What is the dose of insulin in the 50 unit insulin syringe shown in ●Figure 7.19?

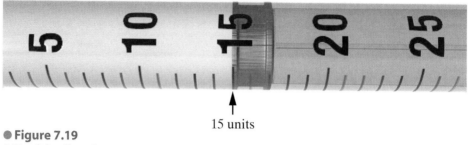

15 units

●**Figure 7.19**
A 50 unit insulin syringe.

The top ring of the plunger is at 15. Because each line represents 1 unit, the dose is 15 units.

Example 7.8

What is the dose of insulin in the 30 unit insulin syringe shown in ●Figure 7.20?

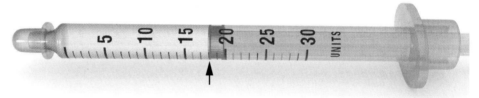

●**Figure 7.20**
A 30 unit Lo-Dose insulin syringe.

The top ring of the plunger is three lines after 15. Because each line represents one unit, the dose is 18 units of insulin.

Example 7.9

The physician prescribed 26 units of Humulin L insulin subcutaneously ac breakfast. Read the label in ●**Figure 7.21** to determine the source of the insulin and place an arrow at the appropriate level of measurement on the insulin syringe in ●**Figure 7.22**.

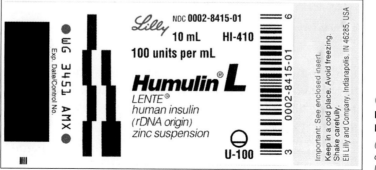

●**Figure 7.21**
Drug label for Humulin L.

(Copyright Eli Lilly and Company. Used with permission.)

The source of the insulin is human (rDNA origin), and the arrow should be placed one line after 25, as shown in Figure 7.22.

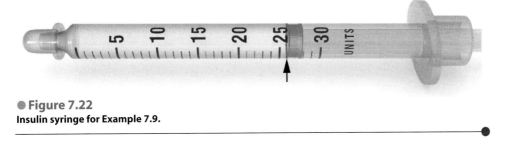

● **Figure 7.22**
Insulin syringe for Example 7.9.

Measuring Two Types of Insulin in One Syringe

Individuals who have IDDM often must have two types of insulin administered at the same time. In order to reduce the number of injections, it is common practice to combine two insulins (usually a rapid-acting with either an intermediate- or a long-acting) in a single syringe. The important points to remember are these:

- The *total volume* in the syringe is the *sum of the two insulin* amounts.

- The smallest capacity syringe containing the dose should be used to measure the insulins because the enlarged scale is easier to read and therefore more accurate.

- The *amount of air equal to the amount of insulin to be withdrawn* from each vial must be injected into each vial.

- You must inject the air into the intermediate- or long-acting insulin before you inject the air into the Regular insulin.

- The *Regular* (rapid-acting) insulin is drawn up *first*; this prevents contamination of the Regular insulin with the intermediate or long-acting insulin.

- The intermediate-acting or long-acting insulins can precipitate; therefore, they must be mixed well before drawing up and administered without delay.

- Only insulins from the same source should be mixed together, for example, Humulin **R** and Humulin **N** are both human insulin and can be mixed.

- If you draw up too much of the intermediate or long-acting insulin, you must discard the entire medication and start over.

The steps of preparing two types of insulin in one syringe are shown in Example 7.10.

Example 7.10

The prescriber ordered 10 units Humulin R insulin and 30 units Humulin N insulin subcutaneously, 30 minutes before breakfast. Explain how you would prepare to administer this in one injection. ●**Figures 7.23** and ● **7.24.**

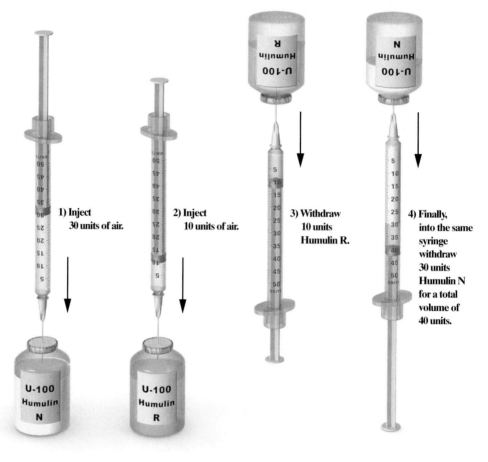

● **Figure 7.23**
Mixing two types of insulin in one syringe.

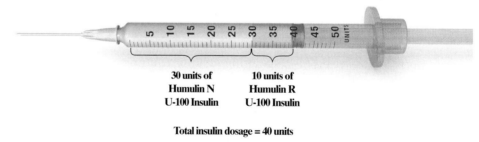

30 units of
Humulin N
U-100 Insulin

10 units of
Humulin R
U-100 Insulin

Total insulin dosage = 40 units

● **Figure 7.24**
Combination of 30 units Humulin N and 10 units of Humulin R.

The total amount of insulin is 40 units (10 + 30). To administer this dose, use a 50 unit Lo-Dose syringe. Inject 30 units of air into the Humulin **N** vial and 10 units of air into the Humulin **R** vial. Withdraw 10 units of the Humulin **R** first and then withdraw 30 units of the Humulin **N**.

Measuring Premixed Insulin

Using premixed insulin (see Table 7.1) eliminates errors that may occur when mixing two types of insulin in one syringe (Figure 7.23).

Example 7.11

Order: Give 35 units of Humulin 70/30 insulin subcutaneously 30 minutes before breakfast. Use the label shown in ● **Figure 7.25** and place an arrow at the appropriate calibration on the syringe.

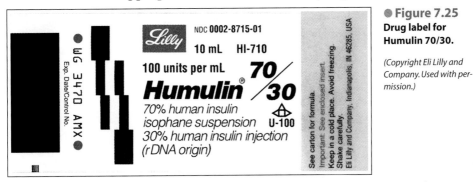

● **Figure 7.25**
Drug label for Humulin 70/30.

(Copyright Eli Lilly and Company. Used with permission.)

In the syringe in ● **Figure 7.26**, the top ring of the plunger is at the 35 unit line.

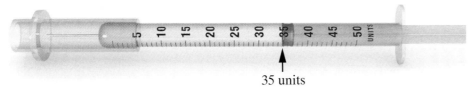

35 units

● **Figure 7.26**
A 50 unit Lo-Dose insulin syringe measuring 35 units.

Prefilled Syringes

A prefilled, single-dose syringe contains the usual dose of a medication. Some prefilled glass cartridges are available for use with a special plunger called a Tubex or Carpuject syringe (● **Figure 7.27**). If a medication order is for the exact amount of drug in the prefilled syringe, the possibility of measurement error by the person administering the drug is decreased.

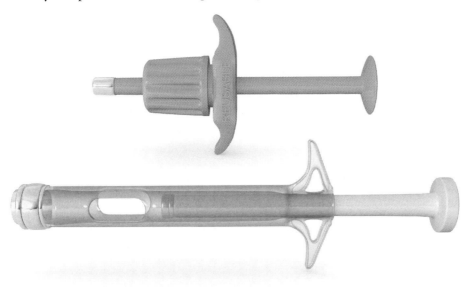

● **Figure 7.27**
Carpuject and Tubex prefilled cartridge holders.

Example 7.12

The prefilled syringe cartridges shown in ● **Figure 7.28** are calibrated so that each line measures 0.1 mL and each has a capacity of 2.5 mL. How many milliliters are indicated by the arrows shown in Figure 7.28?

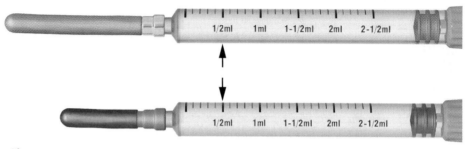

● **Figure 7.28**
Prefilled cartridges (Tubex or Carpuject).

Both cartridges have a total capacity of 2.5 mL, and the arrows are at 0.5 mL.

Example 7.13

How much medication is in the prepackaged cartridge shown in ● **Figure 7.29**?

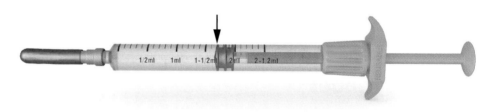

● **Figure 7.29**
Prefilled cartridge in holder.

The top of the plunger is at two lines after the 1.5 mL line. Because each line measures 0.1 mL, the two lines measure 0.2 mL. Therefore, there are 1.7 mL of medication in this prefilled cartridge.

Safety Syringes

In order to prevent the transmission of blood borne infections from contaminated needles, many syringes are now manufactured with various types of safety devices. For example, a syringe may contain a protective sheath that can be used to protect the needle's sterility. This sheath is then pulled forward and locked into place to provide a permanent needle shield for disposal following injection. Others may have a needle that automatically retracts into the barrel after injection. Each of these devices reduces the chance of needle stick injury. ● **Figure 7.30** shows examples of safety syringes.

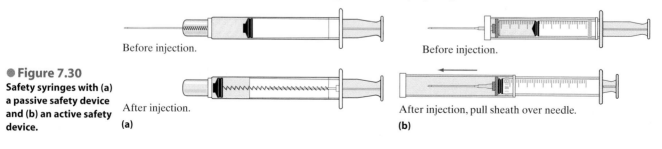

Before injection.

After injection.

(a)

Before injection.

After injection, pull sheath over needle.

(b)

● **Figure 7.30**
Safety syringes with (a) a passive safety device and (b) an active safety device.

Summary

In this chapter, the various types of syringes and needles were discussed. You learned how to measure the amount of liquid in various syringes. The types of insulin, how to measure a single dose, and how to mix two insulins in one syringe were explained. Prefilled, single-dose, and safety syringes were also presented.

- Milliliters (mL), rather than cubic centimeters (cc), are the preferred unit of measure for volume.
- All syringe calibrations must be read at the top ring of the plunger.
- Large-capacity hypodermic syringes (5, 12, 20, 35 mL) are calibrated in increments from 0.2 mL to 1 mL.
- Small-capacity hypodermic syringes (2, 2½, 3 mL) are calibrated in tenths of a milliter (0.1 mL).
- The 1 mL hypodermic (tuberculin) syringe is calibrated in hundredths of a milliliter. It is the preferred syringe for use in measuring a dose of less than 1 milliliter.
- The calibrations on hypodermic syringes differ; therefore, be very careful when measuring medications in syringes.
- Insulin syringes are designed for measuring and administering U-100 insulin. They are calibrated for 100 units per mL.

- Standard insulin syringes have a capacity of 100 units.
- Lo-Dose insulin syringes are used for measuring small amounts of insulin. They have a capacity of 50 units or 30 units.
- For greater accuracy, use the smallest capacity syringe possible to measure and administer doses. However, avoid filling a syringe to its capacity.
- When measuring two types of insulin in the same syringe, Regular insulin is always drawn up in the syringe first.
- The total volume when mixing insulins is the sum of the two insulin amounts.
- Insulin syringes are for measuring and administering insulin only. Tuberculin syringes are used to measure and administer other medications that are less than 1 mL. Confusion of the two can cause a medication error.
- The prefilled single-dose syringe cartridge is to be used once and then discarded.
- Syringes intended for injections should not be used to measure or administer oral medications.
- Use safety syringes to prevent needle stick injuries.

Case Study 7.1

A 55-year-old female with a medical history of obesity, hypertension, hyperlipidemia, and diabetes mellitus comes to the emergency department complaining of anorexia, nausea, vomiting, fever, chills, and severe sharp right upper quadrant pain that radiates to her back and right shoulder. She states that her pain is 9 (on a 0–10 pain scale). Vital signs are: T 100.2 °F, BP 148/94; P 104; R 24. The diagnostic workup confirms gallstones and she is admitted for a cholecystectomy (removal of gall bladder).

Pre-Op Orders:
- NPO
- V/S q4h
- Demerol (meperidine hydrochloride) 75 mg IM stat
- IV D5/RL @ 125 mL/h

- Insert NG (nasogastric) tube to low suction
- Pre-op meds: Demerol (meperidine hydrochloride) 75 mg and Phenergan (promethazine) 25 mg IM 30 minutes before surgery
- Cefuroxime 1.5 g IV 30 minutes before surgery

Post-Op orders:
- Discontinue NG tube
- NPO
- V/S q4h
- IV D5/RL @ 125 mL/h
- Compazine (prochlorperazine) 4 mg IM q4h prn nausea
- Demerol (meperidine hydrochloride) 75 mg and Vistaril (hydroxyzine) 25 mg IM q3h prn pain
- Merrem (meropenem)1g IVPB q8h

1. The label on the meperidine for the stat dose reads 100 mg/mL.
   (a) Draw a line indicating the measurement on each of the following syringes below.
   (b) Which syringe will most accurately measure this dose?
2. Calculate the pre-op dose of the Phenergan and Demerol. Phenergan is available in 25 mg/mL vials. Demerol is available in prepackaged 2 mL syringes labeled 10 mg/mL, 25 mg/mL, 50 mg/mL, 75 mg/mL, and 100 mg/mL.

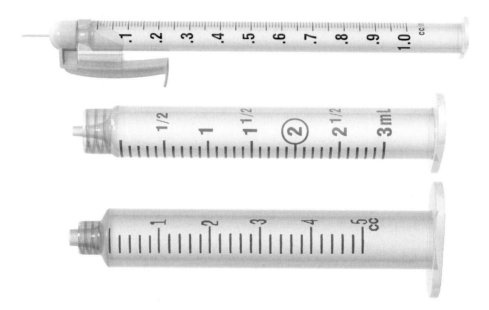

   (a) Which prepackaged syringe of Demerol will you use?
   (b) How many milliliters of Phenergan will you prepare?
   (c) Draw a line on the appropriate syringe below indicating the dose of each of these drugs that you will administer.

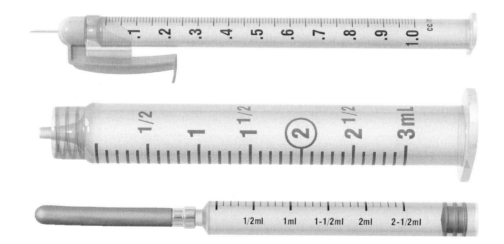

3. The label on the cefuroxime vial states: "add 9 mL of diluent to the 1.5 g vial." Draw a line on the appropriate syringe on the top of the next page indicating the amount of diluent you will add to the vial.

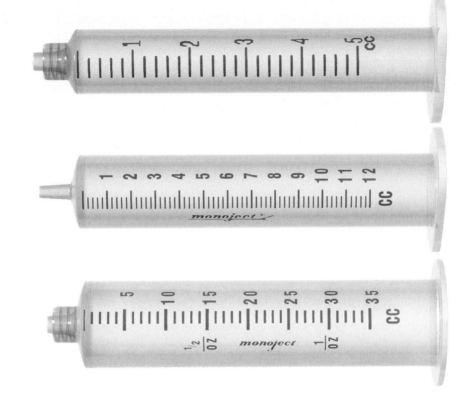

4. The patient is complaining of severe nausea. The Compazine vial is labeled 5 mg/mL. Draw a line on the appropriate syringe below indicating the dose of Compazine.

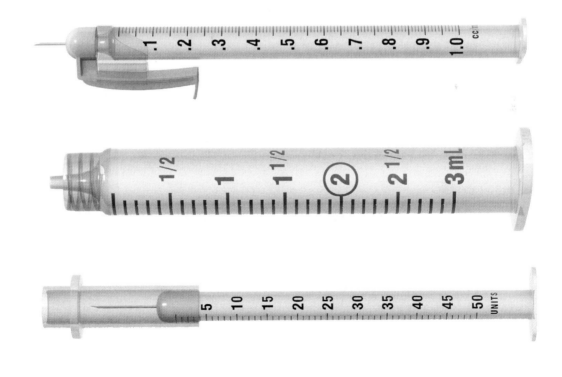

5. The patient is complaining of severe incisional pain of 10 (on a 0–10 pain scale) and has had no pain medication since her surgery. Calculate the dose of the Demerol and Vistaril order. The Vistaril is available in a concentration of 25 mg/mL and 50 mg/mL. The Demerol is available as 100 mg/mL.
   (a) Which vial of Vistaril will you use?
   (b) How many milliliters of Demerol do you need?
   (c) How will you prepare these medications so that you can give the patient a single injection?
   (d) Indicate on the appropriate syringe below the number of milliliters you will administer.

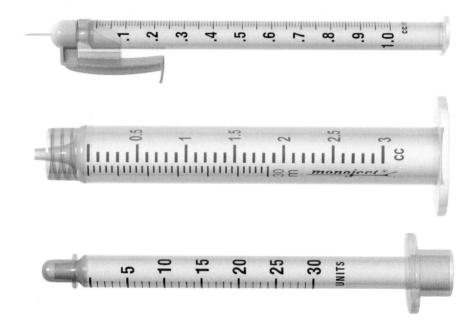

6. The label on the Merrem states 50 mg/mL.
   (a) How many mL will you need?
   (b) Draw a line on the appropriate syringe below indicating the dose of Merem.

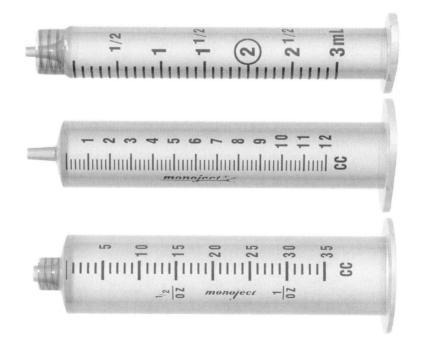

7. The patient has progressed to a regular diet and is ordered Humulin N 13 units and Humulin R 6 units subcutaneous 30 minutes ac breakfast, and Humulin N 5 units and Humulin R 5 units subcutaneous 30 minutes ac dinner.
   (a) How many units will the patient receive before breakfast?
   (b) Indicate on the appropriate syringe below the number of units of each insulin required before breakfast.

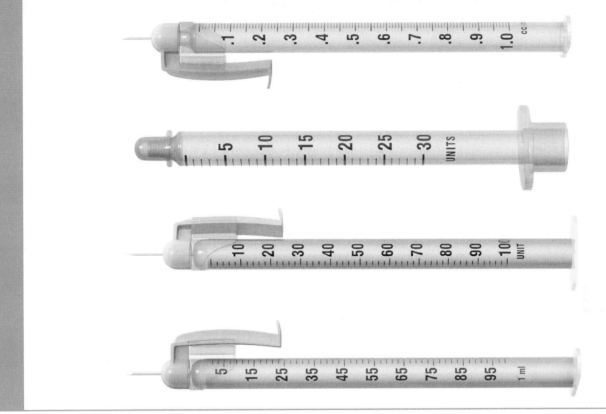

Practice Sets

The answers to *Try These for Practice*, *Exercises*, and *Cumulative Review Exercises* appear in Appendix A at the end of the book. Ask your instructor for answers to the *Additional Exercises*.

Try These for Practice

Test your comprehension after reading the chapter.

In Problems 1 through 4, identify the type of syringe shown in the figure. Place an arrow at the appropriate level of measurement on the syringe for the volume given.

1. _____ syringe; 0.72 mL

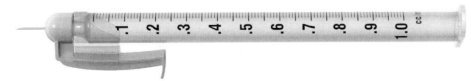

Workspace

2. _____ syringe; 6.8 mL

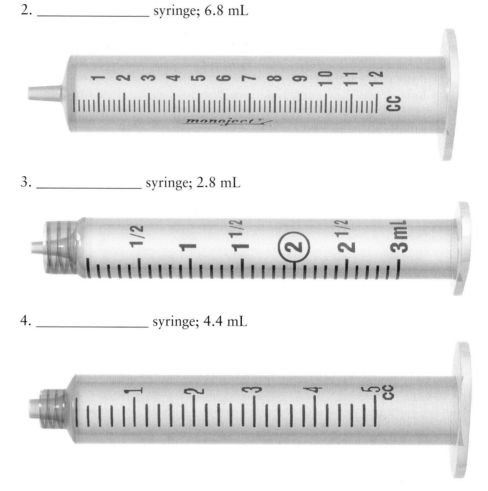

3. _____ syringe; 2.8 mL

4. _____ syringe; 4.4 mL

5. The prescriber ordered 34 units of Regular insulin and 18 units of Humulin N subcutaneously 30 minutes ac breakfast. Read the labels and do the following:

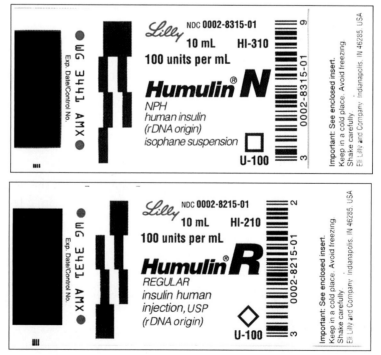

(Copyright Eli Lilly and Company. Used with permission.)

(a) Select the appropriate syringe to administer this dose in one injection.
(b) Place an arrow at the measurement of the Regular insulin.
(c) Place an arrow at the measurement of the Humulin N insulin.
(d) Determine how many units the patient will receive.

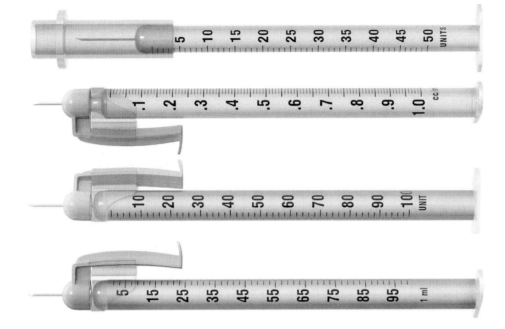

Exercises

Reinforce your understanding in class or at home.

In problems 1 through 14, identify the type of syringe shown in the figure. Then, for each quantity, place an arrow at the appropriate level of measurement on the syringe.

1. _____ syringe; 0.62 mL

2. _____ syringe;. 28 units

3. _____ syringe; 3.6 mL

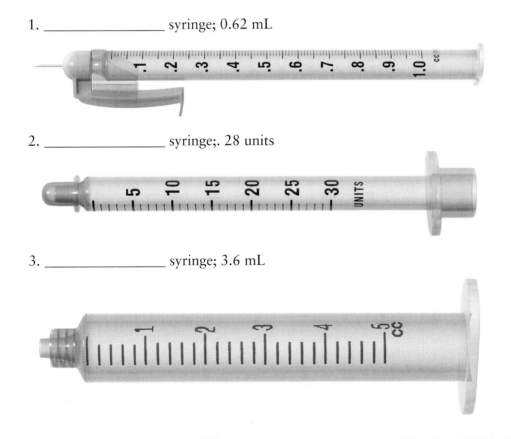

4. _____ syringe; 1.4 mL

5. _____ syringe; 13 mL

6. _____ syringe; 9.6 mL

7. _____ syringe; 32 units

8. _____ syringe; 56 units

9. _____ syringe; 0.37 mL

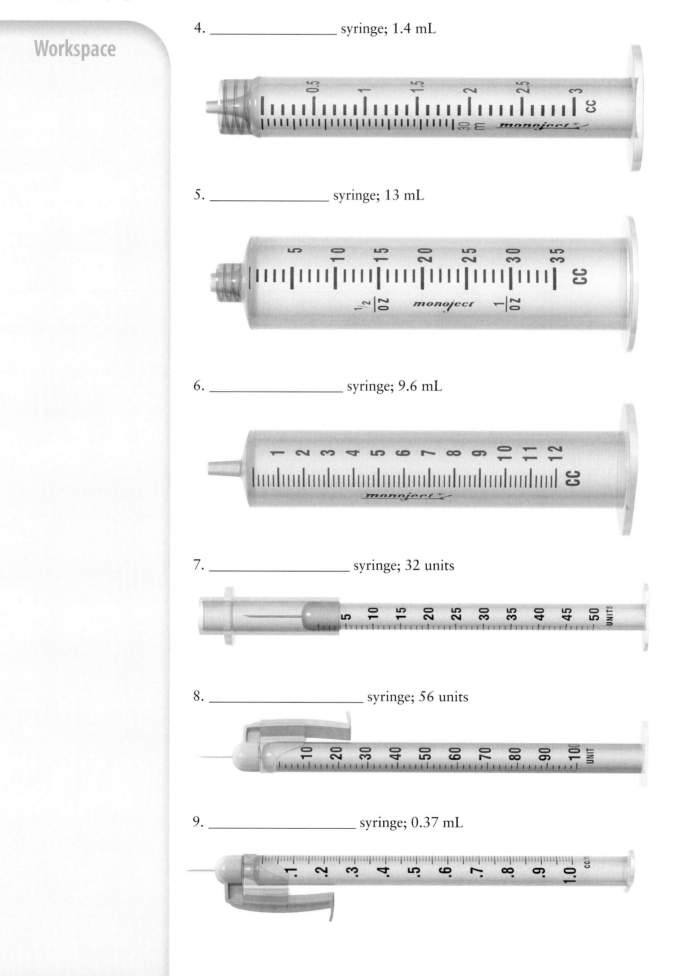

10. _____ syringe; 51 units

11. _____ syringe; 6.6 mL

12. _____ syringe; 0.72 mL

13. _____ syringe; 8.2 mL

14. _____ syringe; 27 mL

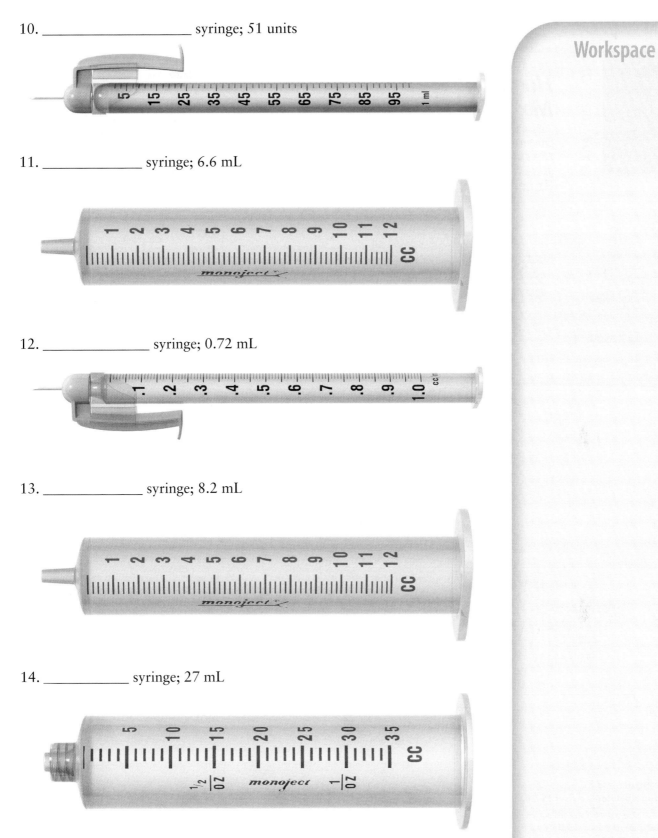

In problems 15 through 20, read the order, use the appropriate label in
● **Figure 7.31** (found at the end of the Exercises), calculate the dosage if necessary, and place an arrow at the appropriate level of measurement on the
syringe.

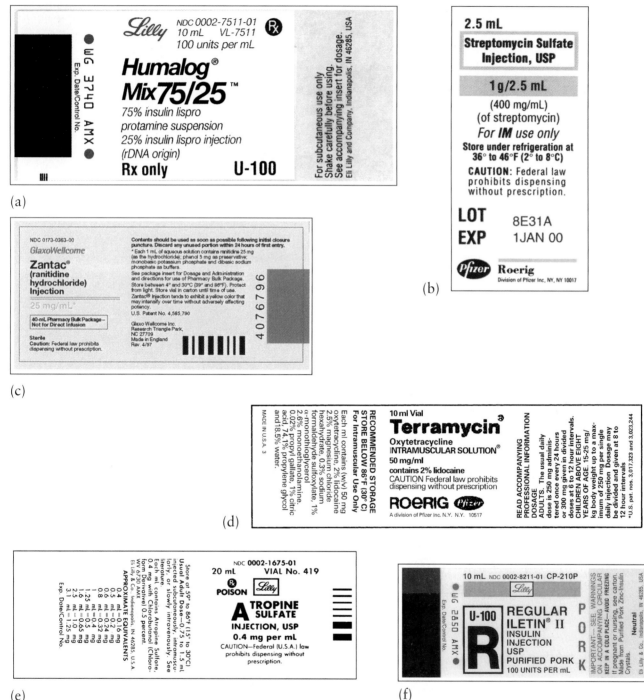

(a)

(b)

(c)

(d)

(e)

(f)

● **Figure 7.31**

Drug labels for *Exercises* 15–20.

(07-31a Copyright Eli Lilly and Company. Used with permission.   07-31b Reg. Trademark of Pfizer Inc. Reproduced with permission.   07-31c Reproduced with permission of GlaxoSmithKline.   07-31d Reg. Trademark Pfizer Inc. Reproduced with permission.   07-31e Copyright Eli Lilly and Company. Used with permission.   07-31f Copyright Eli Lilly and Company. Used with permission.   07-31g Copyright Eli Lilly and Company. Used with permission.)

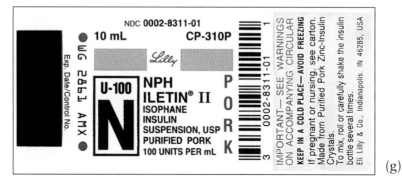

(g)

Workspace

15. Order: Give 26 units of Humalog 75/25 subcutaneously, 30 minutes ac breakfast

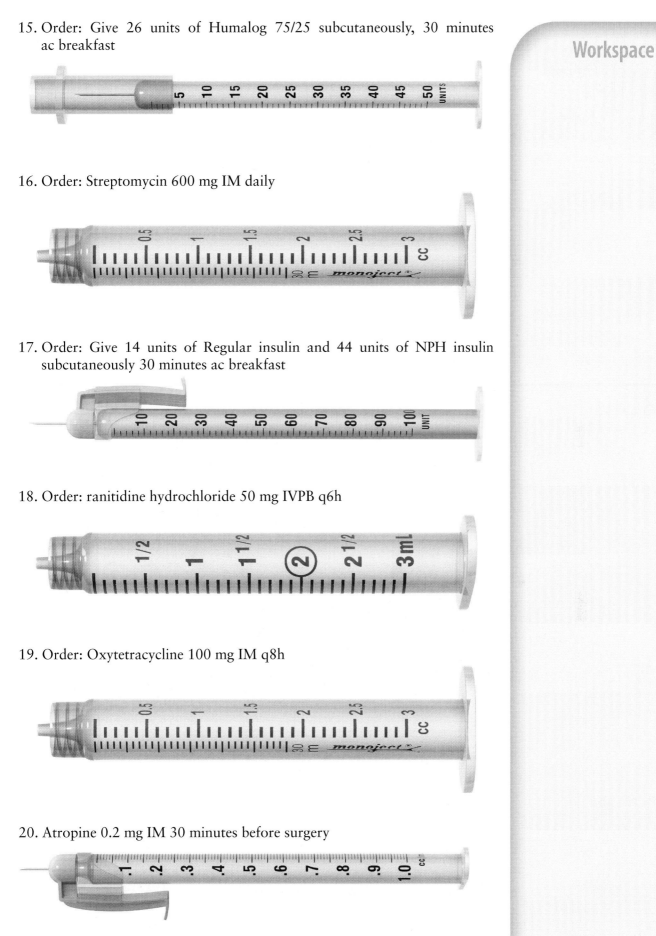

16. Order: Streptomycin 600 mg IM daily

17. Order: Give 14 units of Regular insulin and 44 units of NPH insulin subcutaneously 30 minutes ac breakfast

18. Order: ranitidine hydrochloride 50 mg IVPB q6h

19. Order: Oxytetracycline 100 mg IM q8h

20. Atropine 0.2 mg IM 30 minutes before surgery

Additional Exercises

Now, test yourself!

1. _____ syringe; 42 units

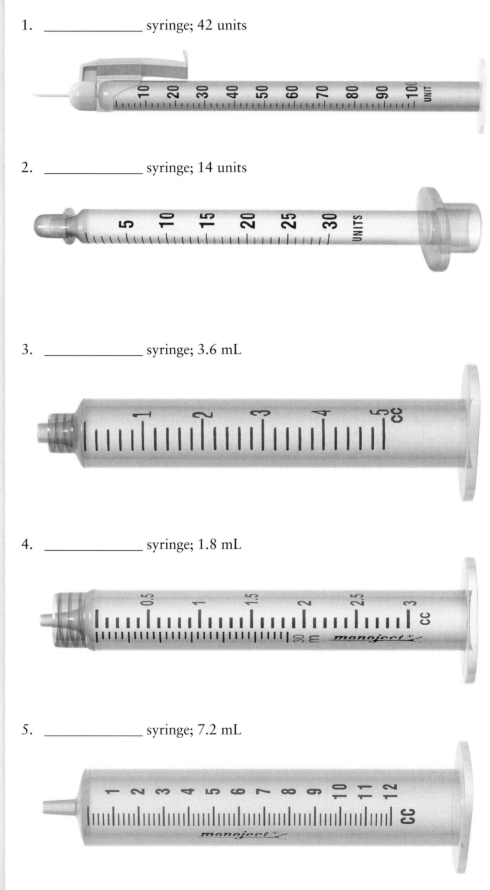

2. _____ syringe; 14 units

3. _____ syringe; 3.6 mL

4. _____ syringe; 1.8 mL

5. _____ syringe; 7.2 mL

6. _____ syringe; 16 mL

7. _____ syringe; 12 units

8. _____ syringe; 54 units

9. _____ syringe; 0.35 mL

10. _____ syringe; 31 units

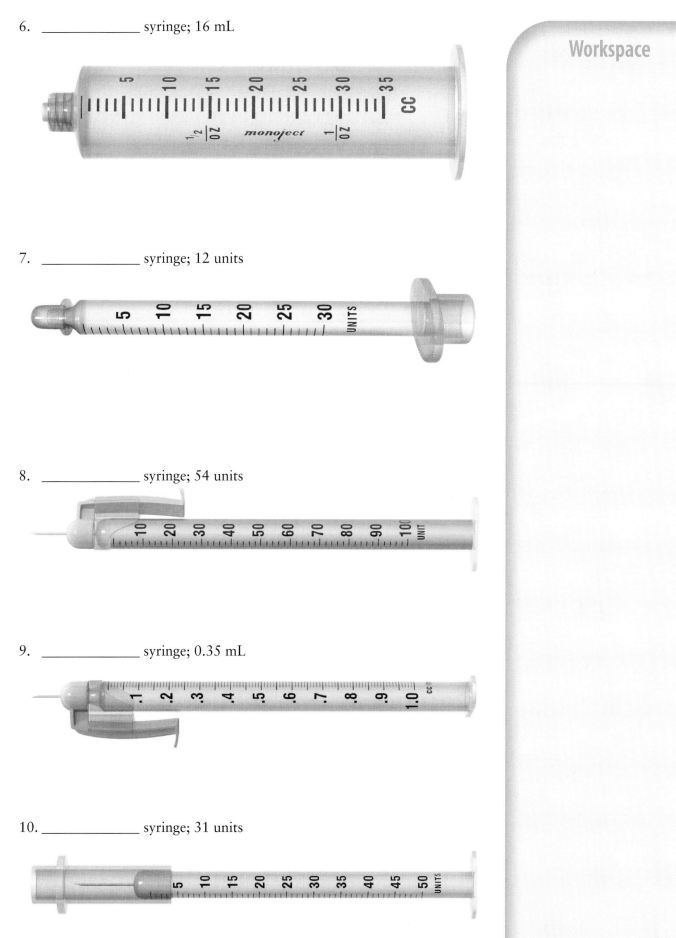

11. _____ syringe; 4.4 mL

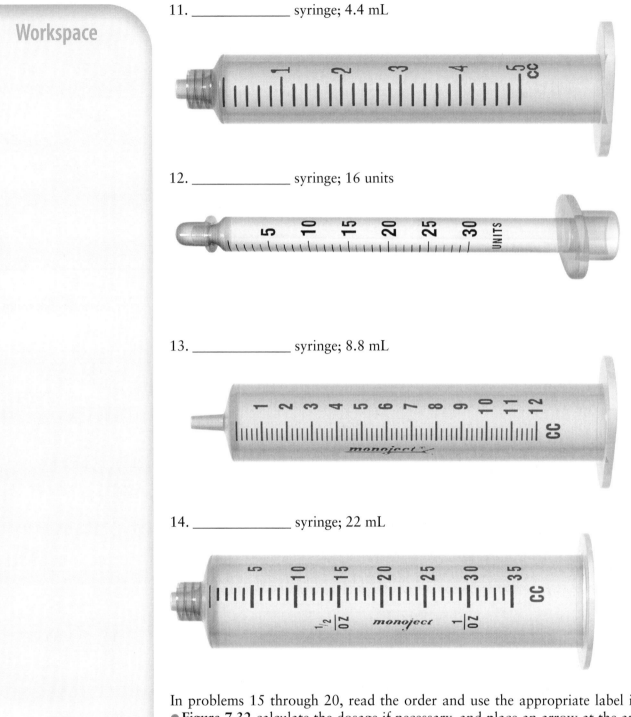

12. _____ syringe; 16 units

13. _____ syringe; 8.8 mL

14. _____ syringe; 22 mL

In problems 15 through 20, read the order and use the appropriate label in ● **Figure 7.32** calculate the dosage if necessary, and place an arrow at the appropriate level of measurement on the syringe.

15. Order: Insulin lispro 8 units subcutaneously 15 minutes ac breakfast

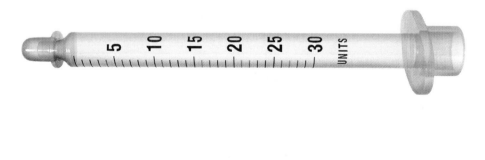

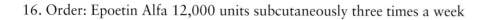

Workspace

16. Order: Epoetin Alfa 12,000 units subcutaneously three times a week

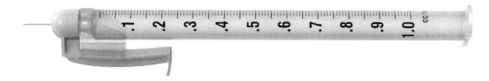

17. Order: Prochlorperazine 9 mg IM, q4h prn vomiting

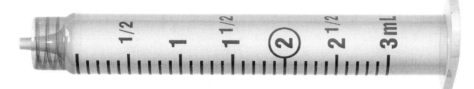

18. Order: filgrastim 750 mcg subcutaneously

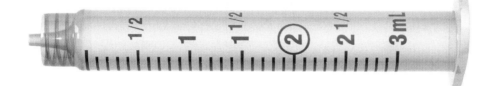

19. Order: Quinidine 400 mg IM q4h prn

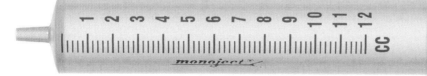

20. Order: Humulin 70/30 U-100 insulin 46 units subcutaneously ac dinner

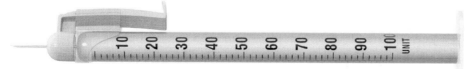

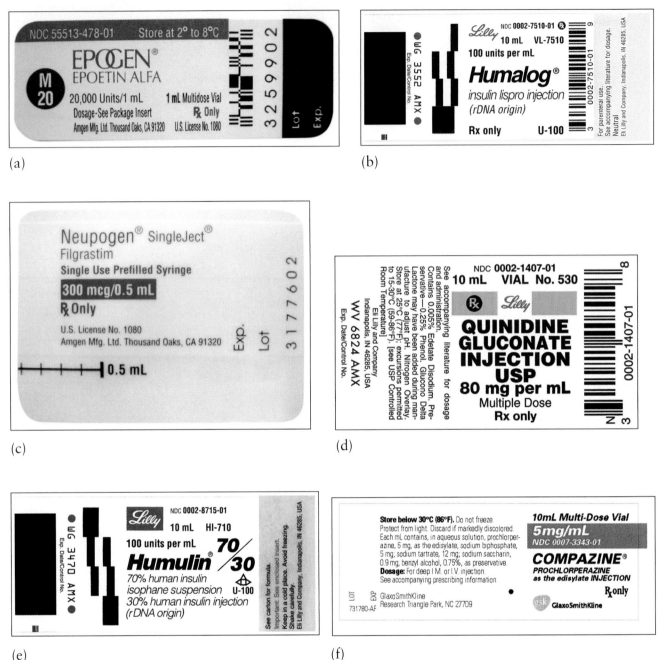

● Figure 7.32
Drug labels for Additional Exercises 15–20.

(07-32a Published with permission of Amgen Inc.   07-32b Copyright Eli Lilly and Company. Used with permission.   07-32c Published with permission of Amgen Inc.   07-32d Copyright Eli Lilly and Company. Used with permission.   07-32e Copyright Eli Lilly and Company. Used with permission.   07-32f Reproduced with permission of GlaxoSmithKline.)

Workspace

Cumulative Review Exercises

Review your mastery of earlier chapters

1. 0.05 g = _____ mg

2. 1,600 mL = _____ L

3. The prescriber ordered Prilosec 40 mg PO daily. Each capsule contains 20 mg. How many capsules will the patient receive in two weeks? _____

4. The order reads morphine sulfate 4 mg subcutaneously q4h prn. What is the maximum number of times the patient may receive this medication in one day? _____

5. The prescriber ordered Biaxin 300 mg PO q12h. The label reads 375 mg/mL. How many milliliters will you administer? _____

6. 1 t = _____ mL

7. The prescriber ordered 120 mL H_2O PO q2h for 10h. How many ounces should the patient receive? _____

8. Convert 4 fluid oz to mL. _____

9. 0.4 mg = gr _____

10. Which of the following has the greatest weight? 0.3 mg, 0.05 mg, 0.125 mg _____

11. The prescriber ordered Amoxicillin 750 mg PO q12h. Each capsule contains 250 mg. How many capsules will you administer to the patient? _____

12. The prescriber ordered 0.3 mg of clonidine hydrochloride. If each tablet contains 0.1 mg, how many tablets will you administer to the patient? _____

13. Read the information on the label in ● **Figure 7.33** and calculate the number of capsules equal to 0.002 g. _____

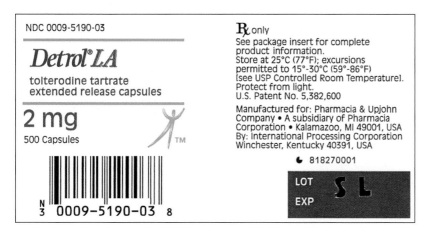

NDC 0009-5190-03

Detrol ® *LA*

tolterodine tartrate
extended release capsules

2 mg
500 Capsules

TM

N
3 0009-5190-03 8

℞ only
See package insert for complete
product information.
Store at 25°C (77°F); excursions
permitted to 15°-30°C (59°-86°F)
[see USP Controlled Room Temperature].
Protect from light.
U.S. Patent No. 5,382,600

Manufactured for: Pharmacia & Upjohn
Company • A subsidiary of Pharmacia
Corporation • Kalamazoo, MI 49001, USA
By: International Processing Corporation
Winchester, Kentucky 40391, USA

● 818270001

LOT   S L

EXP

● **Figure 7.33**
Drug label for Detrol.

14. The prescriber ordered Vistaril 75 mg IM stat. The label reads 50 mg/mL. How many milliliters will you administer? _____

15. Read the label in ●**Figure** 7.34. How many milligrams equal 1 mL? _____

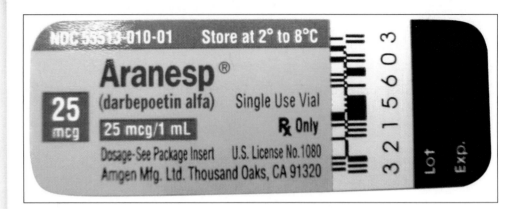

●**Figure 7.34**
Drug label for Aranesp.

(Published with permission of Amgen Inc.)

Preparation of Solutions

Learning Outcomes

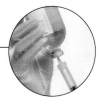

After completing this chapter, you will be able to

1. Describe the strength of a solution both as a ratio and as a percent.
2. Determine the amount of pure drug in a given amount of solution.
3. Determine the amount of solution that would contain a given amount of pure drug.
4. Do the calculations necessary to prepare solutions from pure drugs.
5. Do the calculations necessary to prepare solutions by diluting stock solutions.

I n this chapter you will learn about solutions. Although solutions are generally pre-pared by the pharmacist, healthcare providers should understand the concepts in-volved and be able to prepare solutions.

Drugs are manufactured in both pure and diluted forms. A pure drug contains only the drug and nothing else. A drug is frequently diluted by dissolving a quantity of pure drug in a liquid to form a solution. The pure drug (either dry or liquid) is called the *solute*. The liquid added to the pure drug to form the solution is called the *solvent* or *diluent*. The solvents most commonly used are sterile water and normal saline solution.

Determining the Strength of a Solution

The strength of a solution can be stated as a *ratio* or a *percentage*.

- The ratio 1:2 (read "1 to 2") means that there is 1 part of the drug in 2 parts of solution. This solution is also referred to as a $\frac{1}{2}$ strength solution or a 50% solution.
- The ratio 1:10 (read "1 to 10") means that there is 1 part of the drug in 10 parts of solution. This solution is also referred to as a 10% solution.
- A 5% solution means that there are 5 parts of the drug in 100 parts of solution.
- A $2\frac{1}{2}$% solution means that there are $2\frac{1}{2}$ parts of the drug in 100 parts of solution.

Pure Drugs in Liquid Form

For a pure drug that is in liquid form, the ratio 1:40 means there is 1 milliliter of pure drug in every 40 milliliters of solution. So 40 milliliters of a 1:40 acetic acid solution means that 1 milliliter of pure acetic acid is diluted with water to make a total of 40 milliliters of solution. You would prepare this solution by placing 1 milliliter of pure acetic acid in a graduated cylinder and adding water until the level in the graduated cylinder reaches 40 milliliters. ● **Figure 8.1.**

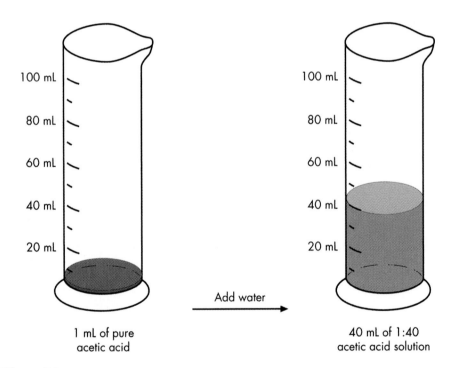

Add water

1 mL of pure
acetic acid

40 mL of 1:40
acetic acid solution

● **Figure 8.1**
Preparing a 1:40 solution from a pure liquid drug.

A 1% solution means that there is 1 part of the drug in 100 parts of solution. So you would prepare 100 mL of a 1% creosol solution by placing 1 milliliter of pure creosol in a graduated cylinder and adding water until the level in the graduated cylinder reaches 100 mL. ● **Figure 8.2.**

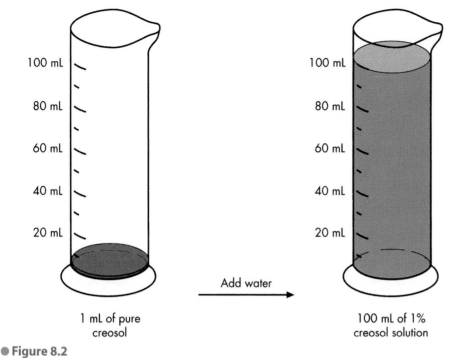

100 mL

80 mL

60 mL

40 mL

20 mL

Add water

1 mL of pure
creosol

100 mL

80 mL

60 mL

40 mL

20 mL

100 mL of 1%
creosol solution

● **Figure 8.2**
Preparing a 1% solution from a pure liquid drug.

Example 8.1

40 mL of an iodine solution contain 14 mL of pure iodine. Express the strength of this solution both as a ratio and a percentage.

The strength of a solution may be expressed as the ratio of the *amount of pure drug in the solution to the total amount of the solution*. The amount of the **solution is always expressed in milliliters,** and because **iodine is a liquid in pure form, the amount of iodine is also expressed in milliliters.**
There are 14 mL of pure iodine in the 40 mL of the solution, so the strength of this solution, expressed as a ratio, is fourteen to forty. The ratio may also be written as *14:40, 14 to 40*, or in fractional form as $\frac{14}{40}$. This fraction could then be simplified to $\frac{7}{20}$, which is equal to 35%.

So, the strength of this iodine solution may be expressed as the ratio 7:20 or the percentage 35%.

Pure Drugs in Dry Form

The ratio 1:20 means 1 part of the pure drug in 20 parts of solution, or 2 parts of the pure drug in 40 parts of solution, or 3 parts in 60, or 4 parts in 80, or 5 parts in 100, and so on. When a pure drug is in *dry* form, the ratio 1:20 means 1 g of pure drug in every 20 mL of solution. So 100 mL of a 1:20 potassium permanganate solution means *5 g* of pure potassium permanganate dissolved in water to make a total of *100 mL* of the solution. A 1:20 solution is the same as a 5% solution. If each tablet is 5 g, then you would prepare this solution by placing 1 tablet of the pure potassium permanganate in a graduated cylinder and adding some water to dissolve the tablet; then add more water until the level in the graduated cylinder reaches 100 mL.

Because a 5% potassium permanganate solution means 5 g of pure potassium permanganate in 100 mL of solution, the strength is written as $\dfrac{5\text{ g}}{100\text{ mL}}$ or $\dfrac{1\text{ g}}{20\text{ mL}}$. ●Figure 8.3.

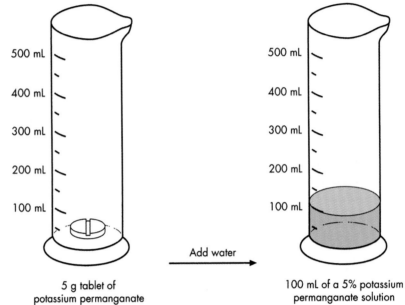

Add water

5 g tablet of potassium permanganate

100 mL of a 5% potassium permanganate solution

●**Figure 8.3**
Preparing a 5% solution from a pure, dry drug.

Example 8.2

One liter of an isotonic normal saline solution contains 9,000 mg of sodium chloride. Express the strength of this solution both as a ratio and as a percentage.

The strength of a solution may be expressed as the ratio of the *amount of pure drug* in the solution to the *total amount of the solution*. Since sodium chloride (NaCl) is a *solid* in pure form, the amount of NaCl (9,000 mg) must be expressed in *grams* (9 g). The *amount of the solution* (1 L) must always be expressed in *milliliters* (1,000 mL).

Since there are 9 g of pure NaCl in 1,000 mL of the solution, the strength of this solution, expressed as a ratio, is *nine to one thousand.*

This ratio may also be written as *9 to 1,000, 9:1,000,* or in fractional form as $\frac{9}{1,000}$. This fraction could be written in decimal form as 0.009, which is equal to 0.9%.
So, the strength of this isotonic normal saline solution may be expressed as the ratio *9:1,000* or the percentage *0.9%.*

Example 8.3

Read the label in ●**Figure 8.4** and verify that the two strengths stated on the label are equivalent.

The two strengths stated on this label are *2 mg/mL and 0.2%.* To show that they are equivalent, take either one of these strengths and show how to change it to the other. For example, if you start with 0.2%, you must change this to 2mg/mL.

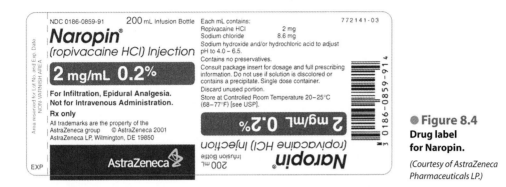

● **Figure 8.4**
Drug label for Naropin.

(Courtesy of AstraZeneca Pharmaceuticals LP.)

A solution whose strength is 0.2% has 0.2 g of pure drug (ropivacaine HCl) in 100 mL of solution. As a fraction, this is $\dfrac{0.2 \text{ g}}{100 \text{ mL}}$

You need to change this fraction to mg/mL. That is,

$$\frac{0.2 \text{ g}}{100 \text{ mL}} = \frac{? \text{ mg}}{\text{mL}}$$

To change the grams in the numerator to milligrams, use the equivalence 1 g = 1,000 mg.

$$\frac{0.2 \text{ g}}{100 \text{ mL}} \times \frac{1{,}000 \text{ mg}}{1 \text{ g}} = \frac{2 \text{ mg}}{\text{mL}}$$

So, the two strengths stated on the label, 2 mg/mL and 0.2%, are equivalent.

Determining the Amount of Pure Drug in a Given Amount of Solution

Dimensional analysis can be used to determine the amount of pure drug in a given amount of a solution of known strength. This is useful in preparing solutions from pure drugs.

The units of measurement for the amount of solution (volume), strength of the solution, and amount of pure drug are listed as follows:

Amount of solution: Use *milliliters*.

Strength: Always write as a fraction for calculations.

For liquids:

$$1{:}40 \text{ acetic acid solution is written as } \frac{1 \text{ mL}}{40 \text{ mL}}$$

$$5\% \text{ acetic acid solution is written as } \frac{5 \text{ mL}}{100 \text{ mL}}$$

For tablets or powder:

$$1{:}20 \text{ potassium permanganate solution is written as } \frac{1 \text{ g}}{20 \text{ mL}}$$

$$12\% \text{ potassium permanganate solution is written as } \frac{12 \text{ g}}{100 \text{ mL}}$$

Amount of pure drug:
>Use *milliliters* for liquids.
>Use *grams* for tablets or powders.

In order to prepare a given amount of a solution of a given strength, you must first determine the amount of pure drug that will be in that solution. The following examples illustrate how this is done.

Example 8.4

How would you prepare 500 mL of a 0.45% sodium chloride solution using 2.25 g sodium chloride tablets?

You need to determine the number of grams of pure sodium chloride needed for this solution.

Given: Amount of solution: 500 mL
            Strength: 0.45%
Find: Amount of pure drug: ? g

Convert the amount of solution (500 mL) to the amount of pure drug.

$$500 \text{ mL} = ? \text{ g}$$

Write the strength of the solution, 0.45%, as the unit fraction $\dfrac{0.45 \text{ g}}{100 \text{ mL}}$.

$$5\cancel{00} \text{ mL} \times \frac{0.45 \text{ g}}{1\cancel{00} \text{ mL}} = 2.25 \text{ g}$$

Since each tablet contains 2.25 g, you would need 1 tablet.
So, you would place 1 tablet into a graduated cylinder, add some water to dissolve the tablet, and then add water until the 500 mL level is reached.

Example 8.5

Read the label in ●**Figure 8.5**. How many grams of dextrose are contained in 30 mL of this solution?

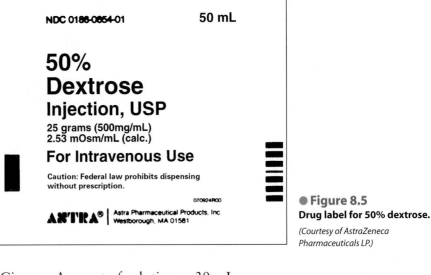

●Figure 8.5
Drug label for 50% dextrose.
(Courtesy of AstraZeneca Pharmaceuticals LP.)

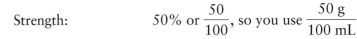

Given: Amount of solution: 30 mL

           Strength: 50% or $\dfrac{50}{100}$, so you use $\dfrac{50 \text{ g}}{100 \text{ mL}}$

Find: Amount of pure drug: ? g

$$30 \text{ mL} \times \frac{50 \text{ g}}{100 \text{ mL}} = ? \text{ g}$$

$$\cancel{30 \text{ mL}} \times \frac{50 \text{ g}}{\cancel{100 \text{ mL}}} = 15 \text{ g}$$

So, 15 g of dextrose are contained in 30 mL of a 50% dextrose solution.

Example 8.6

How would you prepare 2,000 mL of a 1:10 Clorox solution?

Given: Amount of solution: 2,000 mL

Strength: 1:10 or $\dfrac{1}{10}$

Find: Amount of pure drug: ? mL

Because Clorox is a liquid in its pure form, it is measured in milliliters. So, a 1:10 strength means that 1 mL of Clorox is in each 10 mL of the solution.

You want to convert the amount of the solution (2,000 mL) to the amount of the pure Clorox.

$$2,000 \text{ mL} = ? \text{ mL}$$

The preceding expression contains mL on both sides. This can be confusing! To make it clearer, note that on the left side "mL" refers to the volume of the **solution**, whereas on the right side "mL" refers to the volume of the pure **Clorox**.
So, you have the following:

$$2,000 \text{ mL (solution)} = ? \text{ mL (Clorox)}$$

The strength of the solution, 1:10, gives the unit fraction

$$\frac{1 \text{ mL (Clorox)}}{10 \text{ mL (solution)}}$$

$$2,000 \text{ \cancel{mL (solution)}} \times \frac{1 \text{ mL (Clorox)}}{10 \text{ \cancel{mL (solution)}}} = 200 \text{ mL (Clorox)}$$

So, you need 200 mL of Clorox to prepare 2,000 mL of a 1:10 solution. This means that 200 mL of Clorox is diluted with water to 2,000 mL of solution.

Example 8.7

How would you prepare 250 mL of a $\frac{1}{2}$% Lysol solution?

Given: Amount of solution: 250 mL

Strength: $\dfrac{1}{2}$%

Find: Amount of pure Lysol: ? mL

Since Lysol is a liquid in pure form, the amount of Lysol to be found is measured in milliliters.

$\frac{1}{2}\%$ can be written as 0.5% or as $\dfrac{0.5 \text{ mL (Lysol)}}{100 \text{ mL (solution)}}$

Convert the amount of the solution (250 mL) to the amount of Lysol.

$$250 \text{ mL (solution)} = ? \text{ mL (Lysol)}$$

Use the strength of the solution $\dfrac{0.5 \text{ mL (Lysol)}}{100 \text{ mL (solution)}}$ as the unit fraction.

$$250 \; \cancel{\text{mL (solution)}} \times \frac{0.5 \text{ mL (Lysol)}}{100 \; \cancel{\text{mL (solution)}}} = 1.25 \text{ mL (Lysol)}$$

So, you need 1.25 mL of Lysol to prepare 250 mL of a $\frac{1}{2}\%$ Lysol solution. This means that 1.25 mL of Lysol is diluted with water to 250 mL of solution.

Example 8.8

Read the label in ● **Figure 8.6** and determine the number of milligrams of Lidocaine that are contained in 5 mL of this Lidocaine solution.

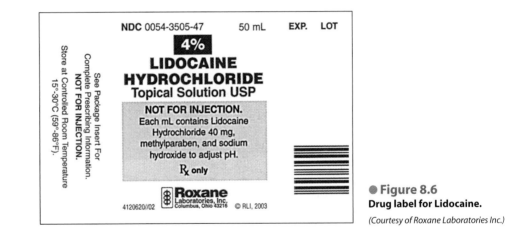

● **Figure 8.6**
Drug label for Lidocaine.

(Courtesy of Roxane Laboratories Inc.)

Given: Amount of solution: 5 mL
         Strength: 4%
Find: Amount of pure drug: ? mg

You want to convert the amount of the solution (5 mL) to the amount of the pure drug (? mg).

$$5 \text{ mL} = ? \text{ mg}$$

Note that Lidocaine is a powder in pure form, so the strength of the 4% solution is expressed in fraction form as $\dfrac{4 \text{ g}}{100 \text{ mL}}$.

This strength can be used to find the amount of Lidocaine in grams.

$$5 \; \cancel{\text{mL}} \times \frac{4 \, \text{\textcircled{g}}}{100 \; \cancel{\text{mL}}} = ? \text{ mg}$$

But you want the answer in milligrams, so the equivalence 1 g = 1,000 mg must also be used. This can be written in one line as follows:

$$5 \; \cancel{mL} \times \frac{4 \; \cancel{g}}{100 \; \cancel{mL}} \times \frac{1,000 \; mg}{\cancel{g}} = 200 \; mg$$

So, 200 milligrams of Lidocaine are contained in 5 milliliters of a 4% Lidocaine solution.

Determining the Amount of Solution That Contains a Given Amount of Pure Drug

In the previous examples, you were **given a volume of solution** of known strength and had to **find the amount of pure drug** in that solution. Now, the process will be reversed. In the following examples, Dimensional Analysis will be used when you will be **given an amount of the pure drug** in a solution of known strength and have to **find the volume of that solution**.

Example 8.9

How many milliliters of a 20% magnesium sulfate solution will contain 40 g of the pure drug magnesium sulfate?

You need to determine the number of milliliters of this solution, which contains 40 g of pure drug.

Given: Amount of pure drug: 40 g
         Strength: 20%
Find: Amount of solution: ? mL

You want to convert the 40 g of pure drug to milliliters of solution.

$$40 \; g = ? \; mL$$

You want to cancel the grams and obtain the equivalent amount in milliliters.

$$40 \; g \times \frac{? \; mL}{? \; g} = ? \; mL$$

In a 20% solution there are 20 g of magnesium sulfate per 100 mL of solution. So, the fraction is

$$\frac{100 \; mL}{20 \; g}$$

$$\overset{2}{\cancel{40}} \; \cancel{g} \times \frac{100 \; mL}{\underset{1}{\cancel{20}} \; \cancel{g}} = 200 \; mL$$

So, 200 mL of a 20% magnesium sulfate solution contains 40 g of magnesium sulfate.

Example 8.10

How many milliliters of a 1:40 acetic acid solution will contain 25 mL of acetic acid?

You need to determine the number of milliliters of this solution, which contains 25 mL of pure drug.

Given: Amount of pure drug: 25 mL (acid)
          Strength: 1:40
Find: Amount of solution: ? mL (solution)

You want to convert the 25 mL of pure acetic acid to milliliters of solution.

$$25 \text{ mL (acid)} = ? \text{ mL (solution)}$$

There may be some confusion in the meaning of the previous line because there are milliliters on both sides of the equal sign. To aid your understanding, the parentheses are included to indicate whether "mL" refers to the amount of pure drug or to the amount of solution.

You want to cancel the milliliters of pure drug and obtain the equivalent amount in milliliters of solution.

$$25 \text{ mL (acid)} \times \frac{? \text{ mL (solution)}}{? \text{ mL (acid)}} = ? \text{ mL (solution)}$$

In a 1:40 acetic acid solution there is 1 mL of pure acetic acid in 40 mL of solution. So, the fraction is

$$\frac{40 \text{ mL (solution)}}{1 \text{ mL (acid)}}$$

$$25 \, \cancel{\text{mL (acid)}} \times \frac{40 \text{ mL (solution)}}{1 \, \cancel{\text{mL (acid)}}} = 1{,}000 \text{ mL (solution)}$$

So, 1,000 mL of a *1:40* acetic acid solution contain 25 mL of acetic acid.

Example 8.11

How many milliliters of Zometa (●**Figure 8.7**) contain 10 mg of the pure drug?

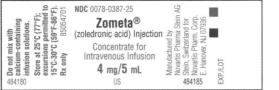

●**Figure 8.7**
Drug label for Zometa.

(Reproduced with the permission of Novartis Pharmaceuticals.)

You need to determine the number of milliliters of the solution, which contains 10 mg of the pure drug.

Given: Amount of pure drug: 10 mg
          Strength: 4 mg/5 mL
Find: Amount of solution: ? mL

You want to convert the amount of the pure drug (10 mg) to the amount of the solution (? mL).

$$10 \text{ mg} = ? \text{ mL}$$

Use the strength of the solution $\dfrac{4 \text{ mg}}{5 \text{ mL}}$ as the unit fraction. In this case, the milligrams need to cancel. So, the fraction must be inverted to have mg in the denominator.

$$10 \text{ mg} \times \frac{5 \text{ mL}}{4 \text{ mg}} = 12.5 \text{ mL}$$

So, 12.5 mL of the Zometa solution contain 10 mg of the pure drug.

Diluting Stock Solutions

A stock solution is one in which a pure drug is already dissolved in a liquid. The strength of each stock solution is written on the label. If the order is for a stronger solution, you will need to prepare a new solution. However, if the order is for a weaker solution, you can dilute the stock solution to the prescribed strength. To find out how much stock solution to take, use the following formula.

$$\frac{\text{Amount prescribed} \times \text{Strength prescribed}}{\text{Strength of stock}} = \text{Amount of stock}$$

Example 8.12

How would you prepare 1 L of a 25% solution from a 50% stock solution? Since this example does not indicate whether the drug in the solution is a solid or a liquid in its pure form, you may choose either *grams* or *milliliters* for the amount of the pure drug, and the choice will have no effect on the answer. *Grams* are chosen in the following solution.

Given: Amount prescribed: 1,000 mL

Strength prescribed: 25% or $\dfrac{25 \text{ g}}{100 \text{ mL}}$

Strength of stock: 50% or $\dfrac{50 \text{ g}}{100 \text{ mL}}$

Find: Amount of stock: ? mL

$$\frac{\text{Amount prescribed} \times \text{Strength prescribed}}{\text{Strength of stock}} = \text{Amount of stock}$$

Substituting the given information into the formula, you get

$$\frac{1,000 \text{ mL} \times \dfrac{25 \text{ g}}{100 \text{ mL}}}{\dfrac{50 \text{ g}}{100 \text{ mL}}} = ? \text{ mL}$$

This complex fraction may be written as a division problem as follows:

$$1,000 \text{ mL} \times \frac{25 \text{ g}}{100 \text{ mL}} \div \frac{50 \text{ g}}{100 \text{ mL}} = ? \text{ mL}$$

This division problem may be changed to a multiplication problem by inverting the last fraction. Now, cancel and multiply.

$$1,000 \text{ mL} \times \frac{25 \text{ g}}{100 \text{ mL}} \times \frac{100 \text{ mL}}{50 \text{ g}} = 500 \text{ mL}$$

So, you would take 500 mL of the 50% stock solution and add water to the level of 1,000 mL.

Example 8.13

How would you prepare 2,500 mL of a 1:10 boric acid solution from a 40% stock solution of this antiseptic?

Given: Amount prescribed: 2,500 mL

Strength prescribed: 1:10 or $\dfrac{1 \text{ mL}}{10 \text{ mL}}$

Strength of stock: 40% or $\dfrac{40 \text{ mL}}{100 \text{ mL}}$

Find: Amount of stock: ? mL

$$\dfrac{2{,}500 \text{ mL} \times \dfrac{1 \text{ mL}}{10 \text{ mL}}}{\dfrac{40 \text{ mL}}{100 \text{ mL}}} = \text{Amount of stock}$$

$$2{,}500 \text{ mL} \times \dfrac{1}{10} \div \dfrac{40}{100} = ? \text{ mL}$$

$$\overset{250}{2{,}500} \text{ mL} \times \dfrac{1}{\underset{1}{10}} \times \dfrac{100}{40} = 625 \text{ mL}$$

So, you would take 625 mL of the 40% stock solution of boric acid and add water to the level of 2,500 mL.

Example 8.14

How would you prepare 500 mL of a 1:25 solution from a 1:4 stock solution of the antiseptic Argyrol?

Given: Amount prescribed: 500 mL

Strength prescribed: 1:25 or $\dfrac{1 \text{ mL}}{25 \text{ mL}}$

Strength of stock: 1:4 or $\dfrac{1 \text{ mL}}{4 \text{ mL}}$

Find: Amount of stock: ? mL

$$\dfrac{500 \text{ mL} \times \dfrac{1 \text{ mL}}{25 \text{ mL}}}{\dfrac{1 \text{ mL}}{4 \text{ mL}}} = \text{Amount of stock}$$

$$500 \text{ mL} \times \dfrac{1}{25} \div \dfrac{1}{4} = ? \text{ mL}$$

$$\overset{20}{500} \text{ mL} \times \dfrac{1}{\underset{1}{25}} \times \dfrac{4}{1} = 80 \text{ mL}$$

So, you would take 80 mL of a 1:4 stock solution of Argyrol and add water to the level of 500 mL.

Summary

In this chapter, you learned that there are 3 quantities associated with a solution: the strength of the solution, the amount of pure drug dissolved in the solution, and the total volume of the solution. If any of 2 of these 3 quantities are known, the other quantity can be found.

- The strength of a solution may be expressed as a ratio or as a percentage.

- The strength of a solution is the ratio of the amount of pure drug dissolved in the solution to the total volume of the solution.

- The volume of the solution should be expressed in milliliters.

- The amount of pure drug dissolved in the solution should be expressed in milliliters if the drug, in its pure form, is a liquid.

- The amount of pure drug dissolved in the solution should be expressed in grams if the drug, in its pure form, is a solid.

- A $\frac{1}{2}$ strength solution is a 50% solution, and should not be confused with a $\frac{1}{2}$% solution.

- To determine the amount of drug in a given amount of solution of known strength, start with the given amount of solution.

- To determine the amount of solution of known strength containing a given amount of drug, start with the given amount of drug.

- To dilute a stock solution, use the following formula:

$$\frac{\text{Amount prescribed} \times \text{Strength prescribed}}{\text{Strength of stock}} = \text{Amount of stock}$$

Case Study 8.1

A 75-year-old female is admitted to a long-term care facility status post-mitral valve replacement. She has a past medical history of osteoarthritis; hypertension; atrial fibrillation; and insulin-dependent diabetes mellitus. Skin assessment reveals a 3 cm wound on the right heel. She is alert and oriented to person, place, time, and recent memory and she rates her pain level as 6 on a scale of 0–10. Vital signs are: T 98.7 °F; P 68; R 18; B/P 124/76.

Her orders are as follows:

- Persantine (dipyridamole) 75 mg PO, q.i.d.
- Cordarone (amiodarone hydrochloride) 400 mg PO daily; notify MD if P less than 60
- Cardizem SR(diltiazem) 180 mg PO daily
- Relafen (nabumetone) 1,000 mg PO daily
- KCL oral solution 20 mEq PO b.i.d.
- Multi-vitamin 1 tab PO daily
- Tylenol 650 mg PO q4h prn T above 101
- Humulin R insulin 10 units and Humulin N insulin 38 units subcutaneous 30 minutes ac breakfast
- Humulin R insulin 10 units and Humulin N insulin 30 units 30 minutes ac dinner
- Pneumovax 0.5 mL IM x 1 dose
- Cleanse right heel with NS solution (0.9% NaCl) and apply a DSD daily
- 1,800 calorie ADA 2 g sodium diet

Refer to the labels in ● **Figure 8.8** when necessary to answer the following questions:

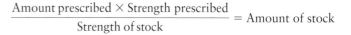

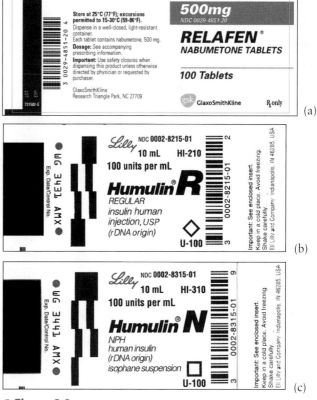

● **Figure 8.8**

Drug labels for Case Study 8.1.

(08-08a Reproduced with permission of GlaxoSmithKline.   08-08b Copyright Eli Lilly and Company. Used with permission.   08-08c Copyright Eli Lilly and Company. Used with permission.)

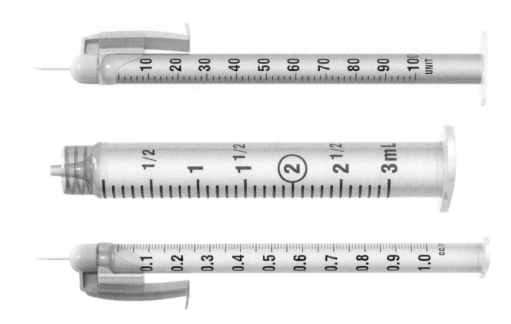

1. The Pneumovax vial contains 2.5 mL. Choose the appropriate syringe from those above and place an arrow at the dose.

2. Cardizem SR is available in 60 mg, and 120 mg tablets. Which strength will you use and how many tablets for the daily dose?

3. The KCL solution label reads 40 mEq/15 mL. How many milliliters will you administer?

4. The dipyridamole is available in 25, 50, and 75 mg tablets. Which strength tablets will you administer and how many?

5. How many tablets of nabumetone will you administer?

6. Describe how you will measure the morning insulin. Select the appropriate syringe from those below and mark the dose of Humulin R and Humulin N.

7. How many grams of sodium chloride (NaCl) are in 1 liter of the saline solution?

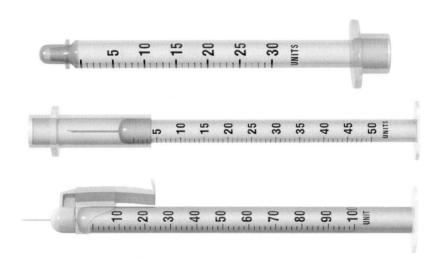

Practice Sets

The answers to *Try These for Practice*, *Exercises*, and *Cumulative Review* appear in Appendix A at the end of the book. Ask your instructor for answers to the *Additional Exercises*.

Try These for Practice

Test your comprehension after reading the chapter.

1. 320 mL of a solution contain 80 mg of a pure drug. Express the strength of this solution as a percent. _____

2. How would you prepare 1 liter of a 10% solution from tablets each containing 5 grams of the pure drug? _____

3. How many milliliters of a 25% potassium permanganate solution contains 20 grams of potassium permanganate? _____

4. How would you prepare 200 mL of a 5% solution from a 20% stock solution? _____

5. Read the label in ● **Figure 8.9** and show how you would determine that two of the strengths mentioned on the label are equivalent (use 500 mcg/2 mL and 0.25 mg/mL). _____

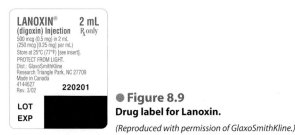

● **Figure 8.9**
Drug label for Lanoxin.

(Reproduced with permission of GlaxoSmithKline.)

Exercises

Reinforce your understanding in class or at home.

1. 750 mL of a solution contain 15 mL of a pure drug. Express the strength of this solution both as a ratio and as a percentage.

2. Two liters of a solution contain 60 g of a pure drug. Express the strength of this solution both as a ratio and as a percentage.

3. How would you prepare 300 mL of a 0.9% sodium chloride solution using sodium chloride crystals?

4. Read the label in ● **Figure 8.10** and determine the number of milligrams of hydroxyzine pamoate that are contained in the vial of Vistaril.

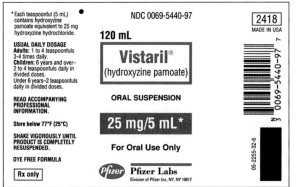

● **Figure 8.10**
Drug label for Vistaril.

(Reg. Trademark of Pfizer Inc. Reproduced with permission.)

5. How many milliliters of Vistaril (see Figure 8.10) contain 20 mg of hydroxyzine pamoate?

6. How would you prepare 400 mL of a 50% solution from a drug that in its pure form is a liquid?

7. How many milliliters of a 6% solution contain 18 g of the pure drug?

8. Read the label in ● **Figure 8.11**. How many milliliters of this Xylocaine solution contain 300 mg of lidocaine HCl?

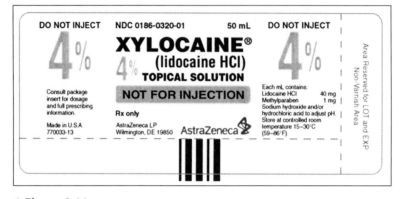

● **Figure 8.11**
Drug label for Xylocaine.
(Courtesy of AstraZeneca Pharmaceuticals LP.)

9. Read the label in ● **Figure 8.12** and verify that the two strengths stated on the Xylocaine label are equivalent.

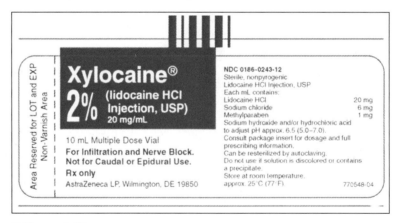

● **Figure 8.12**
Drug label for Xylocaine.
(Courtesy of AstraZeneca Pharmaceuticals LP.)

10. How would you prepare 500 mL of a 1:4 solution from a 1:3 stock solution?

11. How would you prepare 1 L of a 0.45% solution from a 0.9% stock solution?

12. If 600 mL of a solution contain 120 mL of a pure drug, express the strength of this solution both as a ratio and as a percentage.

13. If 1 L of a solution contains 2,000 mL of a pure drug, express the strength of this solution both as a ratio and as a percentage.

14. How would you prepare 800 mL of a 10% solution using tablets each containing 20 g?

15. Read the label in ● **Figure 8.13** and determine how many milligrams of metoprolol tartrate are contained in 12 mL of Lopressor.

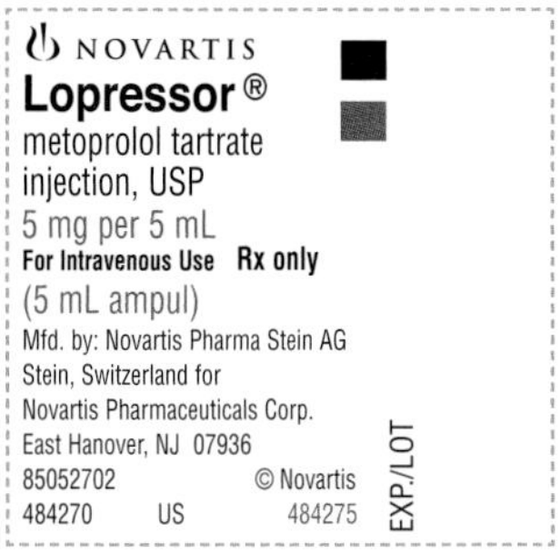

● **Figure 8.13**
Drug label for Lopressor.

(Reproduced with the permission of Novartis Pharmaceuticals)

16. Read the label in Figure 8.13 and determine the number of milliliters of Lopressor that would contain 35 mg of pure metoprolol tartrate.

17. How would you prepare 1,200 mL of a 25% solution from a pure drug in solid form?

18. A drug label states the strength of the solution is 10 mg/mL or 1%. Verify that the two stated strengths are equivalent.

19. How would you prepare 200 mL of a 25% solution from a 35% stock solution?

20. How would you prepare 2 L of a 1:5 solution from a $\frac{1}{2}$ strength stock solution?

Additional Exercises

Now, test yourself!

1. Prepare 2 L of a 1:50 solution of Lysol from a 100% solution.

2. Describe how you would prepare 500 mL of 0.5% Dakin's solution from a 10% solution.

3. Prepare 250 mL of a 3% hydrogen peroxide solution from a 15% solution.

4. Describe how you would prepare 240 mL of a $\frac{1}{2}$ strength solution of Ensure from pure drug Ensure (100%).

5. How many grams of amino acids are contained in 500 mL of an 8.5% amino acid solution?

6. A patient is receiving 250 mL of a 10% Intralipid solution. How many grams of lipids will this patient receive?

_____

7. How many milliliters of a 20% solution of glucose will contain 50 g of a drug?

_____

8. Physician's order:

   Magnesium sulfate 2 g in 10 mL D$_5$W IV push in 10 minutes

   The label on the vial reads 50% magnesium sulfate. How many milliliters will you prepare?

_____

9. A patient has an order for 200 mL of a 2% lidocaine solution. How many milligrams of lidocaine are contained in this order?

_____

10. A patient receives 4 mL of 1% lidocaine as a nerve block. How many grams of lidocaine did the patient receive?

_____

11. Describe how you would prepare 100 mL of 0.9% NaCl from sodium chloride crystals.

_____

12. How many grams of dextrose are contained in 4,000 mL of a 25% dextrose solution?

_____

13. Prepare 240 mL of a $\frac{1}{3}$ solution of Ensure from a can labeled 100% Ensure. Explain how you would do this.

_____

14. Describe how you would prepare 500 mL of a 0.25% solution from a 5% stock solution.

_____

15. Use the information on the label in ● **Figure 8.14** to determine the number of grams of calcium chloride in 2 mL of this solution.

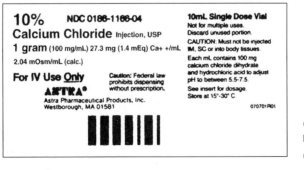

● **Figure 8.14**
Drug label for calcium chloride.
(Courtesy of AstraZeneca Pharmaceuticals LP.)

16. Read the label in ● **Figure 8.15**. Determine how many milliliters of this solution will contain 0.001 g of Epinephrine.

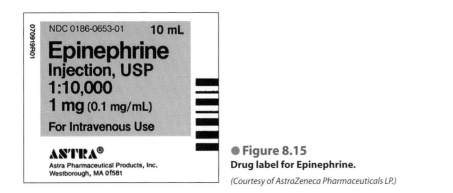

● **Figure 8.15**
Drug label for Epinephrine.
(Courtesy of AstraZeneca Pharmaceuticals LP.)

17. Read the label in ● **Figure 8.16**. How many grams of Mannitol are contained in 25 mL of this solution?

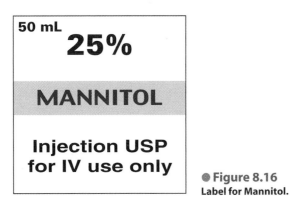

● **Figure 8.16**
Label for Mannitol.

18. How many milliliters of a 1:30 acetic acid solution will contain 20 g of acetic acid?

19. A client must have a foot soak. Prepare 4,000 mL of a 4% solution of potassium permanganate solution from 5 g tablets.

20. Describe how you would prepare 3,500 mL of a 1:1,000 aluminum acetate solution, an antiseptic, from 0.5 g tablets.

Cumulative Review Exercises

Review your mastery of earlier chapters.

1. Read the information on the label in ● **Figure 8.17** and calculate the amount of dextrose in 25 mL.

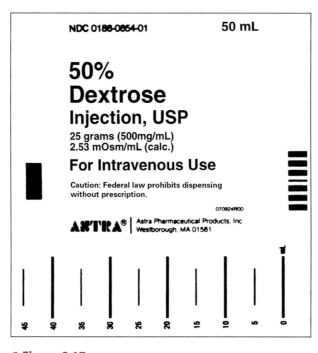

● **Figure 8.17**
Drug label for 50% dextrose.
(Courtesy of AstraZeneca Pharmaceuticals LP.)

2. Physician's order:

> Add 0.06 g of a drug to 1,000 mL of D$_5$W.

Each vial of the drug is labeled 4 mL = 4 mg. How many milliliters of the drug will you add to the D$_5$W?

3. Your patient has an order for a tube feeding of 200 mL of $\frac{3}{4}$ strength Isocal, a nutritional supplement. Each can contains 200 mL of Isocal. How many milliliters of H$_2$O and how many milliliters of Isocal will you need to make a $\frac{3}{4}$ strength solution? (Hint: $\frac{3}{4}$ strength means 75% solution.)

4. gr $\dfrac{1}{120}$ = _____ mg   5. 2 glasses = _____ ounces

6. 0.06 mg = gr _____   7. 0.0006 g = _____ mg

8. 100 mg = gr _____   9. 5 ft 6 in = _____ in

10. The order reads atropine sulfate 0.4 mg sc stat. How many grams will you administer?

11. The order is digoxin 0.25 mg PO q.i.d. Convert this dose to micrograms.

12. You have 2 mL of Epinephrine 1:10,000. How many milligrams of Epinephrine are contained in this solution?

13. A physician orders 0.6 g of a drug PO b.i.d. for three days. How many grams of the drug will the patient receive in three days?

14. The antianxiety drug Tranxene (clorazepate) 15 mg PO at bedtime has been prescribed for a patient. The label reads 7.5 mg per tablet. How many tablets will you give your patient?

15. The order is 600 mg of a drug PO b.i.d. The label reads 0.2 g in 5 mL. How many milliliters will you give your patient?

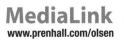

www.prenhall.com/olsen   Animated examples, interactive practice questions with animated solutions, and challenge tests for this chapter can be found on the Prentice Hall Dosage Calculation Tutor that accompanies this text. Additional, unique, interactive resources and activities can be found on the Companion Website.

Parenteral Medications

Learning Outcomes

After completing this chapter, you will be able to

1. Calculate doses for parenteral medications in liquid form.
2. Describe how to reconstitute medications in powder form.
3. Calculate doses of parenteral medications measured in units.

This chapter introduces you to the calculations you will use to prepare and administer parenteral medications safely. Chapter 2 discussed the most common parenteral sites: intramuscular (IM), subcutaneous (subcut), intravenous (IV), intradermal (ID), and intracardiac (IC). This chapter will focus on calculations for administering medications via the subcutaneous and intramuscular routes.

Parenteral Medications

Parenteral medications are those that are injected into the body by various routes. Drugs for parenteral medications may be packaged in a variety of forms, including ampules, vials, and prefilled cartridges or syringes. Prefilled cartridges and syringes were discussed in Chapter 7.

An *ampule* is a glass container that holds a single dose of medication. It has a narrowed neck that is designed to snap open. The medication is aspirated into a syringe by gently pulling back on the plunger, which creates a negative pressure and allows the liquid to be pulled into the syringe (●**Figure 9.1**).

A *vial* is a glass or plastic container that has a rubber stopper on the top. This stopper is covered with a lid that maintains the sterility of the stopper until the vial is used for the first time. Multidose vials contain more than one dose of a medication. Single-dose vials contain a single dose of medication, and many drugs are now prepared in this format to reduce the chance of error. The medication in a vial may be in liquid or powdered form (●**Figure 9.2**).

●**Figure 9.1**
Ampules.

> **NOTE**
>
> Single-dose ampules and vials may contain a little more drug than indicated on the label. Therefore, if the order is for the exact amount of medication stated on the label, it is very important to carefully measure the amount of medication to be withdrawn. Before a fluid can be extracted from a vial, that same volume of air or diluent must be injected into the vial.

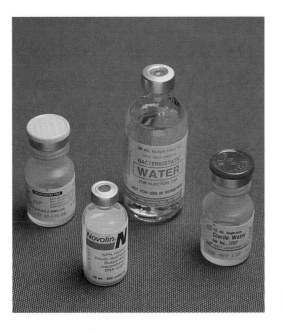

●**Figure 9.2**
Vials.

Parenteral Medications Supplied as Liquids

When parenteral medications are in liquid form, you must calculate the volume of the solution that contains the prescribed amount of the medication. You also need to know the strength of the solution. You will use dimensional analysis to calculate the volume that will be administered.

Example 9.1

The prescriber ordered *Dilaudid-HP (hydromorphone hydrochloride) 4 mg IM q4h prn*. Read the label in ●**Figure 9.3** and calculate how many milliliters of this narcotic analgesic you will administer.

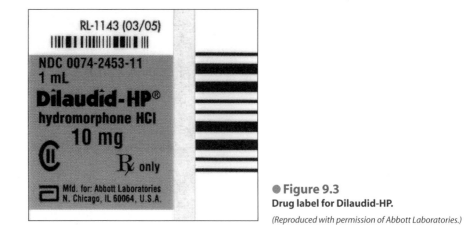

● **Figure 9.3**
Drug label for Dilaudid-HP.

(Reproduced with permission of Abbott Laboratories.)

Begin by determining how many milliliters of the solution in the vial contain the prescribed quantity of the medication prescribed. That is, you want to convert 4 mg to an equivalent in milliliters.

$$4 \text{ mg} = ? \text{ mL}$$

You cancel the milligrams and obtain the equivalent quantity in milliliters.

$$4 \text{ mg} \times \frac{? \text{ mL}}{? \text{ mg}} = ? \text{ mL}$$

The label indicates that there are 10 mg per milliliter, which means that the strength of the solution is 10 mg/1 mL.

So, the unit fraction is $\dfrac{1 \text{ mL}}{10 \text{ mg}}$

$$4 \text{ mg} \times \frac{1 \text{ mL}}{10 \text{ mg}} = 0.4 \text{ mL}$$

So, you would administer 0.4 mL to the patient.

Example 9.2

The prescriber ordered *quinidine gluconate 600 mg IM stat and 400 mg IM q4h prn*. Read the label in ● **Figure 9.4** and calculate the number of milliliters of this antiarrhythmic drug you will administer to the patient immediately.

● **Figure 9.4**
Drug label for quinidine gluconate.

(Copyright Eli Lilly and Company. Used with permission.)

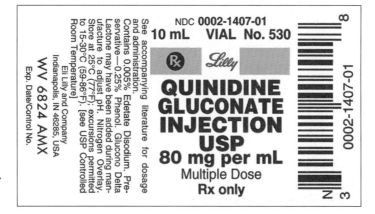

Begin by determining how many milliliters of the liquid in the vial contain the prescribed quantity of the medication (600 mg of quinidine gluconate—the question asks for the stat dose!). That is, you want to convert 600 mg to an equivalent in milliliters.

$$600 \text{ mg} = ? \text{ mL}$$

You cancel the milligrams and obtain the equivalent quantity in milliliters.

$$600 \text{ mg} \times \frac{? \text{ mL}}{? \text{ mg}} = ? \text{ mL}$$

The label reads 80 mg per milliliter, which means the solution strength is 80 mg/1 mL.

So, the unit fraction is $\dfrac{1 \text{ mL}}{80 \text{ mg}}$

$$600 \text{ mg} \times \frac{1 \text{ mL}}{80 \text{ mg}} = \frac{60 \text{ mL}}{8} = 7.5 \text{ mL}$$

So, you would administer 7.5 mL to the patient.

Example 9.3

The prescriber ordered *Compazine (prochlorperazine) 7 mg IM q4h prn*. Read the label in ●**Figure 9.5** and calculate how many milliliters of this antiemetic you will administer to the patient.

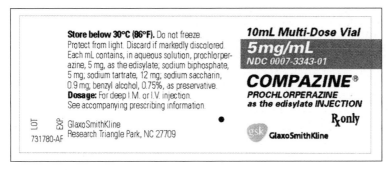

Store below 30°C (86°F). Do not freeze. Protect from light. Discard if markedly discolored. Each mL contains, in aqueous solution, prochlorperazine, 5 mg, as the edisylate; sodium biphosphate, 5 mg; sodium tartrate, 12 mg; sodium saccharin, 0.9 mg; benzyl alcohol, 0.75%, as preservative. **Dosage:** For deep I.M. or I.V. injection. See accompanying prescribing information.

GlaxoSmithKline
Research Triangle Park, NC 27709
LOT EXP
731780-AF

10mL Multi-Dose Vial
5mg/mL
NDC 0007-3343-01
COMPAZINE®
PROCHLORPERAZINE
as the edisylate INJECTION
℞only
gsk **GlaxoSmithKline**

●**Figure 9.5**
Drug label for Compazine.
(Reproduced with permission of GlaxoSmithKline.)

Begin by determining how many milliliters of the liquid in the vial contain the prescribed quantity of the medication. That is, you want to convert 7 mg to an equivalent in milliliters.

$$7 \text{ mg} = ? \text{ mL}$$

You cancel the milligrams and obtain the equivalent quantity in milliliters.

$$7 \text{ mg} \times \frac{? \text{ mL}}{? \text{ mg}} = ? \text{ mL}$$

The label reads 5 milligrams per milliliter.

So, the unit fraction is $\dfrac{1 \text{ mL}}{5 \text{ mg}}$

$$7 \text{ mg} \times \frac{1 \text{ mL}}{5 \text{ mg}} = 1.4 \text{ mL}$$

So, you would administer 1.4 mL to the patient.

Example 9.4

The prescriber ordered *Lanoxin (digoxin) 600 mcg IV push stat*. Read the label in ● **Figure 9.6** and determine how many milliliters of this anti-arrythmic cardiac glycoside you will prepare.

Begin by determining how many milliliters of the solution in the vial contain the prescribed quantity of the medication. That is, you want to convert 600 mcg to an equivalent in milliliters.

$$600 \text{ mcg} = ? \text{ mL}$$

You cancel the micrograms and obtain the equivalent quantity in milliliters.

$$600 \text{ mcg} \times \frac{? \text{ mL}}{? \text{ mcg}} = ? \text{ mL}$$

The label indicates that there are 250 mcg per milliliter.

So, the unit fraction is $\dfrac{1 \text{ mL}}{250 \text{ mcg}}$

$$\overset{12}{\cancel{600}} \text{ mcg} \times \frac{1 \text{ mL}}{\underset{5}{\cancel{250}} \text{ mcg}} = \frac{12 \text{ mL}}{5} = 2.4 \text{ mL}$$

So, you would give the patient 2.4 mL.

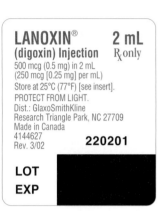

● **Figure 9.6**
Drug label for Lanoxin.

(Reproduced with permission of GlaxoSmithKline.)

LANOXIN®   **2 mL**
(digoxin) Injection   ℞only
500 mcg (0.5 mg) in 2 mL
(250 mcg [0.25 mg] per mL)
Store at 25°C (77°F) [see insert].
PROTECT FROM LIGHT.
Dist.: GlaxoSmithKline
Research Triangle Park, NC 27709
Made in Canada
4144627
Rev. 3/02   **220201**

LOT
EXP

Example 9.5

The prescriber ordered *Tigan (trimethobenzamide hydrochloride) 200 mg IM stat*. You have a 20 mL multidose vial, and the label indicates that the strength is 100 mg/mL. How many milliliters of this antiemetic drug will you prepare?

Begin by determining how many milliliters of the solution in the vial contain the prescribed quantity of the medication. That is, you want to convert 200 mg to an equivalent in milliliters.

$$200 \text{ mg} = ? \text{ mL}$$

You cancel the milligrams and obtain the equivalent quantity in milliliters.

$$200 \text{ mg} \times \frac{? \text{ mL}}{? \text{ mg}} = ? \text{ mL}$$

The label indicates that there are 100 mg per milliliter.

So, the unit fraction is $\dfrac{1 \text{ mL}}{100 \text{ mg}}$

$$200 \text{ mg} \times \frac{1 \text{ mL}}{100 \text{ mg}} = 2 \text{ mL}$$

So, you would give the patient 2 mL.

Parenteral Medications Supplied in Powdered Form

Some parenteral medications are unstable when stored in liquid form, so they are packaged in powdered form. Before they can be administered, the powder in the vial must be diluted with a liquid (*diluent*). This process is referred to as *reconstitution*.

Sterile water and 0.9% sodium chloride (normal saline) are the most commonly used *diluents*. Both the type and amount of diluent to be used must be determined when reconstituting parenteral medications. This information is found on the medication label or package insert. Because many reconstituted parenteral medications can be administered intramuscularly or intravenously, it is essential to verify the route ordered **before** reconstituting the medication.

Drugs dissolve completely in the diluent. Some drugs do not add any volume to the amount of diluent added, while other drugs increase the amount of total volume. This increase in volume is called the *displacement factor*. For example, directions for a 1 g powdered medication may state to add 2 mL of diluent to provide an approximate volume of 2.5 mL. When the 2 mL of diluent is added, the 1 g of powdered drug displaces an additional 0.5 mL for a total volume of 2.5 mL. The available strength after reconstitution is 400 mg/mL. If there are no directions for reconstitution on the label or package insert, consult appropriate resources such as the PDR or the pharmacist.

Some medications are manufactured in a vial that contains a single dose of medication in which the vial has two compartments, separated by a rubber stopper. The top portion contains a sterile liquid (diluent), and the bottom portion contains the medication in powder form. When pressure is applied to the top of the vial, the rubber stopper that separates the medication and diluent is released. This allows the diluent and powder to mix. ●Figure 9.7.

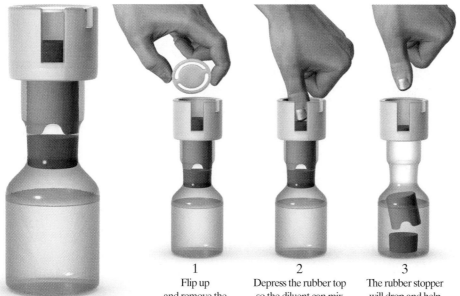

How to use a Mix-O Vial

1
Flip up and remove the protective cover.

2
Depress the rubber top so the diluent can mix into the chamber.

3
The rubber stopper will drop and help mix the drug.

● **Figure 9.7**
How to prepare a mix-o-vial.

NOTE

The label states that when 2.5 mL of diluent is added, the resulting solution has an approximate volume of 3 mL yielding a strength of 330 mg/mL. This is due to the displacement factor of 0.5 mL, which adds 0.5 mL to the total volume.

Example 9.6

The prescriber ordered *Kefzol 265 mg IM q8h*. The directions on the label state: "For IM use, add 2.5 mL of sterile water for injection and shake well. The resulting solution has an approximate volume of 3 mL yielding a strength of 330 mg/mL." Describe how you would prepare this cephalosporin antibiotic. How many milliliters will you administer to the patient?

To prepare the solution, inject 2.5 mL of air into a vial of sterile water for injection and withdraw 2.5 mL of sterile water. Then add the 2.5 mL of sterile water to the Kefzol 1 g vial and shake well. ●**Figure 9.8**.

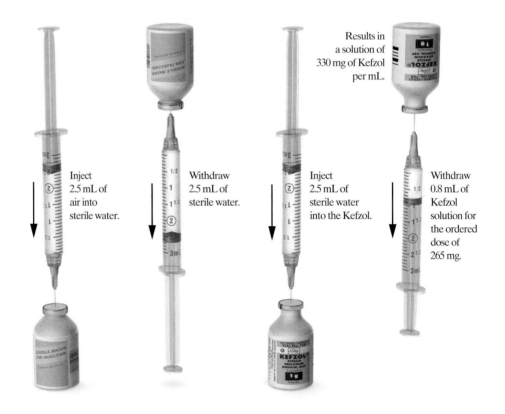

Inject 2.5 mL of air into sterile water.

Withdraw 2.5 mL of sterile water.

Inject 2.5 mL of sterile water into the Kefzol.

Results in a solution of 330 mg of Kefzol per mL.

Withdraw 0.8 mL of Kefzol solution for the ordered dose of 265 mg.

●**Figure 9.8**
Reconstitution of Kefzol.

Now the vial contains a reconstituted solution in which 1 mL = 330 mg

To calculate the number of milliliters to administer the prescribed dose, you need to convert 265 mg to milliliters.

$$265 \text{ mg} \times \frac{? \text{ mL}}{? \text{ mg}} = ? \text{ mL}$$

The vial contains 330 mg per 1 mL, so the unit fraction is $\dfrac{1 \text{ mL}}{330 \text{ mg}}$

$$265 \text{ mg} \times \frac{1 \text{ mL}}{330 \text{ mg}} = 0.803 \text{ mL}$$

So, you would withdraw 0.8 mL (265 mg) from the vial and administer it to the patient.

Example 9.7

The prescriber ordered *Cefotan (cefotetan disodium) 1,500 mg IM q12h*. Read the drug label and portion of the package insert for Cefotan in ●**Figure 9.9** and determine how many milliliters of this cephalosporin antibiotic you would give the patient.

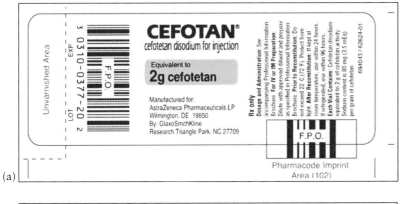

(a)

Vial Size	Amount of Diluent Added (mL)	Approximate Withdrawable Vol (mL)	Approximate Average Concentration (mg/mL)
1 gram	2	2.5	400
2 gram	3	4	500

(b)

●**Figure 9.9**
Drug label and portion of package insert for Cefotan.

(Courtesy of AstraZeneca Pharmaceuticals LP.)

First, prepare the solution. Since the vial contains 2 g, inject 3 mL of air into a vial of sterile water for injection and withdraw 3 mL of sterile water. Add the 3 mL of sterile water to the Cefotan 2 g vial and shake well.

Now the vial contains a solution in which 1 mL = 500 mg

To calculate the amount of this solution, you need to convert the milligrams prescribed to milliliters.

$$1,500 \text{ mg} \times \frac{? \text{ mL}}{? \text{ mg}} = ? \text{ mL}$$

The vial contains 500 mg per 1 mL, so the unit fraction is $\frac{1 \text{ mL}}{500 \text{ mg}}$

$$\overset{3}{\cancel{1,500}} \text{ mg} \times \frac{1 \text{ mL}}{\underset{1}{\cancel{500}} \text{ mg}} = 3 \text{ mL}$$

So, you would withdraw 3 mL and administer it to the patient.

Example 9.8

A prescriber ordered *Pfizerpen (penicillin potassium) 200,000 units IM stat and q6h*. Read the label in ●**Figure 9.10** and calculate how many milliliters of this penicillin antibiotic you will administer to the patient for the stat dose.

● **Figure 9.10**
Drug label for Pfizerpen.

(Reg. Trademark of Pfizer Inc. Reproduced with permission.)

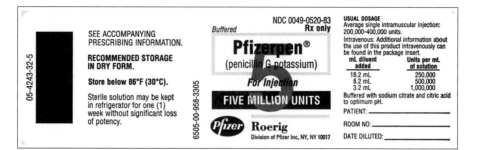

First, reconstitute the solution. The label lists three options: 250,000 units/mL, 500,000 units/mL, and 1,000,000 units/mL. In this example, choose the first option. So 18.2 mL of diluent must be added to obtain a dosage strength of 250,000 units.

Second, inject 18.2 mL of air into a vial of sterile water for injection and then withdraw 18.2 mL of sterile water. Add the sterile water to the Pfizerpen vial and shake well. Now the vial contains a solution in which 1 mL = 250,000 units

To calculate the amount of this solution to be administered, you need to convert units to milliliters.

$$250,000 \text{ units} \times \frac{? \text{ mL}}{? \text{ units}} = ? \text{ mL}$$

The vial contains 250,000 units per 1 milliliter, so the unit fraction is

$$\frac{1 \text{ mL}}{250,000 \text{ units}}$$

$$200{,}000 \text{ units} \times \frac{1 \text{ mL}}{250{,}000 \text{ units}} = \frac{20 \text{ mL}}{25} = 0.8 \text{ mL}$$

So, you would withdraw 0.8 mL from the vial and administer it to the patient.

Example 9.9

The prescriber ordered *Solu-Medrol (methylprednisolone sodium succinate) 200 mg IM q6h.* You have a mix-o-vial of Solu-Medrol 500 mg. The directions on the label state: "Each 4 mL when mixed contains methylprednisolone sodium succinate equivalent to 500 mg methylprednisolone (125 mg per mL)." How many milliliters will you administer?

First, reconstitute the solution. Depress the rubber stopper and allow the diluent into the bottom chamber of the vial and be sure that the powder is dissolved. See Figure 9.7.

Now the vial contains a solution in which 1 mL = 125 mg

To calculate the amount of this solution to be administered, you need to convert mg to milliliters.

$$200 \text{ mg} \times \frac{? \text{ mL}}{? \text{ mg}} = ? \text{ mL}$$

The vial contains 125 mg per 1 mL, so the unit fraction is $\dfrac{1 \text{ mL}}{125 \text{ mg}}$

$$\overset{8}{200} \text{ mg} \times \frac{1 \text{ mL}}{\underset{5}{125} \text{ mg}} = 1.6 \text{ mL}$$

So, you would administer 1.6 mL of Solu-Medrol.

Heparin

Heparin sodium is a potent anticoagulant that inhibits clot formation and blood coagulation. Heparin can be administered subcutaneously or intravenously.

Like insulin, penicillin, and some other medications, heparin is supplied and ordered in units. Heparin is available in single and multidose vials, as well as in commercially prepared IV solutions. Heparin is *never given intramuscularly because of the danger of hematomas*. Heparin is available in a variety of strengths, ranging from 10 units/mL to 40,000 units/mL. Heparin is also available in prepackaged syringes. Lovenox (enoxaprin) and Fragmin (dalteparin sodium) are examples of low molecular weight heparin. They are used to prevent and treat deep vein thrombosis (DVT) following abdominal surgery, hip or knee replacement, unstable angina, or acute coronary syndromes.

Heparin requires close monitoring of the patient's blood work because of the bleeding potential associated with anticoagulant drugs. In order to assure the accuracy of dose measurement, a 1 mL (tuberculin) syringe should be used to administer heparin. Healthcare providers should know and follow agency policies when administering heparin.

ALERT

Heparin flush solutions (for example, Hep-Lock or HepFlush) are used for maintaining the patency of indwelling intravenous catheters. They are available in 10 units/mL and 100 units/mL. Heparin for injection and heparin lock-flush solutions are different drugs and can never be used interchangeably.

Example 9.10

The prescriber ordered *heparin 2,000 units subcutaneously q12h*. The label on the multidose vial reads 5,000 units/mL. How many milliliters will you administer to the patient?

You want to convert units to milliliters.

$$2,000 \text{ units} = ? \text{ mL}$$

You cancel the units and obtain the equivalent amount in milliliters.

$$2,000 \text{ units} \times \frac{? \text{ mL}}{? \text{ units}} = ? \text{ mL}$$

The label on the vial states: "5,000 units per milliliter," so the unit fraction is

$$\frac{1 \text{ mL}}{5,000 \text{ units}}$$

$$2,\cancel{000} \text{ units} \times \frac{1 \text{ mL}}{5,\cancel{000} \text{ units}} = \frac{2 \text{ mL}}{5} = 0.4 \text{ mL}$$

So, you would administer 0.4 mL of heparin to the patient.

Example 9.11

The prescriber ordered *Heparin 2,000 units subcutaneously q12h*. The label on the multidose vial reads 10,000 units/mL. How many milliliters will you administer to the patient?

You want to convert units to milliliters.

$$2,000 \text{ units} = ? \text{ mL}$$

You cancel the units and obtain the equivalent amount in milliliters.

$$2,000 \text{ units} \times \frac{? \text{ mL}}{? \text{ units}} = ? \text{ mL}$$

NOTE

Observe that in examples 9.10 and 9.11 the order for heparin are exactly the same (2,000 units subcutaneously q12h). However, the available dosage strengths are different. In example 9.10 the strength is twice the strength of that in example 9.11. Therefore, only half the amount of solution is needed. The importance of carefully reading the label must always be considered to determine the correct dose.

The label on the vial states: "10,000 units per milliliter," so the unit fraction is $\dfrac{1\ mL}{10{,}000\ units}$

$$2{,}000\ \cancel{units} \times \frac{1\ mL}{10{,}000\ \cancel{units}} = \frac{2}{10} = 0.2\ mL$$

So, you would administer 0.2 mL of heparin to the patient.

Example 9.12

The prescriber ordered *Fragmin (dalteparin sodium) 120 units/kg subcutaneously q12h* for a patient who weighs 92 pounds. See ●**Figure 9.11** and determine how many milliliters of this low molecular weight heparin you will need to administer the dose.

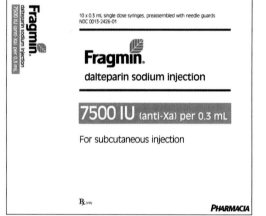

●**Figure 9.11**
Box label for Fragmin single-dose syringes.

Since this example contains a lot of information, it is useful to summarize it as follows:

Given: 92 lb (single unit of measurement)

Known equivalences: 1 kg = 2.2 lb (needed to convert lb to kg)

                       120 units/kg (order)

                       7,500 units/0.3 mL (strength on the drug label)

Volume you want to find: ? mL

You want to convert a single unit of measurement (92 lb) to another single unit of measurement (mL).

$$92\ lb = ?\ mL$$

You want to cancel lb. To do this you must use a unit fraction containing lb in the denominator. Using the equivalence 1 kg = 2.2 lb, this fraction will be $\dfrac{1\ kg}{2.2\ lb}$

$$92\ \cancel{lb} \times \frac{1\ \textcircled{kg}}{2.2\ \cancel{lb}} = ?\ mL$$

Now, on the left side kg is in the numerator. To cancel the kg will require a unit fraction with kg in the denominator, namely, $\dfrac{120\ units}{kg}$

$$92\ \cancel{lb} \times \frac{1\ \cancel{kg}}{2.2\ \cancel{lb}} \times \frac{120\ \textcircled{units}}{kg} = ?\ mL$$

Now, on the left side units is in the numerator. To cancel the units will require a fraction with units in the denominator, namely, $\dfrac{0.3 \text{ mL}}{7{,}500 \text{ units}}$

$$92 \text{ lb} \times \frac{1 \text{ kg}}{2.2 \text{ lb}} \times \frac{120 \text{ units}}{\text{kg}} \times \frac{0.3 \text{ mL}}{7500 \text{ units}} = ? \text{ mL}$$

Only mL remains on the left side. This is what you want. Now multiply the numbers

$$92 \text{ lb} \times \frac{\text{kg}}{2.2 \text{ lb}} \times \frac{120 \text{ units}}{\text{kg}} \times \frac{0.3 \text{ mL}}{7{,}500 \text{ units}} = 0.2007 \text{ mL}$$

Therefore, you would need 0.2 mL.

Summary

In this chapter, you learned how to calculate doses for administering parenteral medications in liquid form, the procedure for reconstituting medications in powdered form, and how to calculate dosages for medications supplied in units.

- Medications supplied in powdered form must be reconstituted following the manufacturer's directions.

- You must determine the best dosage strength for medications ordered when there are several options for reconstituting the medication.

- Label the medication vial with the date, time, and dosage strength after reconstituting a multiple-dose vial.

- When directions on the label are for IM and IV reconstitution, be sure to read the label carefully to determine the necessary amount of diluent to use.

- Heparin is measured in USP units.

- It is especially important that heparin orders be carefully checked with the available dosage strength before calculating the amount to be administered.

- A tuberculin (1 mL) syringe should be used when administering heparin.

- Heparin sodium and heparin flush solutions are different and should never be used interchangeably.

Case Study 9.1

A 64-year-old man is referred by his physician to the hospital for an emergency appendectomy following a CAT scan. The patient reports a past medical history of hypertension, hypercholesterolemia, and BPH (benign prostatic hypertrophy). He is 6 feet tall and weighs 150 lb, has no known drug or food allergies, and is to be transported to the operating room following his admission lab work and physical exam. His vital signs are: T 98.4 °F; B/P 130/86; P 96; R 18.

Pre-op orders:

- NPO
- CBC, serum electrolytes, type and screen

- IV RL @ 125 mL/h
- morphine 2 mg IVP stat
- Transfer to OR

Post-op orders:

- NPO, progress to clear liquids as tolerated
- IV D5/NS @ 125 mL/h
- V/S q4h
- Flagyl (metronidazole) 7.5 mg/kg IVPB q6h
- Avelox (moxifloxacin) 400 mg IV daily for 5 days
- Lopressor (metoprolol) 5 mg IVP q4h, hold for SBP below 110 or HR below 60
- heparin 5,000 units subcutaneously q12h

- Toradol (ketorolac tromethamine) 30 mg IM q6h prn moderate pain

- Percocet 1 tab PO q4h prn pain

- Ambien (zolpidem) 5 mg PO before bedtime

- Avodart (dutasteride) 0.5 mg PO every other day

- Norvasc (amlodipine) 10 mg PO daily

- Vasotec (enalapril maleate) 5 mg PO daily

- Lipitor (atorvastatin calcium) 20 mg PO every day

Refer to the labels in ● **Figure 9.12** when necessary to answer the following questions.

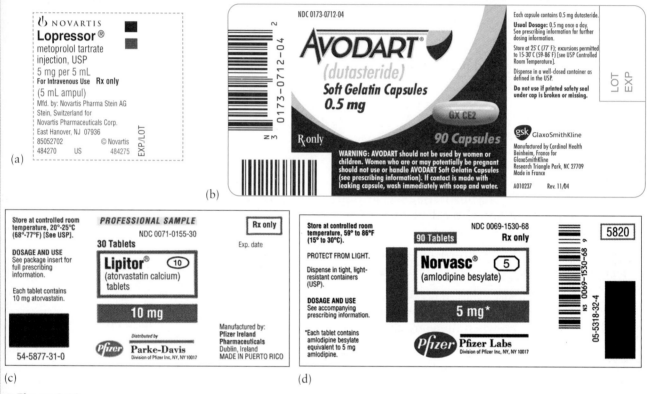

(a)   (b)   (c)   (d)

● **Figure 9.12**

Drug labels for Case Study 9.1.

(09-12a Reproduced with the permission of Novartis Pharmaceuticals.   09-12b Reproduced with permission of GlaxoSmithKline.
09-12c Reg. Trademark of Pfizer Inc. Reproduced with permission.   09-12d Reg. Trademark of Pfizer Inc. Reproduced with permission.)

1. The morphine is supplied in vials labeled 5 mg/mL.
   (a) How many milliliters are needed for the prescribed dose?
   (b) What type of syringe will you use to administer the dose?

2. The heparin vial is labeled 20,000 units/mL.
   (a) How many milliliters will you prepare?
   (b) What type of syringe will you use to administer the dose?

3. How many milliliters are needed to prepare the IV dose of the metoprolol if the label reads 1 mg/mL?

4. What is the number of milligrams of Flagyl to be administered?

5. The Toradol vial is labeled 30 mg/mL. What is the maximum number of milliliters of Toradol that the patient may receive in 24 hours?

6. Avelox is supplied in premixed, ready-to-infuse IV bags of 400 mg in 250 mL. How many milliliters will the patient have received in five days?

7. How many capsules of dutasteride will you administer for each dose?

8. How many tablets of amlodipine will you administer each day?

9. The Vasotec is supplied in 2.5 mg, 5 mg, 10 mg, and 20 mg tablets.
   (a) Which dosage strength will you use?
   (b) How many tablets will you administer?

10. How many tablets of atorvastatin will you administer?

Practice Sets

The answers to *Try These for Practice*, *Exercises* and *Cumulative Review Exercises* appear in Appendix A at the end of the book. Ask your instructor for answers to the *Additional Exercises*.

Try These for Practice

Test your comprehension after reading the chapter.

1. Order:

   Ancef (cefazolin) 750 mg IM q8h for 24 hours.

   The directions on the 1 g vial of Ancef state: "For IM administration add 2.5 mL of sterile water and shake to provide an approximate volume of 3 mL."
   (a) How many milliliters will you administer? _____
   (b) What size syringe will you use? _____

2. Order:

   Librium (chlordiazepoxide hydrochloride) 75 mg IM stat.

   The directions on the 100 mg vial state: "Reconstitute with the 2 mL of special diluent included to provide an approximate volume of 2 mL."
   (a) How many milliliters will you administer? _____
   (b) What size syringe will you use? _____

3. Order:

   Ativan (lorazepam) 0.05 mg/kg IM two hours before surgery.

   The patient weighs 135 pounds, and the label on the 10 mL multidose vial reads: "2 mg per 2 mL."
   (a) How many milligrams will you prepare? _____
   (b) How many milliliters will you administer? _____

4. Order:

   Heparin 8,000 units subcutaneously q12h.

   The vial is labeled 10,000 units/mL.
   (a) How many milliliters will you administer? _____
   (b) What size syringe will you use? _____

5. Order:

   Pipracil (piperacillin sodium) 2 g IM stat with probenecid 1 g PO 30 minutes before giving the Pipracil.

   The package insert for the 2 g Pipracil vial states: "Add 4 mL of diluent to yield 1 g/2.5 mL." The label on the probenecid bottle reads: "0.5 g tablet."
   (a) How many tablets of probenecid will you administer? _____
   (b) How many milliliters of Pipracil contain the prescribed dose? _____

Exercises

Reinforce your understanding in class or at home.

1. The prescriber ordered *ampicillin 750 mg IM q6h*.
   The directions for the 1 g Pipracil vial state, "reconstitute with 3.5 mL of diluent to yield 250 mg/mL." How many milliliters will contain the prescribed dose?

2. The prescriber ordered *Unasyn 1.5 g IM q6h*.
   The package insert for the label in ● **Figure 9.13** states: Add 3.2 mL of sterile water for injection to yield 375 mg/mL (250 mg ampicillin and 125 mg sulbactam/mL). Calculate how many milliliters you will administer.

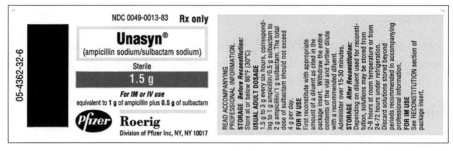

● **Figure 9.13**
Drug label for Unasyn.   *(Reg. Trademark of Pfizer Inc. Reproduced with permission.)*

3. The prescriber ordered *Aranesp 0.49 mcg/kg subcutaneously once per week* for a patient who weighs 155 pounds.
   (a) Read the label in ● **Figure 9.14** and calculate how many milliliters you will administer.
   (b) What size syringe will you use to administer the dose?

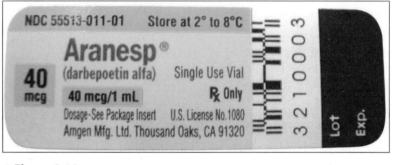

● **Figure 9.14**
Drug label for Aranesp.   *(Published with permission of Amgen Inc.)*

4. The prescriber ordered *Claforan (cefotaxime) 1,200 mg IM q12h*. The directions for the 1 g vial state: "Add 3.2 mL of diluent to yield an approximate concentration of 300 mg/mL. The directions for the 2 g vial state: Add 5 mL of diluent to yield an approximate concentration of 330 mg/mL."
   (a) Which vial will you use?
   (b) How many milliliters will you administer?

5. The prescriber ordered *streptomycin 500 mg IM q12h for 7 days*. Read the label in ● **Figure 9.15** and calculate how many milliliters of this antibiotic you will administer.

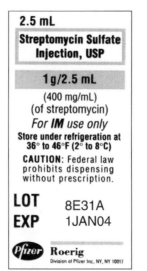

● **Figure 9.15**
Drug label for streptomycin.

(Reg. Trademark of Pfizer Inc. Reproduced with permission.)

6. The prescriber ordered *Stelazine (trifluoperazine hydrochloride) 1.4 mg IM (give deep IM) q6h prn.* The label on the 10 mL multidose vial reads 2 mg/mL injection.
   (a) Calculate the number of milliliters that contain this dose.
   (b) What size syringe will you use?

7. The prescriber ordered *Enbrel (etanercept) 50 mg subcutaneously once a week.* Read the label in ● **Figure 9.16** and calculate how many vials you will use.

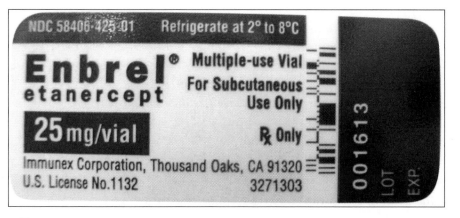

● **Figure 9.16**
Drug label for Enbrel.   *(Published with permission of Amgen Inc.)*

8. The prescriber ordered *Epogen (epoetin alfa) 6,000 units subcutaneously three times a week.* Use the label in ● **Figure 9.17** and do the following:
   (a) Calculate how many milliliters contain this dose.
   (b) Determine what size syringe you will use to administer this medication.

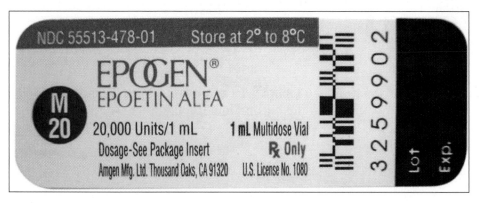

● **Figure 9.17**
Drug label for Epogen.   *(Published with permission of Amgen Inc.)*

9. The prescriber ordered *gentamicin 60 mg IM q12h.* The drug is supplied in a 20 mL multidose vial. The label reads 40 mg/mL. How many milliliters will you administer?

10. The prescriber ordered *morphine sulfate 5 mg subcutaneously q4h prn.* The drug is supplied in a 1 mL vial that is labeled 15 mg/mL.
    (a) How many milliliters will you administer?
    (b) What size syringe will you use?

11. The prescriber ordered *Lasix (furosemide) 30 mg IM stat.* The drug is supplied in a vial labeled 40 mg/mL. How many milliliters will you administer?

12. A patient is to receive *Ativan (lorazepam) 3 mg IM, 2 hours before surgery.* The drug is supplied in a vial labeled 4 mg/mL. How many milliliters will you administer?

13. Use the insulin "sliding scale" below to determine how much insulin you will give to a patient whose blood glucose is 320.

    Order: Give Humulin R Unit-100 insulin subcutaneously for blood glucose levels as follows:

    Glucose less than 160-no insulin
    Glucose 160–220-2 units
    Glucose 221–280-4 units
    Glucose 281–340-6 units
    Glucose 341–400-8 units
    Glucose more than 400-hold insulin and call MD stat

14. The prescriber ordered *heparin 3,500 units subcutaneously q12h.* The label on the vial states 5,000 units/mL.
    (a) How many milliliters will you administer?
    (b) What size syringe will you use?

15. The prescriber ordered *Humulin N 25 units subcutaneously ac breakfast.*

    Use the label in ●**Figure 9.18** to determine the following:
    (a) How many units will you administer?
    (b) What size syringe will you use?

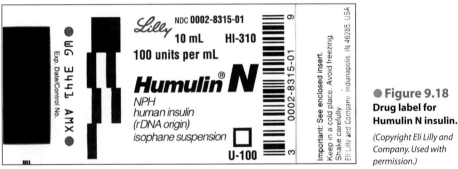

●**Figure 9.18**
Drug label for Humulin N insulin.

(Copyright Eli Lilly and Company. Used with permission.)

16. Read the information in ●**Figure 9.19** and use the highest concentration to determine how many milliliters contain 650,000 units.

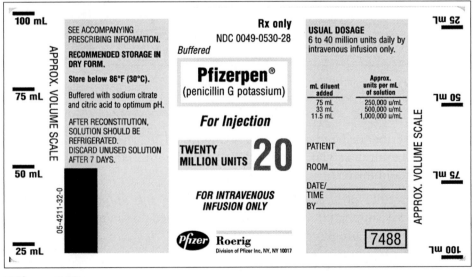

●**Figure 9.19**
Drug label for Pfizerpen.   *(Reg. Trademark of Pfizer Inc. Reproduced with permission.)*

17. A patient is to receive *atropine sulfate 0.2 mg IM 30 minutes before surgery*, The vial is labeled 0.4 mg/mL.
    (a) How many milliliters will you administer?
    (b) What size syringe will you use?

18. The order is *Phenergan (promethazine hydrochloride) 12.5 mg IM q4h prn nausea.* The vial is labeled 50 mg/mL.
    (a) How many milliliters will you administer?
    (b) What size syringe will you use?

19. The order is *Thorazine (chlorpromazine hydrochloride) 40 mg IM q6h prn for agitation.* The vial is labeled 25 mg/mL.
    (a) How many milliliters will you administer?
    (b) What size syringe will you use?

20. Use the information in ● **Figure 9.20** and answer the following:
    (a) How much diluent must be added to the vial to prepare a 250,000 units/mL strength?
    (b) How much diluent must be added to the vial to prepare a 500,000 units/mL strength?
    (c) What is the total dose of this vial?
    (d) The order is *penicillin G 2,000,000 units IM stat.* How will you prepare this dose?

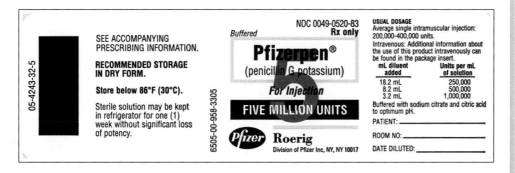

● **Figure 9.20**
Drug label for Pfizerpen.   *(Reg. Trademark of Pfizer Inc. Reproduced with permission.)*

Additional Exercises

Now, test yourself!

1. The prescriber ordered *Brethine (terbutaline sulfate) 0.25 mg subcutaneous stat.* The vial is labeled 1 mg/mL.
   (a) How many milliliters will you administer? _____
   (b) What size syringe will you use? _____

2. Order: *streptomycin 500 mg IM daily for 8 days.* Read the label in ● **Figure 9.21** and calculate how many vials of this antibiotic you would need for your patient over the seven days. _____

3. You need to give 700 mg of a drug IM, and the label reads 250 mg/mL.
   (a) How many milliliters will you need? _____
   (b) What size syringe will you use? _____

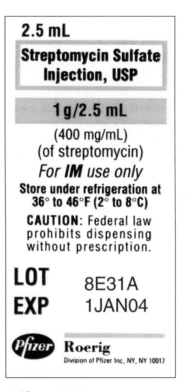

2.5 mL

**Streptomycin Sulfate
Injection, USP**

1 g/2.5 mL

(400 mg/mL)
(of streptomycin)
For IM use only
Store under refrigeration at
36° to 46°F (2° to 8°C)
CAUTION: Federal law
prohibits dispensing
without prescription.

LOT   8E31A
EXP   1JAN04

Pfizer **Roerig**
Division of Pfizer Inc, NY, NY 10017

● **Figure 9.21**
Drug label for streptomycin.

(Reg. Trademark of Pfizer Inc. Reproduced with permission.)

4. A patient is to receive *Inapsine (droperidol) 2.5 mg IM 30 minutes before surgery.* The label reads 5 mg/2 mL.
   (a) How many milliliters will you need? _____
   (b) What size syringe will you use? _____

5. The prescriber ordered *Bactocill (oxacillin sodium) 400 mg IM q4h.*
   The package insert for the 1 g vial states: "Add 5.7 mL of sterile water for injection. Each 1.5 mL contains 250 mg oxacillin."
   (a) How many milliliters will you need? _____
   (b) What size syringe will you use? _____

6. Order: *Claforan (cefotaxime sodium) 750 mg IM q8h.*
   The directions in the package insert for the 1 g vial state: "For IM administration add 3 mL of diluent, approximate withdrawable volume 3.4 mL, approximate concentration 300 mg/mL."
   (a) How many milliliters will you administer? _____
   (b) What size syringe will you use? _____

7. Order: *Lovenox (enoxaprin sodium) 30 mg subcutaneous q12h.*
   The label on the 0.4 mL prefilled syringe reads 40 mg/0.4 mL. How much solution should be discarded to administer the prescribed dose?

   _____

8. Order: *Dilaudid-HP (hydromorphone HCl) 3 mg subcutaneous q4 h prn pain.*
   Read the label in ● **Figure 9.22** and calculate how many milliliters you will administer.

   _____

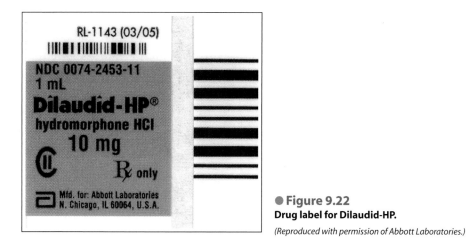

● **Figure 9.22**
Drug label for Dilaudid-HP.

(Reproduced with permission of Abbott Laboratories.)

9. The prescriber ordered *Rocephine (ceftriaxone) 250 mg IM stat.*
The package insert states that when "1.8 mL of diluent is added to a 500 mg vial, 1 mL of solution contains approximately 250 mg of ceftriaxone." How many milliliters will contain the prescribed dose?

_____

10. The prescriber ordered *Energix-B (hepatitis B vaccine) 20 mcg IM stat.* The multidose vial label reads "25 adult doses 20 mcg/mL." How many milliliters will you administer?

_____

11. A patient is to receive *Loxitane (loxapine HCl) 30 mg IM q6h.*
The label reads 50 mg/mL. How many milliliters should the patient receive?

_____

12. The prescriber ordered *Vitamin B (thiamine HCl) 50 mg IM t.i.d.*
The label reads 100 mg/mL. How many milliliters will you administer?

_____

13. Read the label in ● **Figure 9.23**. If you add 45 mL of diluent to the 10 g vial, how many milliliters contain 500 mg?

_____

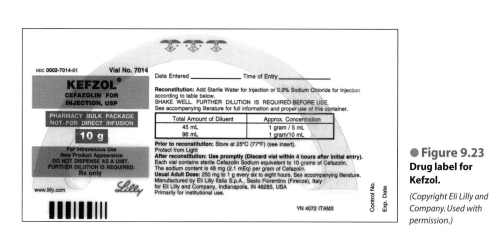

● **Figure 9.23**
Drug label for Kefzol.

(Copyright Eli Lilly and Company. Used with permission.)

14. The prescriber ordered *Demerol (meperidine HCl) 75 mg IM q4h prn pain.* The vial is labeled 100 mg/mL. How many milliliters will you administer?

_____

15. The prescriber ordered *Tigan (trimethobenzamide HCl) 200 mg IM t.i.d. for vomiting.*

    The label on the 20 mL multidose vial reads 100 mg/mL. How many milliliters contain the dose?

    _____

16. Order: *Cogentin (benztropine mesylate) 1 mg IM now.*

    The label on the 2 mL ampule reads 1 mg/mL. How many milliliters is the patient receiving?

    _____

17. The prescriber ordered *cyanocobalamin 30 mcg daily for 5 days, then 200 mcg per month.*

    The label on the vial states 1,000 mcg/mL. How many milliliters contain the daily dose?

    _____

18. Order: *Pentam (pentamidine isethionate) 3 mg/kg IM q.i.d.*

    The label reads: Add 3 mL of sterile water to each 300 mg vial. Calculate how many milliliters you will administer to the patient who weighs 90 pounds.

    _____

19. Order: *Bicillin L-A (penicillin G benzathine) 1.2 million units IM q4 weeks.*

    The label vial reads 2,400,000 units/4 mL. Calculate the number of milliliters you will administer.

    _____

20. Order: *Methergine (methylergonovine maleate) 0.2 mg IM q4h for three doses.*

    The drug label reads 0.2 mg/mL.

    (a) How many milliliters will you administer per dose? _____

    (b) What is the total number of milligrams the patient will receive for the three doses?

    _____

Cumulative Review Exercises

Review your mastery of earlier chapters.

Read the label in ● **Figure 9.24** to answer questions 1 through 4.

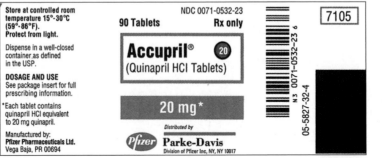

● **Figure 9.24**
Drug label for Accupril.

(Reg. Trademark of Pfizer Inc. Reproduced with permission.)

1. What is the generic name of this drug? _____

2. What is the route of administration? _____

3. What is the name of the manufacturer? _____

4. A patient is to receive 80 mg q12h. How many tablets will he receive every 24 hours? _____

5. The prescriber ordered *Antivert (meclazine HCl) 25 mg PO daily prn vertigo.* Read the label in ●**Figure 9.25** and calculate how many tablets you will administer.

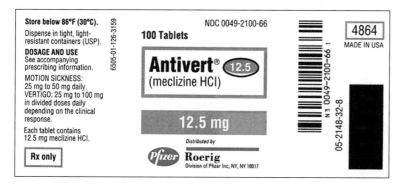

●**Figure 9.25**
Drug label for Antivert.

(Reg. Trademark of Pfizer Inc. Reproduced with permission.)

Read the label in ●**Figure 9.26** to answer questions 6 through 9.

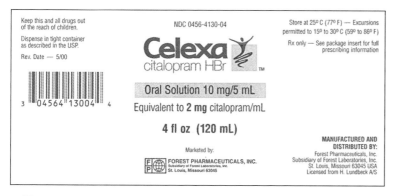

●**Figure 9.26**
Drug label for Celexa.

(Courtesy of Forest Pharmaceuticals, Inc.)

6. What is the trade name of the drug? _____

7. What is the strength of the drug? _____

8. A patient is to receive 20 mg PO daily. How many milliliters will you administer? _____

9. A patient is to receive 20 mg PO daily. How many doses of medication will this container supply? _____

10. The prescriber ordered *Mycobutin (rifabutin) 300 mg PO b.i.d.*
    Read the label in ● **Figure 9.27** and calculate the number of capsules the patient will receive.

R only
Usual Dosage: Two capsules in a single daily administration. For additional prescribing information read package insert.

Dispense in a tight container as defined in the USP.

Keep tightly closed.

Store at 25°C (77°F); excursions permitted to 15°-30°C (59°-86°F) [see USP Controlled Room Temperature].

Each capsule contains: rifabutin, USP 150 mg.

LOT   EXP

NDC 0013-5301-17

Mycobutin.
rifabutin capsules, USP

150 mg

100 Capsules   **PHARMACIA**

N
3   0013-5301-17   2

MADE IN ITALY
Manufactured for:
Pharmacia & Upjohn Company
A subsidiary of Pharmacia Corporation
Kalamazoo, MI 49001, USA

by: Pharmacia Italia S.p.A.
Ascoli Piceno, Italy
819 076 000   100002067 00

● **Figure 9.27**
Drug label for Mycobutin.

11. The label on a reconstituted medication states that the strength is 500,000 units/mL. How many milliliters equal 200,000 units? _____

12. Convert 0.003 g to mg. _____

13. A patient had a clear liquid dinner consisting of 4 oz of apple juice, 8 oz of chicken broth, and 6 oz of hot tea. Calculate the total intake in mL.

14. 89 kg = _____ lb   15.   2.5 L = _____ mL

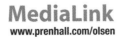

MediaLink
www.prenhall.com/olsen

Animated examples, interactive practice questions with animated solutions, and challenge tests for this chapter can be found on the Prentice Hall Dosage Calculation Tutor that accompanies this text. Additional, unique, interactive resources and activities can be found on the Companion Website.

Unit

Infusions and Pediatric Dosages

Chapter 10

Calculating Flow Rates and Durations of Enteral and Intravenous Infusions

Chapter 11

Calculating Flow Rates for Intravenous Medications

Chapter 12

Calculating Pediatric Dosages

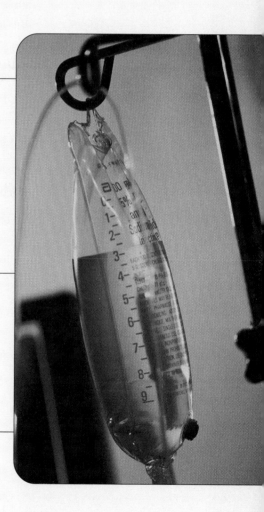

Calculating Flow Rates and Durations of Enteral and Intravenous Infusions

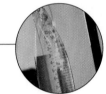

Learning Outcomes

After completing this chapter, you will be able to

1. Describe the basic concepts and standard equipment involved in administering enteral and intravenous (IV) infusions.
2. Calculate the flow rates of enteral and IV infusions.
3. Calculate the durations of enteral and IV infusions.

This chapter introduces the basic concepts and standard equipment involved in intravenous and enteral therapy. You will also learn how to use Dimensional Analysis to calculate flow rates for these infusions and to determine how long it will take for a given amount of solution to infuse (its duration).

Introduction to Intravenous and Enteral Solutions

Fluids can be given to a patient slowly over a period of time through a vein (*intravenous*) or through a tube inserted into the alimentary tract (*enteral*). The rate at which these fluids flow into the patient is very important and must be controlled precisely.

Enteral Feedings

When a patient cannot ingest food or if the upper gastrointestinal tract is not functioning properly, the prescriber may write an order for an *enteral* feeding (*"tube feeding"*). Enteral feedings provide nutrients and other fluids by way of a tube inserted directly into the gastrointestinal system (alimentary tract).

There are various types of tube feedings. A gastric tube may be inserted into the stomach through the nares (**nasogastric**, as shown in ● **Figure 10.1**) or through the mouth (**orogastric**). A longer tube may be similarly inserted, but would extend beyond the stomach into the upper small intestine, jejunum (**nasojejunum** or **orojejunum**).

For long-term feedings, tubes can be inserted surgically or laproscopically through the wall of the abdomen and directly into either the stomach (gastrostomy) or through the stomach and on to the jejunum (jejunostomy). These tubes are sutured in place and are referred to as *percutaneous endoscopic gastrostomy (PEG) tubes* and *percutaneous endoscopic jejunostomy (PEJ) tubes, respectively* (● **Figure 10.2**).

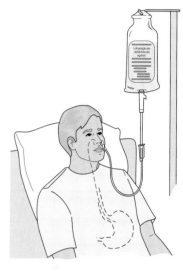

● **Figure 10.1**
A patient with a nasogastric tube.

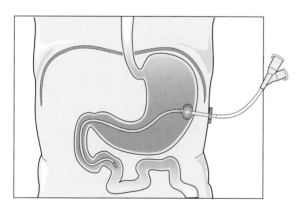

● **Figure 10.2**
A *percutaneous endoscopic jejunostomy (PEJ)* tube.

Enteral feedings may be given *continuously* (over a 24-hour period) or *intermittently* (over shorter periods, perhaps several times a day). There are many enteral feeding solutions, including Boost, Compleat, Ensure, Isocal, Resource, and Sustacal. Enteral feedings are generally administered via pump. ● **Figure 10.3**.

Orders for enteral solutions always indicate a volume of fluid to be infused over a period of time; that is, a flow rate. For example, a tube feeding order might read *Isocal 50 mL/h via nasogastric tube for 6 hours beginning 6 A.M.* This order is for an intermittent feeding in which the name of the solution is Isocal, the rate of flow is 50 mL/h, the route of administration is via nasogastric tube, and the duration is 6 hours.

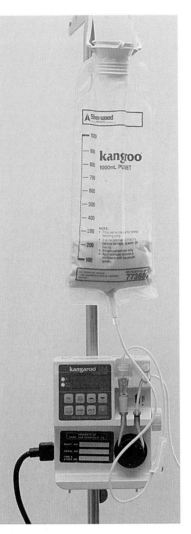

● **Figure 10.3**
Enteral feeding via pump.

(Photographer; Elena Dorfman)

Intravenous Infusions

Intravenous (IV) means *through the veins.* Fluids are administered intravenously to provide a variety of fluids, including blood, water containing nutrients, electrolytes, minerals, and specific medications to the patient. IV fluids can replace lost fluids, maintain fluid and electrolyte balance, or serve as a medium to introduce medications directly into the bloodstream.

Replacement fluids are ordered for a patient who has lost fluids through hemorrhage, vomiting, or diarrhea. *Maintenance fluids* help sustain normal levels of fluids and electrolytes. They are ordered for patients who are at risk of becoming depleted; for example, patients who are NPO (nothing by mouth).

Intravenous infusions may be *continuous* or *intermittent.* Continuous IV infusions are used to replace or maintain fluids or electrolytes. Intermittent IV infusions—for example, IV piggyback (IVPB) and IV push (IVP)—are used to administer drugs and supplemental fluids. *Intermittent peripheral infusion devices* (saline locks or heparin locks) are used to maintain venous access without continuous fluid infusion. Intermittent IV infusions are discussed in Chapter 11.

A healthcare professional must be able to perform the calculations to determine the correct rate at which an enteral or intravenous solution will enter the body (*flow rate*). Infusion flow rates are usually measured in drops per minute (gtt/min) or milliliters per hour (mL/h). It is important to be able to convert each of these rates to the other and to determine how long a given amount of solution will take to infuse.

For example, an IV order might read *IV fluids: D5W 125 mL/h for 8h.* In this case, the order is for an IV infusion in which the name of the solution is 5% dextrose in water, the rate of flow is 125 mL/h, the route of administration is intravenous, and the duration is 8 hours.

Intravenous Solutions

A **saline solution,** which is a solution of *sodium chloride (NaCl)* in sterile water, is commonly used for intravenous infusion. Sodium chloride is ordinary table salt. Saline solutions are available in various concentrations for different purposes. A 0.9% NaCl solution is referred to as **normal saline (NS).** Other saline solutions commonly used include **half-normal saline** (0.45% NaCl), written as $\frac{1}{2}$ NS; and **quarter-normal saline** (0.225% NaCl), written as $\frac{1}{4}$ NS.

Intravenous fluids generally contain dextrose, sodium chloride, and/or electrolytes:

- D5W, D5/W, or 5% D/W is a 5% dextrose solution, which means that 5 g of dextrose are dissolved in water to make each 100 mL of this solution. ● **Figures 10.4a** and **10.4b.**

- NS or 0.9% NaCl is a solution in which each 100 mL contain 0.9 g of sodium chloride. ● **Figures 10.4c** and **10.4d.**

- 5% D/0.45% NaCl is a solution containing 5 g of dextrose and 0.45 g of NaCl in each 100 mL of solution ● **Figure 10.5b.**

- Ringer's lactate (RL), also called lactated Ringer's solution (LRS), is a solution containing electrolytes. ● **Figure 10.5c.**

Additional information on IV fluids can be found in nursing and pharmacology textbooks.

NOTE

Pay close attention to IV abbreviations. *Letters* indicate the solution compounds, whereas *numbers* indicate the solution strength.

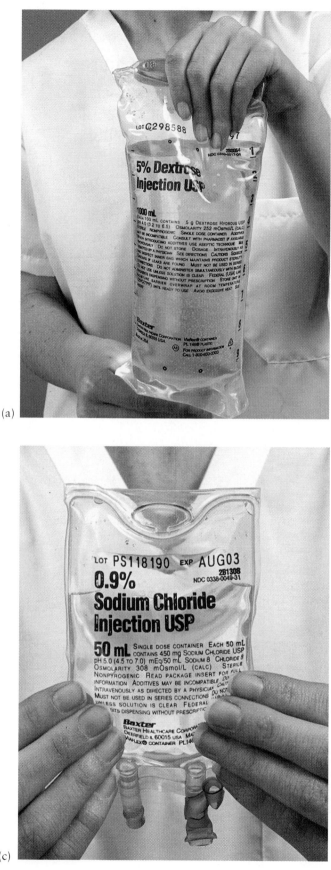

LOT   **EXP**

NDC 0338-0017-04

1

5% Dextrose
Injection USP

2

3

1000 mL
EACH 100 mL CONTAINS   5 g DEXTROSE HYDROUS USP
pH 4.0 (3.2 TO 6.5)   OSMOLARITY 252 mOsmol/L (CALC)
STERILE   NONPYROGENIC   SINGLE DOSE CONTAINER   ADDITIVES
MAY BE INCOMPATIBLE   CONSULT WITH PHARMACIST IF AVAILABLE
WHEN INTRODUCING ADDITIVES USE ASEPTIC TECHNIQUE   MIX
THOROUGHLY   DO NOT STORE   DOSAGE   INTRAVENOUSLY AS
DIRECTED BY A PHYSICIAN   SEE DIRECTIONS   CAUTIONS   SQUEEZE
AND INSPECT INNER BAG WHICH MAINTAINS PRODUCT STERILITY
DISCARD IF LEAKS ARE FOUND   MUST NOT BE USED IN SERIES
CONNECTIONS   DO NOT ADMINISTER SIMULTANEOUSLY WITH BLOOD
DO NOT USE UNLESS SOLUTION IS CLEAR   FEDERAL (USA) LAW
PROHIBITS DISPENSING WITHOUT PRESCRIPTION   STORE UNIT IN
MOISTURE BARRIER OVERWRAP AT ROOM TEMPERATURE
(25°C/77°F) UNTIL READY TO USE   AVOID EXCESSIVE HEAT   SEE
INSERT

4

5

6

7

Baxter
BAXTER HEALTHCARE CORPORATION   VIAFLEX® CONTAINER
DEERFIELD IL 60015 USA   PL 146® PLASTIC
MADE IN USA   FOR PRODUCT INFORMATION
CALL 1-800-933-0303

8

9

(b)

---

abbott 1000 mL   NDC 0074-7983-09

0—   —0

1—   **0.9%**   —1

2—   **Sodium Chloride**   —2
         Injection, USP

3—   —3

—   EACH 100 ML CONTAINS SODIUM CHLORIDE   —
4—   900 mg IN WATER FOR INJECTION.   —4
     ELECTROLYTES PER 1000 mL: SODIUM 154 mEq;
—   CHLORIDE 154 mEq.   —

     308 mOsm/LITER (CALC).   pH 5.6 (4.5—7.0)
5—   ADDITIVES MAY BE INCOMPATIBLE. CONSULT   —5
—   WITH PHARMACIST, IF AVAILABLE. WHEN   —
     INTRODUCING ADDITIVES, USE ASEPTIC
6—   TECHNIQUE, MIX THOROUGHLY AND DO NOT   —6
—   STORE. SINGLE-DOSE CONTAINER. FOR   —
     INTRAVENOUS USE. USUAL DOSE: SEE INSERT.
7—   STERILE, NONPYROGENIC. CAUTION: FEDERAL   —7
—   (USA) LAW PROHIBITS DISPENSING WITHOUT   —
     PRESCRIPTION. USE ONLY IF SOLUTION IS CLEAR
—   AND CONTAINER IS UNDAMAGED. MUST NOT   —
8—   BE USED IN SERIES CONNECTIONS.   —8
                              PATENT PENDING
—   ©ABBOTT 1988   PRINTED IN USA   —
9—   ABBOTT LABORATORIES, NORTH CHICAGO, IL60064, USA   —9

(d)

● **Figure 10.4**

Examples of IV bags and labels.   *(10-04a Al Dodge/Al Dodge.*
10-04b Courtesy of Baxter Healthcare Corporation. All rights reserved.   *10-04c Al*
Dodge/Al Dodge   10-04d Reproduced with permission of Abbott Laboratories)

● **Figure 10.5**
Examples of intravenous fluids.
(Reproduced with permission of Abbott Laboratories.)

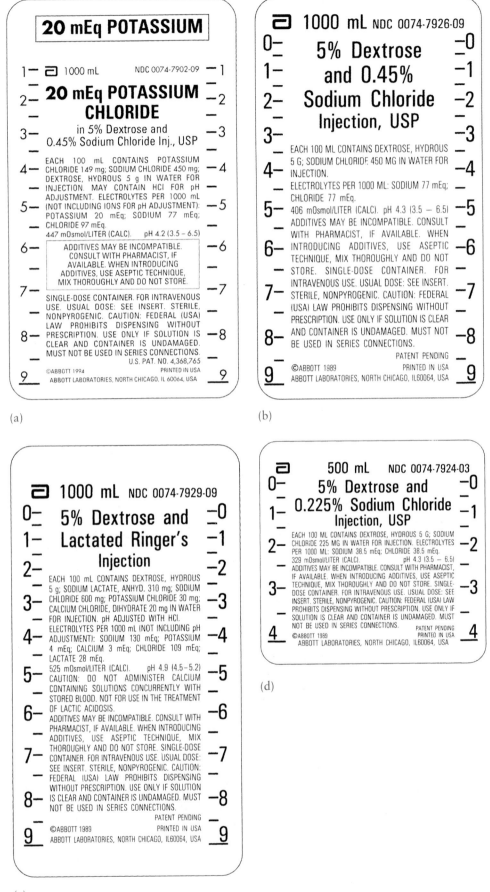

(a)

20 mEq POTASSIUM

1 — 1000 mL   NDC 0074-7902-09 — 1

**20 mEq POTASSIUM
CHLORIDE**

in 5% Dextrose and
0.45% Sodium Chloride Inj., USP

EACH 100 mL CONTAINS POTASSIUM
CHLORIDE 149 mg; SODIUM CHLORIDE 450 mg;
DEXTROSE, HYDROUS 5 g IN WATER FOR
INJECTION. MAY CONTAIN HCl FOR pH
ADJUSTMENT. ELECTROLYTES PER 1000 mL
(NOT INCLUDING IONS FOR pH ADJUSTMENT):
POTASSIUM 20 mEq; SODIUM 77 mEq;
CHLORIDE 97 mEq.
447 mOsmol/LITER (CALC).   pH 4.2 (3.5 – 6.5)

ADDITIVES MAY BE INCOMPATIBLE.
CONSULT WITH PHARMACIST, IF
AVAILABLE. WHEN INTRODUCING
ADDITIVES, USE ASEPTIC TECHNIQUE,
MIX THOROUGHLY AND DO NOT STORE.

SINGLE-DOSE CONTAINER. FOR INTRAVENOUS
USE. USUAL DOSE: SEE INSERT. STERILE,
NONPYROGENIC. CAUTION: FEDERAL (USA)
LAW PROHIBITS DISPENSING WITHOUT
PRESCRIPTION. USE ONLY IF SOLUTION IS
CLEAR AND CONTAINER IS UNDAMAGED.
MUST NOT BE USED IN SERIES CONNECTIONS.
U.S. PAT. NO. 4,368,765
©ABBOTT 1994   PRINTED IN USA
ABBOTT LABORATORIES, NORTH CHICAGO, IL 60064, USA

(b)

1000 mL NDC 0074-7926-09

**5% Dextrose
and 0.45%
Sodium Chloride**
Injection, USP

EACH 100 ML CONTAINS DEXTROSE, HYDROUS
5 G; SODIUM CHLORIDE 450 MG IN WATER FOR
INJECTION.
ELECTROLYTES PER 1000 ML: SODIUM 77 mEq;
CHLORIDE 77 mEq.
406 mOsmol/LITER (CALC). pH 4.3 (3.5 – 6.5)
ADDITIVES MAY BE INCOMPATIBLE. CONSULT
WITH PHARMACIST, IF AVAILABLE. WHEN
INTRODUCING ADDITIVES, USE ASEPTIC
TECHNIQUE, MIX THOROUGHLY AND DO NOT
STORE. SINGLE-DOSE CONTAINER. FOR
INTRAVENOUS USE. USUAL DOSE: SEE INSERT.
STERILE, NONPYROGENIC. CAUTION: FEDERAL
(USA) LAW PROHIBITS DISPENSING WITHOUT
PRESCRIPTION. USE ONLY IF SOLUTION IS CLEAR
AND CONTAINER IS UNDAMAGED. MUST NOT
BE USED IN SERIES CONNECTIONS.
PATENT PENDING
©ABBOTT 1989   PRINTED IN USA
ABBOTT LABORATORIES, NORTH CHICAGO, IL 60064, USA

(c)

1000 mL NDC 0074-7929-09

**5% Dextrose and
Lactated Ringer's**
Injection

EACH 100 mL CONTAINS DEXTROSE, HYDROUS
5 g; SODIUM LACTATE, ANHYD. 310 mg; SODIUM
CHLORIDE 600 mg; POTASSIUM CHLORIDE 30 mg;
CALCIUM CHLORIDE, DIHYDRATE 20 mg IN WATER
FOR INJECTION. pH ADJUSTED WITH HCl.
ELECTROLYTES PER 1000 mL (NOT INCLUDING pH
ADJUSTMENT): SODIUM 130 mEq; POTASSIUM
4 mEq; CALCIUM 3 mEq; CHLORIDE 109 mEq;
LACTATE 28 mEq.
525 mOsmol/LITER (CALC).   pH 4.9 (4.5 – 5.2)
CAUTION: DO NOT ADMINISTER CALCIUM
CONTAINING SOLUTIONS CONCURRENTLY WITH
STORED BLOOD. NOT FOR USE IN THE TREATMENT
OF LACTIC ACIDOSIS.
ADDITIVES MAY BE INCOMPATIBLE. CONSULT WITH
PHARMACIST, IF AVAILABLE. WHEN INTRODUCING
ADDITIVES, USE ASEPTIC TECHNIQUE, MIX
THOROUGHLY AND DO NOT STORE. SINGLE-DOSE
CONTAINER. FOR INTRAVENOUS USE. USUAL DOSE:
SEE INSERT. STERILE, NONPYROGENIC. CAUTION:
FEDERAL (USA) LAW PROHIBITS DISPENSING
WITHOUT PRESCRIPTION. USE ONLY IF SOLUTION
IS CLEAR AND CONTAINER IS UNDAMAGED. MUST
NOT BE USED IN SERIES CONNECTIONS.
PATENT PENDING
©ABBOTT 1989   PRINTED IN USA
ABBOTT LABORATORIES, NORTH CHICAGO, IL60064, USA

(d)

500 mL   NDC 0074-7924-03
**5% Dextrose and
0.225% Sodium Chloride**
Injection, USP

EACH 100 ML CONTAINS DEXTROSE, HYDROUS 5 G; SODIUM
CHLORIDE 225 MG IN WATER FOR INJECTION. ELECTROLYTES
PER 1000 ML: SODIUM 38.5 mEq; CHLORIDE 38.5 mEq.
329 mOsmol/LITER (CALC).   pH 4.3 (3.5 – 6.5)
ADDITIVES MAY BE INCOMPATIBLE. CONSULT WITH PHARMACIST,
IF AVAILABLE. WHEN INTRODUCING ADDITIVES, USE ASEPTIC
TECHNIQUE, MIX THOROUGHLY AND DO NOT STORE. SINGLE-
DOSE CONTAINER. FOR INTRAVENOUS USE. USUAL DOSE: SEE
INSERT. STERILE, NONPYROGENIC. CAUTION: FEDERAL (USA) LAW
PROHIBITS DISPENSING WITHOUT PRESCRIPTION. USE ONLY IF
SOLUTION IS CLEAR AND CONTAINER IS UNDAMAGED. MUST
NOT BE USED IN SERIES CONNECTIONS.
PATENT PENDING
©ABBOTT 1989   PRINTED IN USA
ABBOTT LABORATORIES, NORTH CHICAGO, IL60064, USA

Equipment for IV Infusions

Equipment used for the administration of continuous IV infusions includes the IV solution and IV tubing, a drip chamber, at least one injection port, and a roller clamp. The tubing connects the IV solution to the hub of an IV catheter at the infusion site. The rate of flow of the infusion is regulated by an electronic infusion device (pump or controller) or by gravity. ●Figures 10.6 and 10.9.

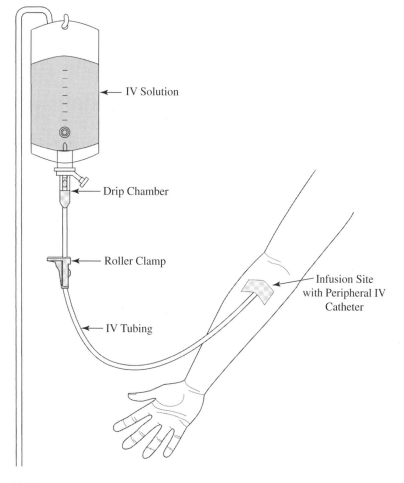

IV Solution

Drip Chamber

Roller Clamp

Infusion Site
with Peripheral IV
Catheter

IV Tubing

●**Figure 10.6**
Primary intravenous line (gravity flow).

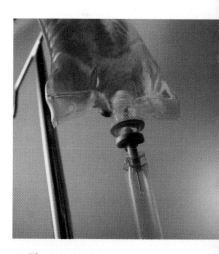

●**Figure 10.7**
Tubing with drip chamber.

(Photodisc/Getty Images)

The drip chamber (Figure 10.6) is located at the site of the entrance of the tubing into the container of intravenous solution. It allows you to count the number of drops per minute that the client is receiving (flow rate).

A roll valve clamp or clip is connected to the tubing and can be manipulated to increase or decrease the flow rate.

The size of the drop that IV tubing delivers is not standard; it depends on the way the tubing is designed. ●**Figure 10.7**. Manufacturers specify the number of drops that equal 1 mL for their particular tubing. This equivalent is called the tubing's *drop factor* (●**Figure 10.8** and Table 10.1). You must know the tubing's drop factor when calculating the flow rate of solutions in drops per minute (gtt/min) or microdrops per minute (μgtt/min or mcgtt/min).

ALERT

Be sure to follow the procedures for eliminating all air in the tubing.

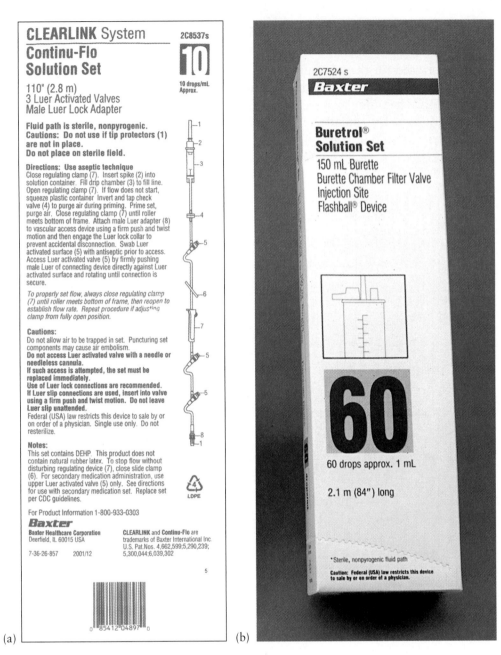

● **Figure 10.8**

Samples of IV tubing containers with drop factors of 10 and 60.

(a)   (b)

Table 10.1 **Common Drop Factors**

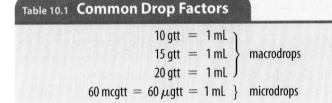

$$
\left.
\begin{array}{l}
10 \text{ gtt} = 1 \text{ mL} \\
15 \text{ gtt} = 1 \text{ mL} \\
20 \text{ gtt} = 1 \text{ mL}
\end{array}
\right\} \text{macrodrops}
$$

$$
60 \text{ mcgtt} = 60\ \mu\text{gtt} = 1 \text{ mL} \} \text{ microdrops}
$$

Note: 60 microdrops = 1 mL is a universal equivalent for IV tubing calibrated in microdrops.

Infusion Pumps

An intravenous infusion can flow solely by the force of gravity or by an electronic infusion device. There are many different types of electronic infusion machines, including controllers and volumetric pumps. ● **Figure 10.9.**

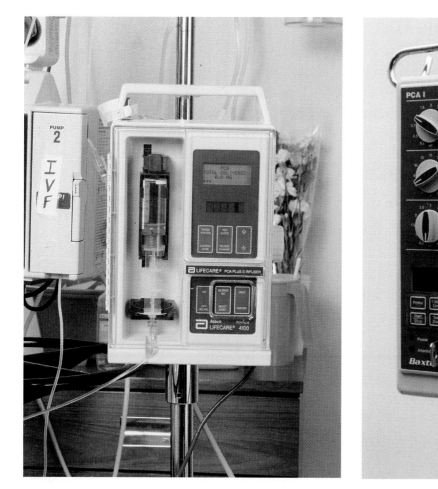

● **Figure 10.9**
Volumetric infusion pump.

● **Figure 10.10**
PCA pump.

These electrically operated devices allow the rate of flow (usually specified in mL/h) to be simply keyed into the device by the user. The pumps can more precisely regulate the flow rate than can the gravity systems. For example, pumps detect an interruption in the flow (constriction) and sound an alarm to alert the nursing staff and the patient, sound an alarm when the infusion finishes, indicate the volume of fluid already infused, and indicate the time remaining for the infusion to finish. "Smart" pumps may contain libraries of safe dosage ranges that will not allow the user to key in an unsafe dosage.

A *Patient Controlled Analgesia (PCA)* pump (●**Figure 10.10**) allows a patient to self-administer pain-relieving drugs whenever the patient needs them without having to wait for the nurse to bring medication. When pain is felt, the patient presses the button on the handset, which is connected to the PCA pump. The pump then delivers the drug down a length of tubing to an injection port.

> **ALERT**
>
> A facility might use many different types of infusion pumps. The healthcare provider must learn how to program all of them. Be sure to use the specific tubing supplied by the manufacturer for each pump.

Calculating the Flow Rate of Infusions

In Exercises 10.1 through 10.10, you will be required to change one rate of flow to another rate of flow. The general method for converting one rate to another rate was introduced in Chapter 3.

Example 10.1

The order is *D₅W 1,250 mL IV q12h*. The tubing is calibrated at 10 drops per milliliter. Calculate the number of drops per minute that you would administer.

Given flow rate: 1,250 mL/12 h

Known equivalences: 10 gtt/mL (drop factor)

                                    1 h = 60 min

Flow rate you want to find: ? gtt/min

You want to convert one flow rate in mL/h to an equivalent flow rate in gtt/min.

$$\frac{1{,}250 \text{ mL}}{12 \text{ h}} = \frac{? \text{ gtt}}{\text{min}}$$

You want to cancel mL. To do this you must use a unit fraction containing mL in the denominator. Using the drop factor, this fraction will be $\dfrac{10 \text{ gtt}}{1 \text{ mL}}$

$$\frac{1{,}250 \text{ mL}}{12 \text{ h}} \times \frac{10 \text{ gtt}}{1 \text{ mL}} = \frac{? \text{ gtt}}{\text{min}}$$

Now, on the left side gtt is in the numerator, which is what you want. But h is in the denominator and it must be cancelled. This will require a unit fraction with h in the numerator, namely, $\dfrac{1 \text{ h}}{60 \text{ min}}$
Now, cancel and multiply the numbers

$$\frac{1{,}250 \text{ mL}}{12 \text{ h}} \times \frac{10 \text{ gtt}}{1 \text{ mL}} \times \frac{1 \text{ h}}{60 \text{ min}} = 17.4 \frac{\text{gtt}}{\text{min}}$$

So, the flow rate is 17 drops per minute.

Example 10.2

The order reads: *IV fluids: 0.9% NaCl 250 mL in 4 hours*. How many microdrops per minute would you administer?

Given flow rate: 250 mL/4 h

Known equivalences: 60 mcgtt/mL (drop factor for microdrops)

                                    1 h = 60 min

Flow rate you want to find: ? mcgtt/min

You want to convert one flow rate in mL/h to an equivalent flow rate in mcgtt/min.

$$\frac{250 \text{ mL}}{4 \text{ h}} = \frac{? \text{ mcgtt}}{\text{min}}$$

You want to cancel mL. To do this you must use a unit fraction containing mL in the denominator. Using the drop factor, this fraction will be $\dfrac{60 \text{ mcgtt}}{1 \text{ mL}}$

$$\frac{250 \text{ mL}}{4 \text{ h}} \times \frac{60 \text{ mcgtt}}{1 \text{ mL}} = \frac{? \text{ mcgtt}}{\text{min}}$$

Now, on the left side mcgtt is in the numerator, which is what you want. But h is in the denominator and it must be cancelled. This will require a fraction with h in the numerator, namely, $\dfrac{1\ h}{60\ min}$

Now, cancel and multiply the numbers

$$\frac{250\ \cancel{mL}}{4\ \cancel{h}} \times \frac{60\ \widehat{mcgtt}}{1\ \cancel{mL}} \times \frac{1\ \cancel{h}}{\cancel{60}\ \widehat{min}} = 62.5\ \frac{mcgtt}{min}$$

So, 63 microdrops per minute would be administered.

Continuous enteral feedings are generally placed on an infusion pump and measured in mL/h.

Example 10.3

A patient must receive a tube-feeding of *Ensure, 240 mL in 90 minutes*. The calibration of the tubing is 20 drops per milliliter. Calculate the flow rate in milliliters per hour.

Given flow rate:	240 mL/90 min
Known equivalences:	20 gtt/mL (drop factor)
	1 h = 60 min
Flow rate you want to find:	? gtt/min

You want to change one flow rate to another,

$$\frac{240\ mL}{90\ min} = \frac{?\ mL}{h}$$

Each side has mL in the numerator which is what you want. You want to cancel min which is in the denominator. To do this you must use a unit fraction containing min in the numerator. This fraction will be $\dfrac{60\ min}{1\ h}$

$$\frac{240\ \widehat{mL}}{90\ \cancel{min}} \times \frac{60\ \cancel{min}}{1\ \widehat{h}} = 160\ \frac{mL}{h}$$

So, the flow rate is 160 mL per hour.

Example 10.4

The prescriber ordered $\frac{1}{4}$ NS 850 mL IV in 8 hours. The label on the box containing the intravenous set to be used for this infusion is shown in ● **Figure 10.11**. Calculate the flow rate in drops per minute.

Given flow rate:	850 mL/8 h
Known equivalences:	10 gtt/mL (drop factor)
	1 h = 60 min
Flow rate you want to find:	? gtt/min

You want to convert the flow rate from milliliters per hour to drops per minute.

$$\frac{850\ mL}{8\ h} = \frac{?\ gtt}{min}$$

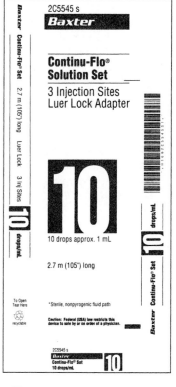

● **Figure 10.11**
Continu-Flo Solution Set box label.

(Courtesy of Baxter Healthcare Corporation. All rights reserved.)

You want to cancel mL. To do this you must use a unit fraction containing mL in the denominator. Using the drop factor, this fraction will be $\dfrac{10 \text{ gtt}}{1 \text{ mL}}$

$$\frac{850 \text{ mL}}{8 \text{ h}} \times \frac{10 \text{ gtt}}{1 \text{ mL}} = \frac{? \text{ gtt}}{\text{min}}$$

Now, on the left side gtt is in the numerator, which is what you want. But h is in the denominator and it must be cancelled. This will require a unit fraction with h in the numerator, namely, $\dfrac{1 \text{ h}}{60 \text{ min}}$

Now cancel and multiply the numbers

$$\frac{850 \text{ mL}}{8 \text{ h}} \times \frac{10 \text{ gtt}}{1 \text{ mL}} \times \frac{1 \text{ h}}{60 \text{ min}} = 17.7 \frac{\text{gtt}}{\text{min}}$$

So, the flow rate is 18 drops per minute.

Example 10.5

(a) The order is *500 mL of 5% D/W to infuse IV in 5 hours*. Calculate the flow rate in drops per minute if the drop factor is 15 drops per milliliter.
(b) When the nurse checks the infusion 2 hours after it started, 400 mL remain to be absorbed in the remaining 3 hours. Recalculate the flow rate in drops per minute for the remaining 400 mL.

(a) Given flow rate: 500 mL/5 h
    Known equivalences: 15 gtt/mL (drop factor)
                              1 h = 60 min

    Flow rate you want to find: ? gtt/min

You want to convert the flow rate from 500 mL in 5 hours to drops per minute.

$$\frac{500 \text{ mL}}{5 \text{ h}} = \frac{? \text{ gtt}}{\text{min}}$$

As in the previous examples, you can do this in one line as follows:

$$\frac{500 \text{ mL}}{5 \text{ h}} \times \frac{\overset{1}{15} \text{ gtt}}{1 \text{ mL}} \times \frac{1 \text{ h}}{\underset{4}{60} \text{ min}} = 25 \frac{\text{gtt}}{\text{min}}$$

So, the flow rate is 25 drops per minute.

(b) When the nurse checks the infusion, 400 mL need to be infused in 3 hours.
So, you now want to convert 400 mL in 3 hours to drops per minute.

$$\frac{400 \text{ mL}}{3 \text{ h}} = \frac{? \text{ gtt}}{\text{min}}$$

In a similar manner to part (a), you can do this in one line as follows:

$$\frac{400 \text{ mL}}{3 \text{ h}} \times \frac{\overset{1}{15} \text{ gtt}}{1 \text{ mL}} \times \frac{1 \text{ h}}{\underset{4}{60} \text{ min}} = 33.3 \frac{\text{gtt}}{\text{min}}$$

So, in order for the infusion to be completed within the 5 hour time period as ordered, the flow rate must be increased to 33 drops per minute.

Example 10.6

The order is *D5W 900 mL IV in 6 hours*. The drop factor is 10 gtt/mL. You would expect that after 3 hours, about 450 mL (half the total infusion of 900 mL) would be left in the bag. However, only 240 mL remain. Recalculate the flow rate in gtt/min so that the infusion will finish on time.

The remainder of the bag (240 mL) must infuse in the remaining time (3 hours).

New flow rate: 240 mL/3 h
Known equivalences: 10 gtt/mL (drop factor)
                                  1 h = 60 min
Flow rate you want to find: ? gtt/min

You want to convert the flow rate from 240 mL in 3 hours to drops per minute.

$$\frac{240 \text{ mL}}{3 \text{ h}} = \frac{? \text{ gtt}}{\text{min}}$$

You can do this in one line as follows:

$$\frac{240 \text{ mL}}{3 \text{ h}} \times \frac{10 \text{ gtt}}{1 \text{ mL}} \times \frac{1 \text{ h}}{60 \text{ min}} = 13.3 \frac{\text{gtt}}{\text{min}}$$

So, the new flow rate would be 13 drops per minute.

Example 10.7

A patient has an order for *Sustacal 240 mL in 2 hours via a feeding tube*. Calculate the rate of flow in
(a) milliliters per hour
(b) milliliters per minute.

(a) The flow rate is 240 mL in 2 hours. No conversion of units of measurement is necessary.

$$\frac{240 \text{ mL}}{2 \text{ h}} \quad \text{can be simplified as follows:}$$

$$\frac{\overset{120}{\cancel{240}} \text{ mL}}{\underset{1}{\cancel{2}} \text{ h}} = \frac{120 \text{ mL}}{\text{h}}$$

So, the flow rate is 120 mL per hour.

(b) Change the flow rate found in part (a) to milliliters per minute. You want to convert the milliliters per hour into milliliters per minute.

$$\frac{120 \text{ mL}}{\text{h}} = \frac{? \text{ mL}}{\text{min}}$$

Do this in one line as follows

$$\frac{120 \text{ mL}}{\text{h}} \times \frac{1 \text{ h}}{60 \text{ min}} = 2 \frac{\text{mL}}{\text{min}}$$

So, the flow rate is 2 mL per minute.

Example 10.8

An IV flow rate is 25 drops per minute. The drop factor is 10 drops per mL. What is the flow rate in milliliters per hour?

Given flow rate: 25 gtt/min

Known equivalences: 10 gtt/mL (drop factor)

                                   1 h = 60 min

Flow rate you want to find: ? mL/h

You want to convert a flow rate in drops per minute to a flow rate in milliliters per hour.

$$\frac{25 \text{ gtt}}{\text{min}} = \frac{? \text{ mL}}{\text{h}}$$

You want to cancel gtt. To do this you must use a unit fraction containing gtt in the denominator. Using the drop factor, this fraction will be $\frac{1 \text{ mL}}{10 \text{ gtt}}$

$$\frac{25 \;\cancel{\text{gtt}}}{\text{min}} \times \frac{1 \text{ mL}}{10 \;\cancel{\text{gtt}}} = \frac{? \text{ mL}}{\text{h}}$$

Now, mL is in the numerator, which is what you want. But min is in the denominator and it must be cancelled. This will require a unit fraction with min in the numerator, namely, $\frac{60 \text{ min}}{1 \text{ h}}$

Now, cancel and multiply the numbers

$$\frac{25 \;\cancel{\text{gtt}}}{\cancel{\text{min}}} \times \frac{1 \;\cancel{\text{mL}}}{10 \;\cancel{\text{gtt}}} \times \frac{60 \;\cancel{\text{min}}}{1 \;\cancel{\text{h}}} = 150 \frac{\text{mL}}{\text{h}}$$

So, the flow rate is 150 mL per hour.

Example 10.9

The prescriber orders D5/0.45% NaCl IV to infuse at 21 drops per minute. If the drop factor is 20 drops per milliliter, how many milliliters per hour will the patient receive?

Given flow rate: 21 gtt/min

Known equivalences: 20 gtt/mL (drop factor)

                                   1 h = 60 min

Flow rate you want to find: ? mL/h

You want to convert a flow rate of 21 drops per minute to a flow rate in milliliters per hour.

$$\frac{21 \text{ gtt}}{\text{min}} = \frac{? \text{ mL}}{\text{h}}$$

You want to cancel gtt. To do this you must use a unit fraction containing *gtt* in the denominator. Using the drop factor, this fraction is $\frac{1 \text{ mL}}{20 \text{ gtt}}$

$$\frac{21 \;\cancel{\text{gtt}}}{\text{min}} \times \frac{1 \text{ mL}}{20 \;\cancel{\text{gtt}}} = \frac{? \text{ mL}}{\text{h}}$$

Now, on the left side *mL* is in the numerator, which is what you want. But *min* is in the denominator and it must be cancelled. This will require a unit fraction with *min* in the numerator, namely, $\dfrac{60 \text{ min}}{1 \text{ h}}$

Now cancel and multiply the numbers

$$\frac{21 \text{ gtt}}{\text{min}} \times \frac{1 \text{ mL}}{20 \text{ gtt}} \times \frac{60 \text{ min}}{1 \text{ h}} = 63 \ \frac{\text{mL}}{\text{h}}$$

So, the flow rate is 63 mL per hour.

Example 10.10

The order reads *125 mL 5% D/W IV in 1 hour*. What is the flow rate in microdrops per minute?

Given flow rate:	125 mL/h
Known equivalences:	60 mcgtt/mL (drop factor for microdrops)
	1 h = 60 min
Flow rate you want to find:	? mcgtt/min

You want to change the flow rate from 125 mL per hour to microdrops per minute.

$$\frac{125 \text{ mL}}{\text{h}} = \frac{? \text{ mcgtt}}{\text{min}}$$

You want to cancel mL. To do this you must use a unit fraction containing mL in the denominator. Using the drop factor, this fraction will be $\dfrac{60 \text{ mcgtt}}{1 \text{ mL}}$

$$\frac{125 \text{ mL}}{\text{h}} \times \frac{60 \text{ mcgtt}}{1 \text{ mL}} = \frac{? \text{ mcgtt}}{\text{min}}$$

Now, on the left side mcgtt is in the numerator, which is what you want. But h is in the denominator and it must be cancelled. This will require a unit fraction with h in the numerator, namely, $\dfrac{1 \text{ h}}{60 \text{ min}}$

Now cancel and multiply the numbers

$$\frac{125 \text{ mL}}{\text{h}} \times \frac{60 \text{ mcgtt}}{1 \text{ mL}} \times \frac{1 \text{ h}}{60 \text{ min}} = 125 \ \frac{\text{mcgtt}}{\text{min}}$$

So, you 125 mL per hour is the same rate of flow as 125 microdrops per minute.

> **NOTE**
>
> In Example 10.10, it is shown that 125 mL per hour is the same flow rate as 125 microdrops per minute because the 60s always cancel. The flow rates of *milliliters per hour* and *microdrops per minute* are equivalent. Therefore calculations are not necessary to change mL/h to μgtt/min.

Calculating the Duration of Flow for IV and Enteral Solutions

In the following three examples, you must determine the length of time it will take to complete an infusion.

Example 10.11

An infusion of 5% D/W is infusing at a rate of 20 drops per minute. If the drop factor is 12 drops per milliliter, how many hours will it take for the remaining solution in the bag (●**Figure 10.12**) to infuse?

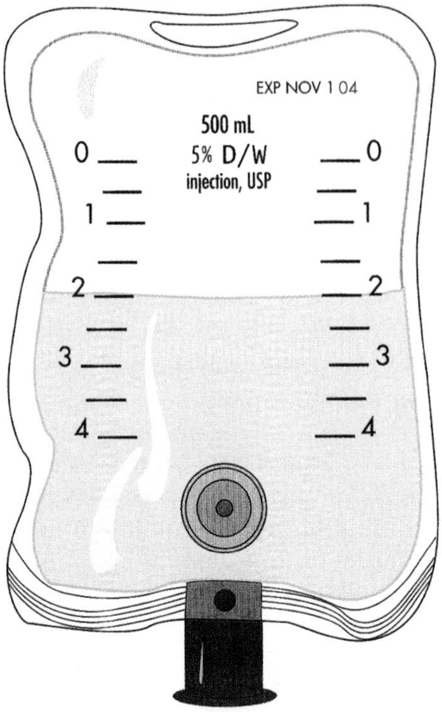

●**Figure 10.12**
5% D/W intravenous solution.

In Figure 10.12 you can see that 500 mL of solution were originally in the bag, and that the patient has received 200 mL. Therefore, 300 mL remain to be infused.

Given: 300 mL (volume to be infused)
Known equivalences: 12 gtt/mL (drop factor)
                                20 gtts/min (flow rate)
                                1 h = 60 min
Find: ? h

You want to convert this single unit of measurement **300 mL** to the single unit of measurement *hours*.

$$300 \text{ mL} = ? \text{ h}$$

You want to cancel mL. To do this you must use a unit fraction containing mL in the denominator. Using the drop factor, this fraction will be $\dfrac{12 \text{ gtt}}{1 \text{ mL}}$

$$300 \, \cancel{\text{mL}} \times \frac{12 \text{ gtt}}{1 \, \cancel{\text{mL}}} = ? \text{ h}$$

Now, on the left side gtt is in the numerator, but you don't want gtt. You need a unit fraction with gtt in the denominator to cancel. Using the flow rate, this fraction is $\dfrac{1 \text{ min}}{20 \text{ gtt}}$

$$300 \, \cancel{\text{mL}} \times \frac{12 \, \cancel{\text{gtt}}}{1 \, \cancel{\text{mL}}} \times \frac{1 \, \text{min}}{20 \, \cancel{\text{gtt}}} = ? \text{ h}$$

Now, on the left side min is in the numerator, but you don't want min. You need a fraction with min in the denominator to cancel, namely,

$$\frac{1\ h}{60\ min}$$

Now cancel and multiply the numbers.

$$\overset{15}{\cancel{300}}\ \cancel{mL} \times \frac{\overset{1}{\cancel{12}}\ \cancel{gtt}}{1\ \cancel{mL}} \times \frac{1\ \cancel{min}}{\underset{1}{\cancel{20}}\ \cancel{gtt}} \times \frac{1\ h}{\underset{5}{\cancel{60}}\ \cancel{min}} = 3\ h$$

So, it will take 3 hours for the remaining solution to infuse.

Example 10.12

A patient is to receive an IV infusion of 500 mL of 5% D/W. The flow rate is 27 drops per minute. If the drop factor is 15 drops per milliliter, how many hours will it take for this infusion to finish?

Given: 500 mL (volume to be infused)

Known equivalences: 15 gtt/mL (drop factor)

                              27 gtt/min (flow rate)

                              1 h = 60 min

Find: ? h

You want to convert this single unit of measurement 500 mL to the single unit of measurement *hours*.

$$500\ mL = ?\ h$$

You want to cancel mL. To do this you must use a unit fraction containing mL in the denominator. Using the drop factor, this fraction will be $\dfrac{15\ gtt}{1\ mL}$

$$500\ \cancel{mL} \times \frac{15\ gtt}{1\ \cancel{mL}} = ?\ h$$

Now, on the left side gtt is in the numerator, but you don't want gtt. You need a unit fraction with gtt in the denominator. Using the flow rate, the fraction is $\dfrac{1\ min}{27\ gtt}$

$$500\ \cancel{mL} \times \frac{15\ \cancel{gtt}}{1\ \cancel{mL}} \times \frac{1\ \boxed{min}}{27\ \cancel{gtt}} = ?\ h$$

Now, on the left side min is in the numerator, but you don't want min. You need a unit fraction with min in the denominator, namely,

$$\frac{1\ h}{60\ min}$$

Now cancel and multiply the numbers.

$$500\ \cancel{mL} \times \frac{\overset{1}{\cancel{15}}\ \cancel{gtt}}{1\ \cancel{mL}} \times \frac{1\ \cancel{min}}{27\ \cancel{gtt}} \times \frac{1\ h}{\underset{4}{\cancel{60}}\ \cancel{min}} = 4.63\ h$$

Now, convert the portion of an hour to minutes—that is, convert 0.63 h to min.

$$0.63 \text{ h} \times \frac{60 \text{ min}}{1 \text{ h}} = 37.8 \text{ min}$$

So, the infusion will take 4 hours and 38 minutes.

Example 10.13

An IV of 1,000 mL of 5% D/0.9% NaCl is started at 8 P.M. The flow rate is 38 drops per minute, and the drop factor is 10 drops per milliliter. At what time will this infusion finish?

Given:	1,000 mL (volume to be infused)
Known equivalences:	10 gtt/mL (drop factor)
	38 gtt/min (flow rate)
	1 h = 60 min
Find:	? h

You must first find how many hours the infusion will take to finish. You want to convert the single unit of measurement 1,000 mL to the single unit of measurement *hours*.

$$1,000 \text{ mL} = ? \text{ h}$$

You want to cancel mL. To do this you must use a unit fraction containing mL in the denominator. This fraction will be $\dfrac{10 \text{ gtt}}{1 \text{ mL}}$

$$1,000 \text{ mL} \times \frac{10 \text{ gtt}}{1 \text{ mL}} = ? \text{ h}$$

Now, on the left side gtt is in the numerator, but you don't want gtt. You need a fraction with gtt in the denominator. Using the flow rate, this fraction is $\dfrac{1 \text{ min}}{38 \text{ gtt}}$

$$1,000 \text{ mL} \times \frac{10 \text{ gtt}}{1 \text{ mL}} \times \frac{1 \text{ min}}{38 \text{ gtt}} = ? \text{ h}$$

Now, on the left side min is in the numerator, but you don't want min. You need a fraction with min in the denominator, namely, $\dfrac{1 \text{ h}}{60 \text{ min}}$

Now, cancel and multiply the numbers.

$$1,000 \text{ mL} \times \frac{\overset{1}{10} \text{ gtt}}{1 \text{ mL}} \times \frac{1 \text{ min}}{38 \text{ gtt}} \times \frac{1 \text{ h}}{\underset{6}{60} \text{ min}} = 4.4 \text{ h}$$

You then convert 0.4 h to min.

$$0.4 \text{ h} \times \frac{60 \text{ min}}{1 \text{ h}} = 24 \text{ min}$$

So, the IV will infuse for 4 hours and 24 minutes. Because the infusion started at 8 P.M., it will finish at 12:24 A.M. on the following day.

Example 10.14

The order reads: *1,000 mL D5W IV over 8 hours*. The drop factor is 10 gtt/mL.

(a) Calculate the flow rate in gtt/min for this infusion.

(b) After 5 hours 700 mL remain to be infused. How must the flow rate be adjusted so that the infusion will finish on time?

(c) If the facility has a policy that flow rate adjustments must not exceed 25% of the original rate, was the adjustment required within the guidelines?

(a) First, convert the flow rate of 1,000 mL in 8 hours to gtt/min. You can do this in one line as follows:

$$\frac{1,000 \text{ mL}}{8 \text{ h}} \times \frac{1 \text{ h}}{60 \text{ min}} \times \frac{10 \text{ gtt}}{\text{mL}} = 20.8 \frac{\text{gtt}}{\text{min}}$$

So, the original flow rate is 21 gtt/min.

(b) After 5 hours, 700 mL remain to be infused in the remaining 3 hours. Now, the new flow rate must be calculated. That is, you must convert the flow rate of 700 mL in 3 hours to gtt/min. You can do this in one line as follows:

$$\frac{700 \text{ mL}}{3 \text{ h}} \times \frac{1 \text{ h}}{60 \text{ min}} \times \frac{10 \text{ gtt}}{\text{mL}} = 38.9 \frac{\text{gtt}}{\text{min}}$$

So, the new flow rate is 39 gtt/min.

(c) Since the facility has a policy that flow rate adjustments must not exceed 25% of the original rate, you must now calculate 25% of the original rate; that is, 25% of 21 gtt/min.

25% of 21 gtt/min = (.25 × 21) gtt/min = 5.25 gtt/min

So, the flow rate may not be changed by more than about 5 gtt/min. Therefore, the original flow rate of 21 gtt/min can be changed to no less than 16 (21 minus 5) gtt/min and no more than 26 (21 plus 5) gtt/min.

Since 39 gtt/min is outside the acceptable range of roughly 16–26 gtt/min, this change is not within the guidelines, and the adjustment may not be made. You must contact the prescriber.

Summary

In this chapter, the basic concepts and standard equipment involved in intravenous and enteral therapy were introduced.

- Fluids can be given to a patient slowly over a period of time through a vein (*intravenous*) or through a tube inserted into the alimentary tract (*enteral*).

- Enteral and IV fluids can be administered continuously or intermittently.

- There is a wide variety of commercially prepared enteral and IV solutions.

- In IV solutions, *letters* indicate solution compounds, whereas *numbers* indicate solution concentration.

- Care must be taken to eliminate the air from, and maintain the sterility of, IV tubing.

- An intravenous infusion can flow solely by the force of gravity or by an electronic infusion device.

- Flow rates are usually given as either mL/h or gtt/min.

- To find the flow rate in *mL/h*, start with the flow rate in gtt/min.
- To find the flow rate in *gtt/min*, start with the flow rate in *mL/h*.
- The drop factor of the IV administration set must be known in order to calculate flow rates.
- *Microdrops/minute* are equivalent to *milliliters/hour*.

- For microdrops, the drop factor is 60 microdrops per milliliter.
- For macrodrops, the usual drop factors are 10, 15, or 20 drops per milliliter.
- To calculate the duration of an IV infusion, start with the volume of the solution in the bag.
- Know the policy of the facility regarding readjustment of flow rates.

Case Study 10.1

A 54-year-old female is transferred from a nursing home and admitted to the hospital with a diagnosis of right-upper-lobe pneumonia. She has a past medical history of lung cancer, hypertension, depression, and anxiety disorder. Her vital signs are as follows: B/P 150/86; P 90; R 30; T 101 °F. Her orders include the following:

- IV fluids: D5/0.45 NaCl 1,000 mL q8h
- Zithromax (azithromycin) 500 mg IVPB daily
- Sustacal $\frac{3}{4}$ strength 800 mL via PEG to run 0100 to 0800 daily
- Xanax (alprazolam) 0.5 mg via PEG t.i.d.
- Zoloft (sertraline) 50 mg PO at bedtime
- Cozaar (losartan potassium) 25 mg via PEG daily
- Fluconazole 200 mg, oral suspension, via PEG stat, then 100 mg daily for 7 days
- Colace (docusate sodium) 100 mg, oral suspension, via PEG b.i.d.
- Lasix (furosemide) 40 mg, oral suspension via PEG b.i.d.
- Tylenol (acetaminophen) 600 mg, oral suspension, via PEG q4h prn temperature above 101.8 °F

Read the labels in ●**Figure 10.13**, when necessary, to answer the following questions.

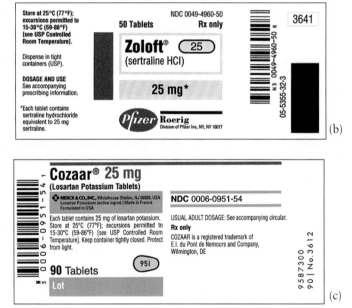

(b)

(c)

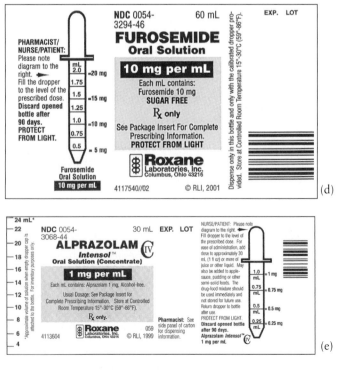

(d)

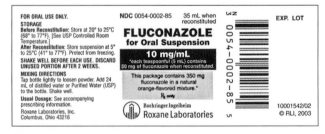

(a)

●**Figure 10.13**
Drug labels for Case Study 10.1. *(10-13a Courtesy of Roxane Laboratories Inc. 10-13b Reg. Trademark of Pfizer Inc. Reproduced with permission. 10-13c The labels for the products Cozaar 25 mg are reproduced with permission of Merck & Co., Inc., copyright owner. 10-13d Courtesy of Roxane Laboratories Inc. 10-13e Courtesy of Roxane Laboratories Inc.)*

(e)

1. What is the rate of flow for the IV solution in mL per hour?

2. What is the rate of flow for the IV in drops/min? Drop factor is 15 gtt/mL?

3. The IV infusion was started at 1900h. When will it be completed?

4. What is the amount of dextrose and sodium chloride in the IV solution?

5. The directions printed on the azithromycin IV bag label read "500 mg in D5W 100 mL, infuse via pump over 60 minutes." What is the pump setting in mL/h?

6. Sustacal is available in 10-ounce cans.
   (a) How many cans will you need to prepare the strength ordered?
   (b) Calculate the rate of flow in mL/h.

7. How many milliliters of alprazolam will you administer?

8. How many milliliters of fluconazole will you prepare for the stat dose?

9. The label on the docusate sodium reads 60 mg/15 mL. How many milliliters contain the prescribed dose?

Practice Sets

The answers to *Try These for Practice*, *Exercises*, and *Cumulative Review Exercises* appear in Appendix A at the end of the book. Ask you instructor for answers to the *Additional Exercises*.

Try These for Practice

Test your comprehension after reading the chapter.

1. The prescriber ordered:

   500 mL 5% D/W IV for 8h

   Calculate the flow rate in gtt/min when the drop factor is 10 drops per milliliter.

   _____

2. The prescriber ordered:

   1,000 mL 0.9% NaCl IV in 8h

   The flow rate is 31 drops per minute. When the nurse assessed the infusion, 425 mL had infused in 4 hours. Calculate the new flow rate in gtt/min if the drop factor is 15 drops per milliliter. _____

3. The prescriber ordered:

   500 mL 5% D/W IV in 4h

   Calculate the flow rate in milliliters per hour. _____

4. An IV of D/5/0.45% NaCl is infusing at a rate of 27 drops per minute. The drop factor is 15 gtt/mL. How many milliliters per hour is the patient receiving? _____

5. Order: *Pulmocare 400 mL over 6 hours via PEG.* Determine the pump setting in mL/h. _____

Workspace

Exercises

Reinforce your understanding in class or at home.

1. The physician ordered *750 mL of NS IV for 8 hours*. Calculate the flow rate in drops per minute. The drop factor is 10 gtt = 1 mL.

2. The patient is to receive *375 mL of RL over 3 hours*. Set the rate on the infusion pump in milliliters per hour.

3. The physician ordered: *Ensure 50 mL per hour via feeding tube*. The drop factor is 10 drops per milliliter. Calculate the flow rate in drops per minute.

4. Ordered: *1,000 mL D5W to infuse at 125 mL/h*. The tubing is calibrated at 15 gtt/mL. How long will this infusion take to finish?

5. A patient is to receive 500 mL 5%D/0.45%NaCl IV in 3 hours. Calculate the flow rate in microdrops per minute.

6. The order reads *1,500 mL D_5W IV over 12 hours*. The drop factor is 20 gtt/mL.
   (a) Find the flow rate in gtt/min for this infusion.
   (b) If after 3 hours 1,200 mL remain to be infused, how must the flow rate be adjusted so that the infusion will finish on time?
   (c) If the facility has a policy that flow rate adjustments must not exceed 25% of the original rate, is the adjustment required in part (b) within the guidelines?

7. Order: *750 mL Ringer's Lactate IV in 8 hours*. Calculate the flow rate in drops per minute if the drop factor is 15 gtt/mL.

8. An IV infusion of 750 mL Ringer's Lactate began at noon. It has been infusing at the rate of 125 mL/h. At what time is it scheduled to finish?

9. A patient has an order for a total parenteral nutrition (TPN) solution 1,000 mL in 24 hours. At what rate in mL/h should the pump be set?

10. An IV is infusing at 90 mL/h. The IV tubing has a drop factor of 20 gtt/mL. Calculate the flow rate in gtt/min.

11. Order: *1,000 mL NS IV over 6 hours*. Calculate and set the flow rate in mL/h for the electronic controller.

12. Calculate the infusion time for an IV of 500 mL that is ordered to run at 40 mL/h.

13. The order reads *750 mL of NS IV. Infuse over a 24 h period*. Set the flow rate on the infusion pump in milliliters per hour.

14. An IV of 800 mL is to infuse over 8 hours at the rate of 20 gtt/min. After 4 hours and 45 minutes, only 300 mL had infused. Recalculate the flow rate in gtt/min. The set calibration is 15 gtt/mL.

15. The order reads *10 AM: 1,000 mL D₅W IV in 8 hours*. The IV was stopped at 4:30 P.M. for 45 minutes with 90 mL of fluid remaining. Determine the new flow rate setting for the infusion pump in mL/h so that the infusion finishes on time.

16. An IV bag has 350 mL remaining. It is infusing at 35 gtt/min, and a 15 gtt/mL set is being used. How long will it take to finish?

17. An IV solution is infusing at 32 microdrops per minute. How many milliliters of this solution will the patient receive in 6 hours?

18. A patient must have a tube feeding of 1,000 mL Ensure for 10 hours. The drop factor is 15 gtt/mL. After 5 hours, a total of 650 mL has infused. Recalculate the new gtt/min flow rate to complete the infusion on schedule.

19. An IV is infusing at a rate of 30 drops per minute. The drop factor is 15gtt/mL. Calculate the flow rate in milliliters per hour.

20. An IV of 500 mL is to infuse 20 gtt/min. If the drop factor is 10 gtt/mL, how long would it take to finish?

_____

Additional Exercises

Now, test yourself!

1. The physician ordered *3,000 mL of 5% Dextrose and Lactated Ringer's solution IV q24h*. Calculate the flow rate in drops per minute. The drop factor is 10 gtt = 1 mL.

_____

2. The order reads: *D5W 250 mL per 8 hours IV*. Calculate the flow rate in microdrops per minute.

_____

3. The patient is to receive *1,000 mL of 0.9% NaCl IV*. It begins at 0600h. It is infusing at 45 gtt/min, and the drop factor is 10 gtt/mL. At what time will the infusion finish?

_____

4. The physician ordered the enteral solution, *Sustacal, via feeding tube 75 milliliters per hour*. The drop factor is 18 drops per milliliter. Calculate the flow rate in milliliters per hour.

_____

5. A patient is to receive *100 mL D5/0.45% NaCl IV in 60 minutes*. Calculate the flow rate in microdrops per minute.

_____

6. The order reads *650 mL D5W q8h IV*. Set the flow rate on the infusion pump in milliliters per hour.

_____

7. The medication order is *300 mL D5W IV in 3 hours*. Calculate the flow rate in drops per minute. The drop factor is 12 gtt/mL.

_____

8. A patient is to receive *500 mL of D10W over 5 hours*. After 2 hours there is 200 mL remaining in the bag. Recalculate the flow rate in microdrops per minute so that the infusion finishes on time.

_____

9. A patient has an order for a solution of *2,500 mL of 5% D/W in 24 hours*. Set the rate on the infusion pump in milliliters per hour.

_____

10. The order reads *850 mL D5/0.45% NaCl q6h IV*. The drop factor is 15 gtt/mL. Calculate the flow rate in drops per minute.

11. There is 550 mL of normal saline in an IV bag. It is 0800h. If the flow rate is 53 drops per minute, and the drop factor is 30 gtt/mL, at what time should this IV finish?

12. An intravenous solution is infusing at a rate of 17 drops per minute. The drop factor is 10 drops per milliliter. How many milliliters per hour is the patient receiving?

13. The order reads *250 mL of 2 $\frac{1}{2}$% D/W IV. Infuse over a 24 h period*. After 12 hours, there is 150 mL left in the bag. Reset the flow rate on the infusion pump in milliliters per hour.

14. An IV solution is infusing at a rate of 50 microdrops per minute.
    (a) How many milliliters per hour is the patient receiving? _____
    (b) How many milliliters will the patient receive in 24 hours? _____

15. The order reads *1,000 mL D5/W IV in 8 h*. The infusion pump is set at 125 mL/h. The IV was stopped for 1 h with 625 mL remaining. Calculate the new flow rate.

16. The flow rate for an intravenous solution of 750 mL is 150 microdrops per minute. How long will this infusion take to finish?

17. The patient has an order for *1,250 mL D5/0.45% NaCl in 15 hours IV*. The drop factor is 10 gtt/mL, and the flow rate is 14 drops per minute. Seven hours later, 500 mL remained in the IV bag. If it is necessary to recalculate the flow rate, what will the new flow rate be in milliliters per hour?

18. A patient must have a tube feeding of 1,000 mL Ensure for 10 hours. The drop factor is 20 gtt/mL.
    (a) Calculate the setting for the pump in milliliters per hour.

    (b) If each can of Ensure contains 200 mL, how many cans of Ensure will you need?

19. An IV is infusing at a rate of 31 drops per minute. The drop factor is 15gtt/mL. Calculate the flow rate in milliliters per hour.

_____

20. An IV solution is infusing at 40 microdrops per minute. How many milliliters of this solution will the patient receive in 18 hours?

_____

Cumulative Review Exercises

Review your mastery of earlier chapters.

1. You have a sodium chloride solution with a concentration of 0.45%. How many milligrams of sodium chloride are in 1 mL?

_____

2. The order reads *Compleat-B 480 mL via PEG q12h*. At how many mL/h will you set the pump?

_____

3. The prescriber orders 2,500 mL of 20% D/W to infuse in 16 hours. Set the rate on the infusion pump at milliliters per hour.

_____

4. An IV of 1,000 mL of 5% D/W is to infuse at a rate of 30 drops per minute for 10 hours. After 4 hours, the patient had received 600 mL. The drop factor is 15 drops per milliliter. Recalculate the flow rate in gtt/min.

_____

5. Calculate the BSA of a patient who is 5 feet 10 inches and weighs 200 pounds.

_____

6. The patient has a BSA of 1.6 m^2. The medication order is 0.8 mg/m^2. The drug is supplied in 1.2 mg capsules. How many capsules will you prepare?

_____

7. An intravenous solution is infusing at 80 microdrops per minute. How many milliliters per hour is the patient receiving? _____

8. You are to prepare 0.75 g of cefuroxime IM stat for your patient. The label reads 250 mg/mL. How many milliliters will you prepare for your patient?

_____

9. Your patient weighs 101 pounds. The prescriber has ordered 6.6 mL per kilogram of a drug PO t.i.d. The label reads 300 mL per capsule. How many capsules will you prepare?

_____

10. The order reads *1,500 mL lactated Ringer's solution IV for 24h*. How many milliliters per hour will the patient receive?

_____

11. 4 T = _____ tsp

12. 6 mg = _____ gr

13. 10 mL = _____ mcgtt

14. $\frac{1}{2}$ lb = _____ oz

15. 1 oz = _____ mL

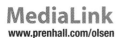

Chapter

Calculating Flow Rates for Intravenous Medications

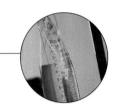

Learning Outcomes

After completing this chapter, you will be able to

1. Describe intravenous medication administration.
2. Calculate the rate of flow of intravenous piggyback medications.
3. Calculate the flow rate of intravenous solutions based on the amount of drug per minute or per hour.
4. Determine the amount of drug a patient will receive IV per minute or per hour.
5. Calculate IVPB flow rates based on body weight.
6. Calculate IVPB flow rates based on body surface area.
7. Calculate the infusion time of an IVPB solution.
8. Calculate the rate of flow for a medication requiring titration.

This chapter extends the discussion of intravenous infusions to include administration of intravenous medications. You will also learn how to calculate the flow rates for IVs based on body weight or BSA.

Intravenous Administration of Medications

Intravenous administration of medications provides rapid access to a patient's circulatory system, thereby presenting potential hazards. Errors in medication, dose, or dosage strength can prove fatal. Therefore, *caution must be taken in the calculation, preparation, and administration of IV medications.*

Typically, a *primary* IV line provides continuous fluid to the patient. *Secondary* lines can be attached to the primary line at injection ports, and these lines are often used to deliver *continuous or intermittent* medication intravenously. A secondary line is referred to as a *piggyback* or *intravenous piggyback (IVPB)*. With intermittent IVPB infusions, the bags hold generally 50–250 mL of fluid containing dissolved medication and usually require 20–60 minutes to infuse. Like a primary line, an IVPB infusion may use a manually controlled gravity system or an electronic pump.

A *heplock, or saline lock,* is an infusion port attached to an indwelling needle or cannula in a peripheral vein. Intermittent IV infusions can be administered through these ports via IV lines connected to these ports. An *IV push, or bolus (IVP),* is a direct injection of medication either into the heplock/saline lock or directly into the vein.

Syringe pumps can also be used for intermittent infusions. A syringe with the medication is inserted into the pump. The medication is delivered at a set rate over a short period of time.

A *volume-control* set is a small container, called a burette, that is connected to the IV line. Burettes are often used in pediatric or geriatric care, where accurate volume control is critical. The danger of overdose is limited because of the small volume of solution in the burette. Burettes will be discussed in Chapter 12.

Intravenous Piggyback Infusions

Patients can receive a medication through a port in an existing IV line. This is called *intravenous piggyback (IVPB)*; ●**Figure 11.1**. The medication is in a secondary bag. Notice in Figure 11.1 that the secondary bag is higher than the primary bag so that the pressure in the secondary line will be greater than the pressure in the primary line. Therefore, the secondary medication infuses first. Once the secondary infusion is completed, the primary line begins to flow. Be sure to keep both lines open. If you close the primary line, when the secondary IVPB is completed the primary line will not flow into the vein.

A typical IVPB order might read: *cimetidine 300 mg IVPB q6h in 50 mL NS infuse over 30 min.* This is an order for an IV piggyback infusion in which 300 mg of the drug cimetidine diluted in 50 mL of a normal saline solution must infuse in 30 minutes. So, the patient receives 300 mg of cimetidine in 30 minutes via a secondary line, and this dose is repeated every 6 hours.

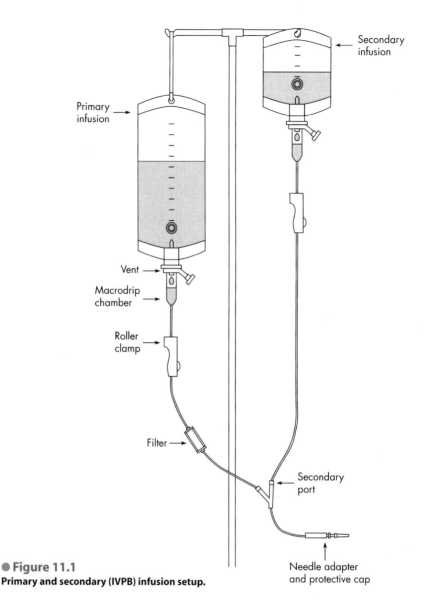

Primary infusion

Secondary infusion

Vent

Macrodrip chamber

Roller clamp

Filter

Secondary port

Needle adapter and protective cap

● **Figure 11.1**
Primary and secondary (IVPB) infusion setup.

Example 11.1

The prescriber ordered: *Ancef 1 g IVPB q4h*

The package insert information is as follows: Add 50 mL sterile water to the bag of Ancef 1 g and infuse in 30 min. The tubing is labeled 20 drops per milliliter. Calculate the flow rate in drops per minute for this antibiotic.

The patient receives 50 mL in 30 minutes. You want to change this flow rate from mL per minute to an equivalent flow rate in drops per minute.

$$\frac{50 \text{ mL}}{30 \text{ min}} \longrightarrow ? \frac{\text{gtt}}{\text{min}}$$

Using the drop factor of 20 gtt/mL, you can do this on one line as follows:

$$\frac{50 \text{ mL}}{30 \text{ min}} \times \frac{20 \text{ gtt}}{1 \text{ mL}} = \frac{100 \text{ gtt}}{3 \text{ min}} = 33.3 \frac{\text{gtt}}{\text{min}}$$

So, the flow rate is 33 drops per minute.

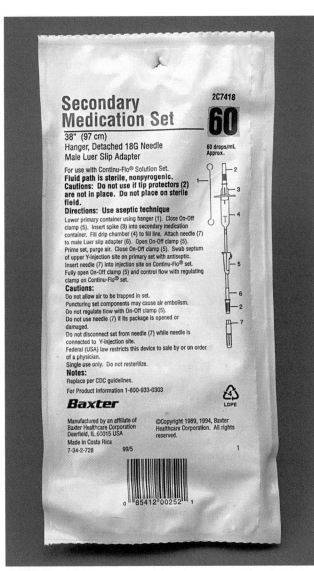

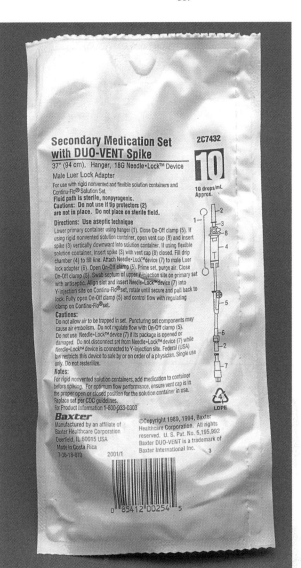

(a)

(b)

● Figure 11.2
Packages of secondary IV tubing.

(Courtesy of Baxter Healthcare Corporation. All rights reserved. Photos by Al Dodge.)

Example 11.2

The order is Mefoxin 1 g IVPB q6h in 50 mL over 30 minutes. Read the label for the premixed Mefoxin in ● **Figure 11.3** and find the drip rate if the drop factor is 10 gtt/mL. The package insert indicates that the Mefoxin should be infused in 30 minutes.

The label states: 1 g in 50 mL. This entire solution must be infused in 30 minutes.

You want to change the flow rate from 50 mL per 30 minutes to an equivalent flow rate in drops per minute.

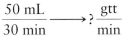

$$\frac{50 \text{ mL}}{30 \text{ min}} \longrightarrow ? \frac{\text{gtt}}{\text{min}}$$

● Figure 11.3
Drug label for Mefoxin.

(The labels for the products Mefoxin 1g are reproduced with permission of Merck & Co., Inc., copyright owner.)

Using the drop factor of 10 gtt/mL, you can do this on one line as follows:

$$\frac{50 \; \cancel{mL}}{30 \; min} \times \frac{10 \; gtt}{\cancel{mL}} = \frac{50 \; gtt}{3 \; min} = 16.67 \; \frac{gtt}{min}$$

So, the flow rate is 17 drops per minute.

Example 11.3

The medication order reads: *1,000 mL 5% D/W with 1,000 mg of a drug at* 1 mg/min. Calculate the flow rate in drops per minute if the drop factor is 15 drops per milliliter.

In this example, the prescriber has specified the amount of solution and its strength (1,000 mL of 5% D/W containing 1,000 mg of the drug) and also the rate at which the patient receives the drug (1 mg/min). This "flow rate" is not the usual volume per time (mL/h or gtt/min), but it is in terms of weight of drug per time (mg/min).

Given flow rate: 1 mg/min (notice that a flow rate always has "time" in the denominator)

Known equivalences: 1,000 mg/1,000 mL (strength)

                          15 gtt/mL (drop factor)

Flow rate you want to find: ? gtt/min

You want to convert the flow rate from milligrams per minute to an equivalent flow rate in drops per minute.

$$1 \frac{mg}{min} \longrightarrow ? \frac{gtt}{min}$$

You want to cancel mg. To do this you must use a unit fraction containing mg in the denominator. Using the strength, this fraction will be $\frac{1,000 \; mL}{1,000 \; mg}$.

$$\frac{1 \; \cancel{mg}}{min} \times \frac{1,000 \; \textcircled{mL}}{1,000 \; \cancel{mg}} = \frac{? \; gtt}{min}$$

Now, on the left side mL is in the numerator, and it must be cancelled. This will require a unit fraction with mL in the denominator. Using the drop factor, this fraction will be $\frac{15 \; gtt}{mL}$.

Now cancel and multiply the numbers

$$\frac{1 \; \cancel{mg}}{1 \; min} \times \frac{1,000 \; \cancel{mL}}{1,000 \; \cancel{mg}} \times \frac{15 \; gtt}{1 \; \cancel{mL}} = 15 \; \frac{gtt}{min}$$

So, you would administer 15 gtt/min.

Example 11.4

The prescriber writes an order for 1,000 mL of 5% D/W with 10 units of a drug. Your patient must receive 30 mU of this drug per minute. Calculate the flow rate in microdrops per minute.

NOTE

1 unit = 1,000 milliunits (mU)

Given flow rate: 30 mU/min (notice that a flow rate always has "time" in the denominator)

Known equivalences: 10 units/1,000 mU (strength)
                         60 gtt/mL (standard microdrop drop factor)
                         1 unit = 1,000 mU

Flow rate you want to find: ? mcgtt/min

You want to change the flow rate from milliunits per minute to microdrops per minute.

$$30\,\frac{mU}{min} = ?\,\frac{mcgtt}{min}$$

You want to cancel mU. To do this you must use a unit fraction containing mU in the denominator. Using the equivalence 1 mU = 1,000 units, this fraction will be $\frac{1\ unit}{1,000\ mU}$.

$$\frac{30\ \cancel{mU}}{min} \times \frac{1\ \text{unit}}{1,000\ \cancel{mU}} = ?\,\frac{mcgtt}{min}$$

Now, on the left side unit is in the numerator, and it must be cancelled. This will require a unit fraction with unit in the denominator. Using the strength, this fraction will be $\frac{1,000\ mL}{10\ units}$.

$$\frac{30\ \cancel{mU}}{min} \times \frac{1\ \cancel{unit}}{1,000\ \cancel{mU}} \times \frac{1,000\ \text{mL}}{10\ \cancel{units}} = ?\,\frac{mcgtt}{min}$$

Now, on the left side mL is in the numerator, and it must be cancelled. This will require a unit fraction with mL in the denominator. Using the drop factor, this fraction will be $\frac{60\ mcgtt}{mL}$.

Now, cancel and multiply the numbers

$$\frac{30\ \cancel{mU}}{min} \times \frac{1\ \cancel{unit}}{\cancel{1,000}\ \cancel{mU}} \times \frac{\cancel{1,000}\ \cancel{mL}}{10\ \cancel{units}} \times \frac{60\ mcgtt}{\cancel{mL}} = 180\,\frac{mcgtt}{min}$$

So, you will administer 180 mcgtt/min.

Example 11.5

Calculate the flow rate in milliliters per hour if the medication order reads: Add 10,000 units of heparin to 1,000 mL 5% D/W IV. Your patient is to receive 1,250 units of this anticoagulant per hour via an infusion pump.

You want to change the flow rate from units per hour to milliliters per hour.

$$\frac{1,250\ units}{1\ h} \longrightarrow ?\,\frac{mL}{h}$$

Using the strength of the solution (10,000 units/1,000 mL) you do this on one line as follows:

$$\frac{1{,}250 \ \cancel{units}}{1 \ h} \times \frac{1{,}\cancel{000} \ mL}{10{,}\cancel{000} \ \cancel{units}} = \frac{1{,}250 \ mL}{10 \ h} = 125 \frac{mL}{h}$$

So, your patient will receive 125 mL per hour. ●

In Examples 11.6, 11.7, and 11.8, you are given the flow rate in milliliters per hour, and you need to determine the amount of medication the patient will receive in a given amount of time.

Example 11.6

Calculate the number of units of Regular insulin a patient is receiving per hour if the order is *500 mL NS with 300 units of Regular insulin and it is infusing at the rate of 12.5 mL per hour via the pump.*

You want to convert the flow rate from mL per hour to units per hour.

$$\frac{12.5 \ mL}{h} \xrightarrow{\quad} ? \frac{units}{h}$$

Using the strength of the solution (300 units/500 mL) you do this in one line as follows:

$$\frac{12.5 \ \cancel{mL}}{h} \times \frac{3\cancel{00} \ units}{5\cancel{00} \ \cancel{mL}} = \frac{37.5 \ units}{5 \ h} \quad or \quad 7.5 \frac{units}{h}$$

So, the patient is receiving 7.5 units per hour. ●

Example 11.7

Order: *heparin 40,000 units continuous IV in 1,000 mL of D5W infuse at 30 mL/h.* Find the flow rate in units/day and determine if it is in the safe dose range—the normal heparinizing range is between 20,000 to 40,000 units per day.

You want to convert the flow rate from milliliters per hour to units per day.

$$\frac{30 \ mL}{1 \ h} \xrightarrow{\quad} ? \frac{units}{day}$$

Using the strength of the solution (40,000 units/1,000 mL) and that there are 24 hours in a day, you do this on one line as follows:

$$\frac{30 \ \cancel{mL}}{\cancel{h}} \times \frac{40{,}\cancel{000} \ units}{1{,}\cancel{000} \ \cancel{mL}} \times \frac{24 \ \cancel{h}}{day} = 28{,}800 \frac{units}{day}$$

So, your patient is receiving 28,800 units of heparin per day. This rate is within the safe dosage range of 20,000 to 40,000 units per day. ●

Example 11.8

Your patient is receiving an IV of 1,000 mL of NS with 1,000 mg of the bronchodilator aminophylline. The flow rate is 50 mL/h. How many milligrams per hour is your patient receiving?

You want to convert the flow rate from milliliters per hour to milligrams per hour.

$$\frac{50 \text{ mL}}{1 \text{ h}} \longrightarrow ? \frac{\text{mg}}{\text{h}}$$

Using the strength of the solution (1,000 mg/1,000 mL) you do this on one line as follows:

$$\frac{50 \text{ mL}}{1 \text{ h}} \times \frac{1{,}000 \text{ mg}}{1{,}000 \text{ mL}} = 50 \frac{\text{mg}}{\text{h}}$$

So, your patient is receiving 50 mL of aminophylline per hour.

Calculating Flow Rates Based on Body Weight

In Chapter 6 you calculated dosages based on *body weight alone*. Suppose a patient weighing 100 kg is to receive a drug at the rate of **2 micrograms per kilogram** (2 mcg/kg). You could convert the single unit of measurement (kg) into the single unit of measurement (mcg), and the patient would receive 200 mcg of the drug as the following computation shows:

$$100 \text{ kg} \times \frac{2 \text{ mcg}}{\text{kg}} = 200 \text{ mcg}$$

In this chapter you will see that some IV medications are not only prescribed based on the patient's body weight, but the amount of drug the patient receives also depends on time. For example, an order might indicate that a drug is to be administered at the rate of **2 micrograms per kilogram per minute** (2 mcg/kg/min). This means that *each minute* the patient is to receive 2 mcg of the drug for every kilogram of body weight. Therefore, the amount of medication the patient receives is based on *both body weight and time*.

For computational purposes this new type of rate (compound rate) is written as

$$\frac{2 \text{ mcg}}{\text{kg} \times \text{min}}$$

Suppose that a patient weighing 100 kg is receiving a drug at the rate of 2 mcg/kg/min. If you multiply the weight of this patient (a single unit of measurement) by the compound rate, you obtain a rate which depends only on *time* as follows:

$$100 \text{ kg} \times \frac{2 \text{ mcg}}{\text{kg} \times \text{min}} = \frac{200 \text{ mcg}}{\text{min}}$$

So, the patient is receiving the drug at the rate of 200 mcg/min.

Example 11.9

The prescriber ordered: *250 mL 5% D/W with 60 mg Aredia 0.006 mg/kg/min IVPB*. The patient weighs 75 kg, and the drop factor is 20 gtt/mL. Calculate the flow rate for this antihypercalcemic drug in drops per minute.

Given: 75 kg (weight of the patient)

Known equivalences: 0.006 mg/kg/min (order)

              60 mg/mL (strength)

              20 gtt/mL (drop factor)

Find: ? gtt/min (flow rate)

As shown , multiplying the weight of the patient by the order will yield a rate based on *time*. This rate can then be converted to the desired flow rate (drops per minute). So you want to start with the weight of the patient (kilograms) and convert to drops per minute.

$$75 \text{ kg} = \text{gtt/min}$$

You want to cancel kg. To do this you must use a fraction containing kg in the denominator. Using the order, this fraction will be $\dfrac{0.006 \text{ mg}}{\text{kg} \times \text{min}}$.

$$75 \text{ kg} \times \frac{0.006 \text{ mg}}{\text{kg} \times \text{min}} = ? \frac{\text{gtt}}{\text{min}}$$

Now, on the left side mg is in the numerator, but you don't want mg. You need a fraction with mg in the denominator. Using the strength of the solution, the fraction is $\dfrac{250 \text{ mL}}{60 \text{ mg}}$.

$$75 \text{ kg} \times \frac{0.006 \text{ mg}}{\text{kg} \times \text{min}} \times \frac{250 \text{ mL}}{60 \text{ mg}} = ? \frac{\text{gtt}}{\text{min}}$$

Now, on the left side mL is in the numerator, but you don't want mL. To cancel the mL you need a fraction with mL in the denominator. Using the drop factor, the fraction is $\dfrac{20 \text{ gtt}}{\text{mL}}$.

Now cancel and multiply the numbers.

$$75 \text{ kg} \times \frac{0.006 \text{ mg}}{\text{kg} \times \text{min}} \times \frac{250 \text{ mL}}{60 \text{ mg}} \times \frac{20 \text{ gtt}}{\text{mL}} = 37.5 \frac{\text{gtt}}{\text{min}}$$

So, the flow rate is 38 gtt/min.

Titrating Medications

Sometimes medications must be *titrated*. That is, the dose of the medication must be adjusted until the desired therapeutic effect (e.g., blood pressure maintenance) is achieved. The following example includes a drug that is titrated.

Example 11.10

Order: *Intropin (dopamine) 2 mcg/kg/min IVPB, titrate to maintain SBP above 90, increase by 5 mcg/kg/min q 10–30 minutes. Maximum dose 20 mcg/kg/min. Monitor BP and HR q 2–5 minutes during titration.* The label on the 500 mL medication bag states 800 mcg/mL, and the patient weighs 175 pounds.

(a) How many mcg/min of Intropin should the patient receive initially?

(b) Calculate the initial pump setting in mL/h.

(a) You want to convert the weight of the patient (175 pounds) to micrograms of Intropin per minute.

$$175 \text{ lb} \longrightarrow ? \frac{\text{mcg}}{\text{min}}$$

Using 1 kg = 2.2 lb and the order (2 mcg/kg/min), you can do this on one line as follows:

$$175 \text{ lb} \times \frac{1 \text{ kg}}{2.2 \text{ lb}} \times \frac{2 \text{ mcg}}{\text{kg} \times \text{min}} = 159 \frac{\text{mcg}}{\text{min}}$$

So, initially the patient will receive 159 mcg/min.

(b) Now, convert $159 \dfrac{\text{mcg}}{\text{min}}$ to $\dfrac{\text{mL}}{\text{h}}$.

Using the strength of the solution (800 mcg/mL) and 1 h = 60 min you can do this on one line as follows:

$$\frac{159 \text{ mcg}}{\text{min}} \times \frac{1 \text{ mL}}{800 \text{ mcg}} \times \frac{60 \text{ min}}{\text{h}} = 11.96 \frac{\text{mL}}{\text{h}}$$

So, the pump would initially be set at 12 mL/h.

Calculating Flow Rates Based on Body Surface Area

As you know, certain medications are ordered based on body surface area (BSA). Chapter 6 discussed how to determine BSA. The following examples show how to calculate flow rates for this type of medication order.

Example 11.11

The order is *100 mg/m² IVPB in 50 mL NS*. The patient has BSA of 1.55 m². The package insert indicates that the infusion should be given in 30 minutes. The label on the vial indicates that the strength of the reconstituted drug is 38 mg/mL.

(a) How many mg of the drug would the patient receive?
(b) How many mL of the drug would you need to take from the vial?
(c) What is the total volume (in mL) to be infused?
(d) What is the flow rate in mL/h?
(e) If the drop factor is 10 gtt/mL, what is the rate of flow in gtt/min?

(a) You want to change the size of the patient (in m²) to the number of milligrams of the drug.

$$1.55 \text{ m}^2 \longrightarrow ? \text{ mg}$$

$$1.55 \text{ m}^2 \times \frac{100 \text{ mg}}{\text{m}^2} = 155 \text{ mg}$$

NOTE

Verify the institution's policy concerning IV medications that are reconstituted for administration. Determine whether in the calculations, the total volume to be infused must include the volume of the added reconstituted medication. For example, in Example 11.11 if the volume of the reconstituted drug added to the IVPB bag (4.1 mL) had been ignored in the calculations, the answer to part (d) would have been ($50\text{ mL}/\frac{1}{2}\text{h}$) 100 mL/h instead of 108.2 mL/h.

So, the patient would receive 155 mg of the drug.

(b) You want to convert the amount of drug (in mg) to the volume of drug (in mL).

$$155\text{ mg} \longrightarrow ?\text{ mL}$$

The label indicates that the strength of the reconstituted the drug is 38 mg/mL.

$$155\ \cancel{\text{mg}} \times \frac{1\text{ mL}}{38\ \cancel{\text{mg}}} = 4.1\text{ mL}$$

Since your patient should receive 4.1 mL of the drug, 4.1 mL should be withdrawn from the vial.

(c) Since the 4.1 mL of the drug must be added to the 50 mL bag, the total volume to be infused will be (50 + 4.1) 54.1 mL.

(d) Since the entire volume must infuse in 30 minutes ($\frac{1}{2}$ hour), the flow rate, in milliliters per hour, is $\dfrac{54.1\text{ mL}}{\frac{1}{2}\text{h}} = 108.2\dfrac{\text{mL}}{\text{h}}$.

(e) Since the drop factor is 10 gtt = 1 mL, the flow rate found in part (d) can be converted to gtt/min as follows:

$$\frac{108.2\ \cancel{\text{mL}}}{\cancel{\text{h}}} \times \frac{10\text{ gtt}}{\cancel{\text{mL}}} \times \frac{1\ \cancel{\text{h}}}{60\text{ min}} = 18.03\frac{\text{gtt}}{\text{min}}$$

So, the flow rate, in drops per minute, is 18 gtt/min.

NDC 0009-7529-01
5 mL
CAMPTOSAR®
irinotecan hydrochloride injection
100 mg/5 mL
(20 mg/mL)
—on basis of trihydrate
INTRAVENOUS USE ONLY
See package insert for complete product information.
Store at controlled room temperature 15° to 30°C (59° to 86°F).
Protect from freezing.
Pharmacia & Upjohn Company
A subsidiary of Pharmacia Corporation
Kalamazoo, MI 49001
816904205
LOT/EXP

● **Figure 11.4**
Drug label for Camptosar.

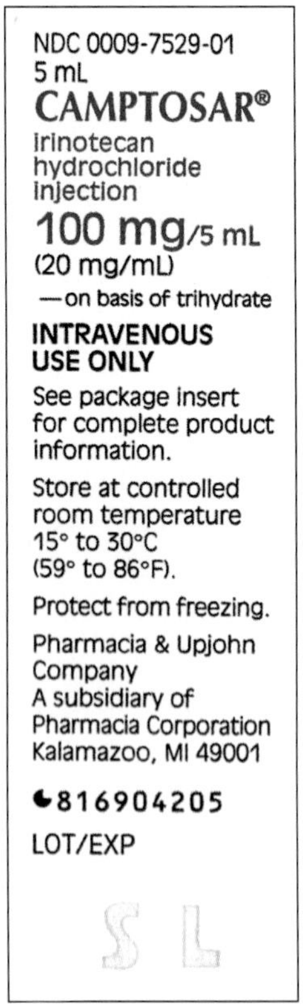

Example 11.12

Order: *Camptosar 125 mg/m² IVPB in 250 mL of NS over 90 minutes once weekly for 4 weeks.* The patient has a BSA of 1.67 m^2. Read the label for this antineoplastic drug in ● **Figure 11.4** and determine the pump setting in milliliters per hour.

First change the size of the patient (BSA) to the number of milliliters needed to be taken from the Camptosar vial.

$$1.67\text{ m}^2 \longrightarrow ?\text{ mL}$$

From the order, you need to use 125 mg/m^2; and from the label, the concentration of the Camptosar is 100 mg/5 mL.

$$1.67\ \cancel{\text{m}^2} \times \frac{125\ \cancel{\text{mg}}}{\cancel{\text{m}^2}} \times \frac{5\text{ mL}}{100\ \cancel{\text{mg}}} = 10.4\text{ mL}$$

So, 10.4 mL is taken from the Camptosar vial and is added to the 250 mL bag. This means that the total volume of the infusion is (250 + 10.4) 260.4 mL, and the patient would receive 260.4 mL of Camptosar in 90 minutes.

Now, change the flow rate of $\dfrac{260.4 \text{ mL}}{90 \text{ min}}$ to mL/h.

$$\dfrac{260.4 \text{ mL}}{90 \text{ min}} \times \dfrac{60 \text{ min}}{\text{h}} = 173.6 \text{ mL/h}$$

So, the pump is set at 174 mL/h.

Example 11.13

Order: Infuse *50 mL IVPB in $\frac{1}{2}$ hour*. After 20 minutes, it is discovered that 30 mL still remain to be infused. Recalculate the rate of flow in *gtt/min* if the drop factor of the administration set is *20 gtt/mL*.

Since the remaining volume (30 mL) must infuse in the remaining time (10 minutes), the flow rate is 30 mL/10 minutes.
You want to change 30 mL/10 minutes to gtt/minute. Since the drop factor is 20 gtt/mL:

$$\dfrac{30 \text{ mL}}{10 \text{ min}} \times \dfrac{20 \text{ gtt}}{\text{mL}} = 60 \dfrac{\text{gtt}}{\text{min}}$$

So, the flow rate is $60 \dfrac{\text{gtt}}{\text{min}}$.

Example 11.14

The prescriber ordered Vancomycin 1.5 g in 200 mL of D_5W. Infuse in 60 minutes, the label reads: 1.5 g of Vancomycin. The vial available is used with a reconstitution device similar to that shown in ● **Figure 11.5**. The tubing is labeled 15 drops per milliliter. Calculate the flow rate in drops per minute.
You want to change the flow rate from milliliters per minute to gtt/min.

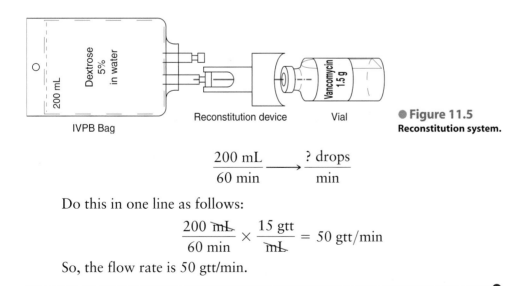

IVPB Bag   Reconstitution device   Vial

● **Figure 11.5**
Reconstitution system.

$$\dfrac{200 \text{ mL}}{60 \text{ min}} \longrightarrow \dfrac{? \text{ drops}}{\text{min}}$$

Do this in one line as follows:

$$\dfrac{200 \text{ mL}}{60 \text{ min}} \times \dfrac{15 \text{ gtt}}{\text{mL}} = 50 \text{ gtt/min}$$

So, the flow rate is 50 gtt/min.

There are reconstitution systems that enable the healthcare provider to reconstitute a powdered drug and place it into an IVPB bag without using a syringe. One such device is shown in Figure 11.5. With this device, when the IVPB bag is squeezed, fluid is forced into the vial, dissolving the powder. The system is then placed in a vertical configuration with the vial on top and the IVPB bag on the bottom. The IVPB bag is then squeezed and released, thereby creating a negative pressure, which allows the newly reconstituted drug to flow into the IVPB bag.

Another reconstitution device is the ADD-Vantage system, which employs an IV bag containing intravenous fluid. The bag is designed with a special port, which will accept a vial of medication. When the vial is placed into the bag port, the contents of the vial and the fluid mix to form the desired solution.

Example 11.15

A patient who weighs 55 kg is receiving a medication at the rate of 30 mL/h. The concentration of the medication is 400 mg in 500 mL of D5W. The recommended dose range for the drug is 2–5 mcg/kg/min. Is the patient receiving a safe dose?

Method 1 Convert the safe dose range of 2–5 mcg/kg/min to mL (of the drug)/hour.

First, use the minimum recommended dose (2 mcg/kg/h) and start with the weight of the patient to determine how many mL/h the patient should minimally receive as follows:

$$55 \text{ kg} \times \frac{2 \text{ mcg}}{\text{kg} \times \text{min}} \times \frac{60 \text{ min}}{\text{h}} \times \frac{1 \text{ mg}}{1,000 \text{ mcg}} \times \frac{500 \text{ mL}}{400 \text{ mg}} = 8.3 \frac{\text{mL}}{\text{h}} \text{ Min}$$

Now, use the maximum recommended dose (5 mcg/kg/h) and start with the weight of the patient to determine how many mL/h the patient should maximally receive as follows:

$$55 \text{ kg} \times \frac{5 \text{ mcg}}{\text{kg} \times \text{min}} \times \frac{60 \text{ min}}{\text{h}} \times \frac{1 \text{ mg}}{1,000 \text{ mcg}} \times \frac{500 \text{ mL}}{400 \text{ mg}} = 20.6 \frac{\text{mL}}{\text{h}} \text{ Max}$$

So, the safe dose range for this patient is 8.3–20.6 mL/h. Since the patient is receiving 30 mL/h, the patient is not receiving a safe dose, but is receiving an overdose.

Method 2 Convert the 30 mL/h, which the patient is receiving, to mcg/kg/min and then compare this to the safe dose range of 2–5 mcg/kg/min.

This may be a mathematically more sophisticated approach, but it requires fewer calculations.

Realize that what you are looking for, mcg/kg/min, is in the form of amount of drug/weight of patient/time.

An amount of drug (30 mL) is being administered to a (55 kg) patient over a period of time (1 hour). So, the patient is receiving 30 mL/55kg/1h.

You want to change 30 mL/55kg/1h to mcg/kg/min, which can be done in one line as follows:

$$\frac{30 \text{ mL}}{55 \text{ kg} \times 1 \text{ h}} \times \frac{1 \text{ h}}{60 \text{ min}} \times \frac{400 \text{ mg}}{500 \text{ mL}} \times \frac{1,000 \text{ mcg}}{1 \text{ mg}} = 7.3 \frac{\text{mcg}}{\text{kg} \times \text{min}}$$

The safe dose range for this patient is 2–5 mcg/kg/min, and since the patient is receiving 7.3 mcg/kg/min, the patient is not receiving a safe dose, but an overdose.

NOTE

Whenever your calculations indicate that the prescribed dose is not within the safe range, you should verify the order with the prescriber.

Summary

In this chapter, the IV medication administration process was discussed. IVPB and IVP infusions were described, and orders based on body weight and body surface area were illustrated.

- A secondary line is referred to as an IV piggyback.
- IV push, or bolus, medications can be injected into a heplock/saline lock or directly into the vein.
- The IV bag that is hung highest will infuse first.
- An order containing *mg/kg/min* directs that each minute, the patient must receive the stated number of milligrams of medication for each kilogram of the patient's body weight.

- For calculation purposes write mg/kg/min as $\dfrac{mg}{kg \times min}$.
- When calculating rates of flow of infusions based on body weight or BSA, start with the patient's size, as measured by weight or BSA.
- When looking for *mg/kg/min*, start with the amount of *drug/weight/time*.
- When titrating medications, the dose is adjusted until the desired therapeutic effect is achieved.

Case Study 11.1

A woman is admitted to the labor room with a diagnosis of preterm labor. She states that she has not seen a physician because this is her third baby and she "knows what to do while she is pregnant." Her initial workup indicates a gestational age of 32 weeks, and she tests positive for Chlamydia and Strep-B. Her vital signs are: T 100 °F; P 98; R 18; B/P 140/88; and the fetal heart rate is 140–150. The orders include the following:

- NPO
- IV fluids: D5/RL 1,000 mL q8h
- Electronic fetal monitoring
- Vital signs q4h
- dexamethasone 6 mg IM q12h for 2 doses
- Brethine (terbutaline sulfate) 0.25 mg subcutaneous q30 minutes for 2h
- Rocephin (ceftriaxone sodium) 250 mg IM stat

- Penicillin G 5 million units IVPB stat; then 2.5 million units q4h
- Zithromax (azithromycin) 500 mg IVPB stat and daily for 2 days

1. Calculate the rate of flow for the D5/RL in mL/h.
2. The label on the dexamethasone reads 8 mg/mL. How many milliliters will you administer?
3. The label on the terbutaline reads 1 mg/mL. How many milliliters will you administer?
4. The label on the ceftriaxone states to reconstitute the 1 g vial with 2.1 mL of sterile water for injection, which results in a strength of 350 mg/mL. How many milliliters will you administer?
5. The instructions state to reconstitute the penicillin G (use the minimum amount of diluent), add to 100 mL D5W, and infuse in one hour. The drop factor is 15. What is the rate of flow in gtts/min? See the label in ● **Figure 11.6**

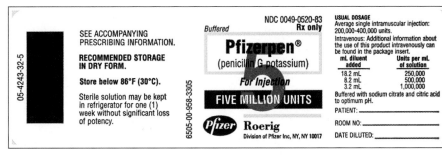

● **Figure 11.6**
Drug label for penicillin G.   *(Reg. Trademark of Pfizer Inc. Reproduced with permission.)*

6. The instructions for the azithromycin state to reconstitute the 500 mg vial with 4.8 mL until dissolved, and add to 250 mL of D5W and administer over at least 60 minutes. What rate will you set the infusion pump if you choose to administer the medication over 90 minutes?

7. The patient continues to have uterine contractions, and a new order has been written: *magnesium sulfate 4g IV bolus over 20 minutes, then 1g/h.*

   The label on the IV bag states magnesium sulfate 40 g in 1,000 mL.
   (a) What is the rate of flow in mL/h for the bolus dose?
   (b) What is the rate of flow in mL/h for the maintenance dose?

The patient continues to have contractions and her membranes rupture. The following orders are written:
- Discontinue the magnesium sulfate.
- Pitocin (oxytocin) 10 units/1,000 mL RL, start at 0.5 mU/min increase by 1 mU/min q20 minutes.
- Stadol (butorphanol tartrate) 1 mg IVP stat.

8. What is the rate of flow in mL/h for the initial dose of Pitocin?

9. The Pitocin is infusing at 9 mL/h. How many mU/h is the patient receiving?

10. The vial of butorphanol tartrate is labeled 2 mg/mL. How many milliliters will you administer?

Workspace

Practice Sets

The answers to *Try These for Practice, Exercises,* and *Cumulative Review Exercises* appear in Appendix A at the end of the book. Ask your instructor for answers to the *Additional Exercises.*

Try These for Practice

Test your comprehension after reading the chapter.

1. Order: *Tagamet (cimetidine) 300 mg IVPB q6h in 50 mL NS infuse over 30 min.* The drop factor is 15 gtt/mL. Find the flow rate in gtt/min.

2. The order is for a continuous infusion of theophylline at a rate of 25 mg/h. It is diluted in 5% dextrose to produce a concentration of 500 mg per 500 mL. Determine the rate of the infusion in mL/h.

3. A 500 mL D5W solution with 2 g of Pronestyl (procainamide HCl) is infusing at 15 mL/h via a volumetric pump. How many mg/h is the patient receiving?

4. Order: *Dobutrex (dobutamine) 250 mg in 250 mL of D5W at 3.5 mcg/kg/min.* Determine the flow rate in mcgtt/min for a patient who weighs 120 pounds.

5. A patient is receiving heparin 1,200 units/hour. The directions for the infusion are, add *"25,000 units of heparin in 250 mL of solution."* Determine the flow rate in mL/h.

Exercises

Reinforce your understanding in class or at home.

1. The patient is to receive 20 mEq of KCl (potassium chloride) in 100 mL of IV fluid at the rate of 10 mEq/h. What is the flow rate in microdrops per minute?

2. A maintenance dose of *Levophed (norepinephrine bitartrate) 2 mcg/min IVPB* has been ordered to infuse using an 8 mg in 250 mL of D5W solution. What is the pump setting in mL/h?

3. The patient is receiving lidocaine at 40 mL/h. The concentration of the medication is 1 g per 500 mL of IV fluid. How many mg/min is the patient receiving?

4. Order: *dopamine 400 mg in 250 mL D5W at 3 mcg/kg/min IVPB*. Calculate the flow rate in mL/h for a patient who weighs 91 kg.

5. A drug is ordered 180 mg/m^2 in 500 mL NS to infuse over 90 minutes. The BSA is 1.38 m^2. What is the flow rate in mL/h?

6. How long will a 550 mL bag of intralipids take to infuse at the rate of 25 mL/h?

7. The patient is receiving heparin at 1,000 units/hour. The IV has been prepared with 24,000 units of heparin per liter. Find the flow rate in mL/h.

8. Order: *Humulin R 50 units in 500 mL NS infuse at 1 mL/min IVPB*. How many units per hour is the patient receiving?

9. An IVPB of 50 mL is to infuse in 30 minutes. After 15 minutes, the IV bag contains 40 mL. If the drop factor is 20 gtt/mL, recalculate the flow rate in gtt/min.

10. The patient is receiving *Nipride (nitroprusside) 50 mg in 250 mL of D5W* for hypertension. The rate of flow is 20 mL/h. If the patient weighs 75 kg, determine the dosage in micrograms/kilogram/minute the patient is receiving.

11. Order: *Coumadin (warfarin sodium) 4 mg IVP stat administer over 1 minute*. The available 5 mg of Coumadin is in a vial with directions that state to dilute with 2 mL of sterile water:
    (a) How many mg will the patient receive?
    (b) How many mL will you administer?
    (c) How many mL/min will be infused?

12. The patient is to receive Aldomet (methyldopa) 500 mg IVPB dissolved in 100 mL of IV fluid over 60 minutes. If the drop factor is 15 gtt/mL, determine the rate of flow in gtt/min.

13. The patient is to receive Isuprel (isoproterenol) at a rate of 4 mcg/min. The concentration of the Isuprel is 2 mg per 500 mL of IV fluid. Find the pump setting in mL/h.

14. The patient is receiving aminophylline at the rate of 20 mL/h. The concentration of the medication is 500 mg/1,000 mL of IV fluid. How many mg/h is the patient receiving?

15. Nipride 3 mcg/kg/min has been ordered for a patient who weighs 82 kg. The solution has a strength of 50 mg in 250 mL of D5W. Calculate the flow rate in mL/h.

16. A medication is ordered at 75 mg/m^2 IVP. The patient has BSA of 2.33 m^2. How many milliliters of the medication will be administered if the vial is labeled 50 mg/mL?

17. A liter of D5/$\frac{1}{4}$NS with 10 units of Regular insulin is started at 9:55 A.M. at a rate of 22 gtt/mim. If the drop factor is 20 gtt/min, when will the infusion finish?

18. Mefoxin 2 g in 100 mL NS IVPB. Infuse in 1 hour. After 30 minutes, 70 mL remain in the bag. Reset the flow rate on the pump in mL/h.

19. Order: *heparin sodium 40,000 units IV in 500 mL of $\frac{1}{2}$ NS to infuse at 1,200 units/hour.* What is the flow rate in mL/h?

20. The patient is receiving Dobutrex (dobutamine) at a rate of 18 mcgtt/min. The concentration is 250 mg/250 mL of IV fluid. Determine the dosage in microdrops/kilogram/minute that the 150-pound patient is receiving.

Additional Exercises

Now, test yourself!

1. Physician's order:
   Dobutamine (Dobutrex) 500 mg in 500 mL D₅W, 6 mcg/kg/min IVPB. Weight 145 lb.
   (a) Set the flow rate on the infusion pump in milliliters per hour. _____
   (b) If the above infusion begins at 6 A.M., when will it be completed? _____

2. Order: *Amiodarone 160 mg in 20 mL D₅W IVPB; infuse over 10 minutes.* The label reads 50 mg/mL. The drop factor is 60 mcgtt/mL. Calculate the flow rate in mcgtt/min. _____

3. The dose of amiodarone (Cordarone) in Question 2 is increased to 720 mg in 24 hours in 500 mL D₅W. Set the rate on the infusion pump in milliliters per hour. _____

4. Pamidronate disodium (Aredia), an antihypercalcemic drug, 0.09 g IV has been prescribed. The label reads: Add 10 mL to a 90 mg vial.
   (a) How many milliliters contain the prescribed dose?_____
   (b) Add the correct amount of Aredia to 1,000 mL of 0.45% NaCl and infuse in 24 hours. Set the flow rate on the infusion pump in milliliters per hour._____

5. Order: *lidocaine HCl IV drip 0.75 mg/kg in 500 mL D5W.* The patient weighs 150 pounds.
   (a) How many milliliters of lidocaine 2% will be needed to prepare the IV solution? _____
   (b) Calculate the flow rate in mL/h in order for the patient to receive 5 mg/h. _____

6. Order: *Diltiazem (Cardizem) 0.25 mg/kg IV push over 2 min.* The label on the vial reads 5 mg/mL. The patient weighs 210 pounds.
   (a) How many milligrams of Cardizem will the patient receive?_____
   (b) How many milliliters contain the dose of medication?_____

7. Physician's order:
   Phenytoin (Dilantin) 500 mg IV push over 10 min
   The label on the vial reads 50 mg/mL.
   (a) How many milliliters will you prepare? _____
   (b) Calculate the flow rate in microdrops per minute. _____

8. The loading dose of digoxin is 0.25 mg IV push q6h for 4 doses. The label on the ampule reads 0.5 mg/mL. How many milliliters contain this dose?_____

9. The prescriber ordered cefuroxime 18 mg/kg IVPB in 200 mL NS. Infuse in 1.5 hours. The patient weighs 80 kg. The label on the vial states that after reconstitution the strength is 3 g/32 mL.
   (a) How many milligrams of cefuroxime will the patient receive?_____

   (b) How many milliliters of cefuroxime will you add to the 200 mL of NS?
   _____

   (c) Calculate the flow rate in milliliters per hour._____

10. Adenocor, (adenosine) 6 mg IV push over 1-2 seconds has been prescribed for your patient. The label on the vial reads 3 mg/mL. How many milliliters will you prepare? _____

11. The order for *cefuroxime is 500 mg in 100 mL D$_5$W IVPB q8h; infuse in 20 min*. The vial states: "add 77 mL of sterile water, and the concentration is 750 mg/8 mL."
   (a) How many milliliters of cefuroxime contain this dose? _____
   (b) Calculate the flow rate in milliliters per minute. _____

12. Your patient has developed bradycardia, and Atropine gr $\frac{1}{60}$ IV push stat is ordered. The label reads 0.5 mg/mL. How many milliliters will you administer? _____

13. Ritodrine HCL (Yutopar) 150 mg added to 500 mL D$_5$W has been ordered for a patient who is having premature uterine contractions.
   (a) Calculate the flow rate in microdrops per minute over a 15-hour period.
   _____

   (b) Change the flow rate to milliliters per hour. _____

14. A patient has been admitted to the ER with a diagnosis of lead poisoning. The physician orders edetate calcium disodium (calcium EDTA) 1.5 g/m^2 IV. The BSA is 2.0 m^2. The label on the vial reads 200 mg/mL. Add the prescribed amount of drug to 250 mL D$_5$W and infuse at a rate of 11 mL/h. At what time will the infusion finish if it begins at 10 A.M.?
   _____

15. The order is *cefuroxime 1.5 g added to 100 mL NS infuse in 60 minutes IVPB*. The strength of the cefuroxime is 750 mg per 8 mL.
   (a) How many milliliters of cefuroxime will you add to the normal saline solution?
   (b) Calculate the milligrams per minute the patient is receiving.

16. The order is Narcan maxolone (a narcotic antidote) 2 mg IV push. The vial reads 0.4 mg/mL. How many milliliters will you give the patient?
   _____

17. Prescriber order:
   Sufentanil 6 mcg/kg IVPB in 100 mL D$_5$W, infuse over 30 minutes. Weight 172 lb. The label states that the concentration is 50 mcg/mL. Each ampule contains 1 mL.
   (a) How many milliliters contain the prescribed dose? _____

   (b) How many ampules of this drug will you need? _____

   (c) How many microdrops are infused per minute?_____

18. The prescriber ordered *morphine sulfate 50 mg to be added to 250 mL of NS IVPB. Infuse in 5 hours.* The strength of the morphine is 1 mg/mL.

    (a) How many milliliters contain the prescribed dose? _____

    (b) Calculate the flow rate in milliliters per hour. _____

    (c) After 90 minutes, the patient had breakthrough pain, and the physician increased the morphine to 15 mg/h. Recalculate the flow rate. _____

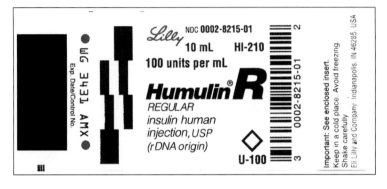

● **Figure 11.7**
Drug label for Regular insulin.

(Reproduced with permission of GlaxoSmithKline.)

19. The prescriber ordered a continuous IV insulin drip of *500 units of Regular insulin added to 250 mL 0.45% NaCl q12h.* Read the information on the label in ● **Figure 11.7.**

    Calculate the flow rate in units per hour. _____

20. You have an infusion of heparin 50,000 units in 500 mL D$_5$W. The patient is receiving 1,500 units/h. What is the setting on the pump? _____

Cumulative Review Exercises

Review your mastery of earlier chapters.

1. The patient weighs 130 pounds. The medication order for a drug is 150 mcg/kg of body weight. The label reads 2 mg/mL. How many milliliters of solution are equal to the medication order? _____

2. The prescriber ordered 0.04 mg of Methergine (methylergonovine maleate) PO q6h. How many tablets will you prepare if the label reads 0.02 mg/tab? _____

3. The patient must receive 1,500,000 units of penicillin IM, and the vial contains 20,000,000 units (in powdered form). The directions are as follows: Add 38.7 mL to vial; 1 mL = 500,000 units. How many milliliters will equal 1,500,000 units? _____

4. A patient must receive 0.5 mg of scopolamine IM, a parasympathetic antagonist. The label on the ampule reads 0.3 mg/mL. How many milliliters will you administer to this patient? _____

5. The prescriber ordered *cefprozil 200 mg PO q12h for 10 days.* The bottle is labeled 100 mg/5 mL. How many milliliters of this antibiotic will you give your patient?_____

6. If you have a vial labeled 120 mg/mL, how many milliliters would equal 1.2 g? _____

7. If tablets are 250 mg each, how many tablets equal 0.5 g? _____

8. The prescriber has requested that you give 40 mEq of potassium chloride (K-Lor) PO to a patient from a bottle labeled 10 mEq/5 mL. How many milliliters are needed? _____

9. 2,400 mL = _____ L

10. 0.6 mg = gr _____

11. 23 mL/h = _____ mcgtt/min

12. 5 pt = _____ qt

13. 500 mcg = _____ mg

14. 1 T = _____ t

15. 45 mL = _____ oz

MediaLink
www.prenhall.com/olsen   Animated examples, interactive practice questions with animated solutions, and challenge tests for this chapter can be found on the Prentice Hall Dosage Calculation Tutor that accompanies this text. Additional, unique, interactive resources and activities can be found on the Companion Website.

Calculating Pediatric Dosages

Learning Outcomes

After completing this chapter, you will be able to

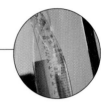

1. Determine if a pediatric dose is within the safe dose range.
2. Calculate pediatric oral and parenteral dosages based on body weight.
3. Calculate pediatric oral and parenteral dosages based on body surface area.
4. Calculate daily fluid maintenance.

Because the metabolism and body mass of children are different from those of adults, pediatric medication dosages are usually less than adult dosages. In this chapter, you will be applying dimensional analysis to the calculation of pediatric dosages.

Pediatric dosages are generally rounded down, instead of rounded off, because of the danger overdose poses to infants and children.

Safe Pediatric Drug Dosages

For many years, pediatric dosage calculations used formulas such as Fried's rule, Young's rule, and Clark's rule. These formulas were based on the weight of the child in pounds, or on the age of the child in months, and the normal adult dose of a specific drug. By using these formulas, one could determine how much should be prescribed for a particular child.

At the present time, the most accurate method of determining an appropriate pediatric dose is based on body weight. Body surface area is also used, especially in pediatric oncology and critical care. You must be able to determine whether the amount of a prescribed pediatric dosage is within the safe range. In order to do this, you must compare the child's ordered dosage to the recommended safe dosage as found in a reputable drug resource. First, determine the recommended dose or dosage range found on the package insert, in the hospital formulary, in the *Physician's Desk Reference (PDR)*, in the *United States Pharmacopeia*, or in a pharmacology text.

Administration of Oral and Parenteral Medications

When prescribing medications for the pediatric population, the oral route is preferred. However, if a child cannot swallow, or the medication is ineffective when given orally, the parenteral route is used.

Oral Medications

The developmental age of the child must be taken into consideration when determining the device to administer oral medication. For example, an older child may be able to swallow a pill or drink a liquid medication from a cup. An oral syringe, calibrated dropper, or measuring spoon may be selected when giving medication to an infant or younger child. ●**Figures 12.1** and **12.2**

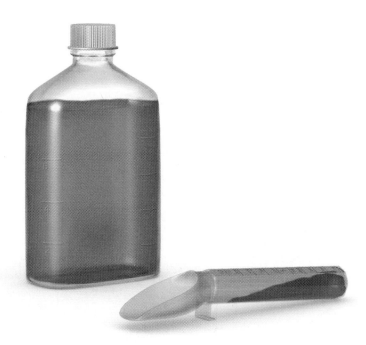

● **Figure 12.1**
Measuring spoon.

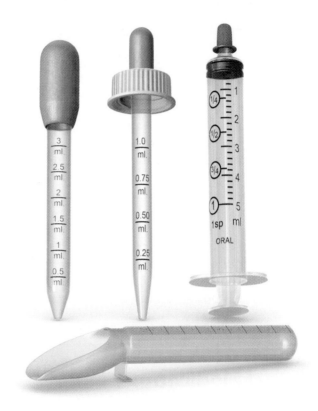

● **Figure 12.2**
Liquid medication administration.

Parenteral Medications

Subcutaneous or intramuscular routes may be necessary depending on the type of medication to be administered. Because of the small muscle mass of children, usually not more than 1 mL is injected.

Calculating Drug Dosages by Body Weight

Drug manufacturers sometimes recommend a dosage based on the weight of the patient. Body weight is most frequently used when prescribing drugs for infants and children.

Example 12.1

The medication order reads:
erythromycin 10mg/kg PO q8h
Read the label in ● **Figure 12.3**. The child weighs 40 kg. How many milliliters of the drug will you administer to this child?

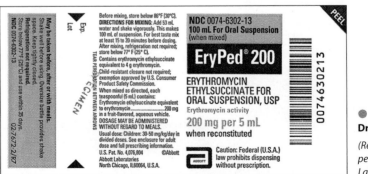

● **Figure 12.3**
Drug label EryPed 200.

(Reproduced with permission of Abbott Laboratories.)

You want to convert the body weight to the dose in milliliters.

$$40 \text{ kg} \longrightarrow ? \text{ mL}$$

Do this problem on one line as follows:

$$40 \text{ kg} \times \frac{? \text{ mg}}{? \text{ kg}} \times \frac{? \text{ mL}}{? \text{ mg}} = ? \text{ mL}$$

Because the order is 10 mg/kg, the first unit fraction is $\dfrac{10 \text{ mg}}{1 \text{ kg}}$.

Because the strength is 200 mg/5 mL, the second unit fraction is $\dfrac{5 \text{ mL}}{200 \text{ mg}}$.
You cancel the kilograms and milligrams and obtain the dose in milliliters.

$$40 \cancel{\text{ kg}} \times \frac{10 \cancel{\text{ mg}}}{\cancel{\text{kg}}} \times \frac{5 \text{ mL}}{200 \cancel{\text{ mg}}} = 10 \text{ mL}$$

So, the child should receive 10 mL of erythromycin.

Example 12.2

The order is for Ceftin (cefuroxime) 15mg/kg PO q12h. How many milligrams of this antibiotic would you administer to a child who weights 25 kg?

You want to convert body weight to a dose in milligrams.

$$25 \text{ kg} \longrightarrow ? \text{ mg}$$

$$25 \text{ kg} \times \frac{? \text{ mg}}{? \text{ kg}} = ? \text{ mg}$$

Because the order is 15 mg/kg the unit fraction is $\dfrac{15 \text{ mg}}{\text{kg}}$.

You cancel the kilograms and obtain the dose in milligrams.

$$25 \cancel{\text{ kg}} \times \frac{15 \text{ mg}}{\cancel{\text{kg}}} = 375 \text{ mg}$$

So, the child would receive 375 mg of cefuroxime.

Example 12.3

The prescriber ordered:

Zithromax (azithromycin) 15 mg /kg PO stat

Read the information on the label in ●**Figure 12.4**. The child weighs 18 kg. How many milliliters would contain this dose?

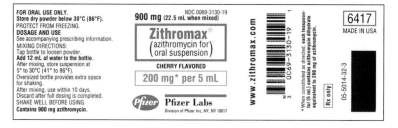

●**Figure 12.4**
Drug label for Zithromax.   *(Reg. Trademark of Pfizer Inc. Reproduced with permission.)*

You want to convert the body weight to a dose in milliliters.

$$18 \text{ kg} \longrightarrow ? \text{ mL}$$

Do this on one line as follows:

$$18 \text{ kg} \times \frac{? \text{ mg}}{? \text{ kg}} \times \frac{? \text{ mL}}{? \text{ mg}} = ? \text{ mL}$$

Because the order is 15 mg/kg, the first unit fraction is $\dfrac{15 \text{ mg}}{\text{kg}}$

Because the strength is 200 mg per 5 mL the second unit fraction is $\dfrac{5 \text{ mL}}{200 \text{ mg}}$.

$$18 \text{ \cancel{kg}} \times \frac{15 \text{ \cancel{mg}}}{\cancel{kg}} \times \frac{5 \text{ mL}}{200 \text{ \cancel{mg}}} = 6.75 \text{ mL}$$

So, you would prepare 6.7 mL of zithromax.

Example 12.4

The recommended dosage for neonates receiving *Tazidime (ceftazidime)* is 30mg/kg IM every 12 hours. If an infant weighs 2,600 grams how many milligrams of Tazidime would the neonate receive in one day?

You want to convert the body weight to a dose in milligrams.

$$2,600 \text{ g (body weight)} \longrightarrow ? \text{ mg (drug)}$$

Do this on one line as follows:

$$2,600 \text{ g} \times \frac{? \text{ kg}}{? \text{ g}} \times \frac{? \text{ mg}}{? \text{ kg}} = ? \text{ mg}$$

Because 1 kg = 1,000 g, the first unit fraction is $\dfrac{1 \text{ kg}}{1,000 \text{ g}}$.

Because the recommended dosage is 30 mg/kg, the second equivalent fraction is $\dfrac{30 \text{ mg}}{1 \text{ kg}}$.

$$2,600 \text{ \cancel{g}} \times \frac{1 \text{ \cancel{kg}}}{1,000 \text{ \cancel{g}}} \times \frac{30 \text{ mg}}{\cancel{kg}} = 78 \text{ mg} \text{ per dose}$$

Since the neonate receives two doses per day, the total daily dose is 156 mg.

Example 12.5

The order reads:

morphine sulfate 0.3 mg IM stat

The recommended dose is 0.01 milligram per kilogram. Is the ordered dose safe for a child who weighs 31 kg?

You want to convert the body weight to the recommended dose in milligrams.

$$31 \text{ kg} \longrightarrow ? \text{ mg}$$

$$31 \text{ kg} \times \frac{? \text{ mg}}{? \text{ kg}} = ? \text{ mg}$$

Because the recommended dose is 0.01 mg/kg, the unit fraction is $\dfrac{0.01 \text{ mg}}{\text{kg}}$

You cancel the kilograms and obtain the dose in milligrams.

$$31\text{ kg} \times \frac{0.01 \text{ mg}}{1 \text{ kg}} = 0.31 \text{ mg}$$

The recommended dose is 0.31 mg, whereas the ordered dose is 0.3 mg. So, 0.3 mg is a safe dose of morphine sulfate for this child.

Example 12.6

The order reads Kantrex (kanamycin sulfate) 30 mg IM q 12h for a child who weighs 9 lb. The recommended dosage for adults or children is 15 mg/kg/day in two equally divided doses. The vial is labeled 75 mg/2 mL.

(a) What is the recommended dosage in mg/day, and is the order safe?

(b) How many milliliters would you administer for one dose?

(a) You want to convert the body weight in pounds to kilograms and then convert the body weight in kilograms to the recommended dose in milligrams per day.

$$9 \text{ lb (body weight)} \longrightarrow \text{kg (body weight)} \longrightarrow \text{mg (drug)}$$

Do this on one line as follows:

$$\frac{9 \text{ lb}}{1} \times \frac{? \text{ kg}}{? \text{ lb}} \times \frac{? \text{ mg}}{? \text{ kg} \times \text{d}} = \frac{? \text{ mg}}{\text{d}}$$

Because 1 kg = 2.2 lb, the first unit fraction is $\dfrac{1 \text{ kg}}{2.2 \text{ lb}}$.

Because the recommended dosage is 15mg/kg per day, the second unit fraction is $\dfrac{15 \text{ mg}}{\text{kg} \times \text{day}}$.

$$\frac{9 \text{ lb}}{1} \times \frac{1 \text{ kg}}{2.2 \text{ lb}} \times \frac{15 \text{ mg}}{\text{kg} \times \text{day}} = 61.3 \frac{\text{mg}}{\text{day}}$$

Since the patient receives 2 doses per day:

$$\frac{61.3 \text{ mg}}{\text{day}} \times \frac{\text{day}}{2 \text{ doses}} = 30.6 \frac{\text{mg}}{\text{dose}}$$

Because the recommended dose is 30.6 mg, and the ordered dose is 30 mg, then the order is safe.

You want to convert the ordered drug dosage in milligrams (mg) to milliliters (mL).

$$\text{mg (drug)} \longrightarrow \text{mL (drug)}$$

Do this on one line as follows:

$$30 \text{ mg} \times \frac{? \text{ mL}}{? \text{ mg}} = ? \text{ mL}$$

Because the vial label says 75 mg/2 mL, the unit fraction is $\dfrac{2\text{mL}}{75 \text{ mg}}$.

$$\frac{30 \text{ mg}}{1} \times \frac{2 \text{ mL}}{75 \text{ mg}} = 0.8 \text{ mL}$$

So, you would administer 0.8 mL for one dose.

Calculating Drug Dosages by Body Surface Area

Drug manufacturers may recommend a pediatric dosage based on body surface area (BSA).

Example 12.7

If a child has a BSA of 0.75 m^2, and the medication order is for Cosmegen (dactinomycin) 0.5 mg/m^2 daily for 5 days IVP, what dose (in milligrams) of this antineoplastic drug should the child receive?

You want to convert the body surface area to a dose in milligrams.

$$0.75 \text{ m}^2 \longrightarrow \text{? mg}$$

$$0.75 \text{ m}^2 \times \frac{\text{? mg}}{\text{? m}^2} = \text{? mg}$$

Because the order is 0.5 mg/m^2, the unit fraction is $\dfrac{0.5 \text{ mg}}{\text{m}^2}$.

You cancel the square meters and obtain the dose in milligrams.

$$\frac{0.75 \text{ m}^2}{1} \times \frac{0.5 \text{ mg}}{1 \text{ m}^2} = 0.375 \text{ mg}$$

So, 0.37 mg of Cosmegen should be administered.

Example 12.8

The prescriber has ordered 15 mg/m^2 of Cortef (hydrocortisone cypionate) PO. The child weighs 40 kg and is 45 inches tall. Read the label in ● Figure 12.5 and determine how many milliliters this child should receive.

You want to find the body surface area and convert it to a dose in milliliters.

Using the BSA formula, the child has a BSA of approximately 1.11 m^2.

$$1.11 \text{ m}^2 \longrightarrow \text{mL}$$

$$\text{m}^2 \times \frac{\text{? mg}}{\text{? m}^2} \times \frac{\text{? mL}}{\text{? mg}} = \text{? mL}$$

Because the order is 15 mg/m^2, the first unit fraction is $\dfrac{15 \text{ mg}}{\text{m}^2}$

Because the strength on the label is 10 mg/5 mL, the second unit fraction is $\dfrac{5 \text{ mL}}{10 \text{ mg}}$.

You cancel the square meters and milligrams to obtain the dose in milliliters.

$$1.11 \text{ m}^2 \times \frac{15 \text{ mg}}{\text{m}^2} \times \frac{5 \text{ mL}}{10 \text{ mg}} = 8.3 \text{ mL}$$

So, the child should receive 8.3 mL of Cortef.

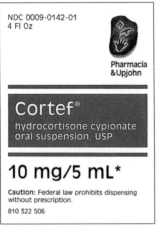

NDC 0009-0142-01
4 Fl Oz

Pharmacia
&Upjohn

Cortef®
hydrocortisone cypionate
oral suspension, USP

10 mg/5 mL*

Caution: Federal law prohibits dispensing without prescription.
810 322 506

● Figure 12.5
Drug label for Cortef.

Example 12.9

Valium (diazepam) 3.75 mg was ordered for a child with status epilepticus. The package insert says that the recommended dose is 0.2–0.5 mg/kg IVP slowly every 2–5 minutes up to a maximum of 5 mg. The child weighs 33 lbs, and the label on the vial reads 5 mg/mL.

(a) Is the ordered dose within the safe range?

(b) How many milliliters would you administer?

(a) You want to convert the body weight in *pounds* to *kilograms*; then convert the body weight in *kilograms* to a recommended dose in *milligrams*.

$$33 \text{ lb (body weight)} \longrightarrow ? \text{ kg (body weight)} \longrightarrow ? \text{ mg (drug)}$$

Do this on one line as follows:

$$33 \text{ lb} \times \frac{? \text{ kg}}{? \text{ lb}} \times \frac{? \text{ mg}}{? \text{ kg}} = ? \text{ mg}$$

Because 1 kg = 2.2 lb, the first unit fraction is $\frac{1 \text{ kg}}{2.2 \text{ lb}}$.

Because the recommended dosage is 0.2 mg to 0.5 mg/kg per day, you need to find the minimum and the maximum recommended doses in milligrams for this patient. Use the unit fractions $\frac{0.2 \text{ mg}}{\text{kg}}$ and $\frac{0.5 \text{ mg}}{\text{kg}}$

$$\frac{33 \text{ lb}}{1} \times \frac{1 \text{ kg}}{2.2 \text{ lb}} \times \frac{0.2 \text{ mg}}{\text{kg}} = 3 \text{ mg} \qquad 3 \text{ mg is the minimum dose}$$

$$\frac{33 \text{ lb}}{1} \times \frac{1 \text{ kg}}{2.2 \text{ lb}} \times \frac{0.5 \text{ mg}}{\text{kg}} = 7.5 \text{ mg} \qquad 7.5 \text{ mg is the maximum dose}$$

The safe dose range for this patient is 3–7.5 mg.
Because the ordered dose of 3.75 mg is between 3 mg and 7.5 mg, it is a safe dose.

(b) You want to convert the ordered dosage in milligrams to the liquid daily dose in milliliters.

$$3.75 \text{ mg (drug)} \longrightarrow ? \text{ mL (drug)}$$

Do this on one line as follows:

$$3.75 \text{ mg} \times \frac{? \text{ mL}}{? \text{ mg}} = ? \text{ mL}$$

Because the vial label says that 5 mg/mL, the unit fraction is $\frac{1 \text{ mL}}{5 \text{ mg}}$.

$$\frac{3.75 \text{ mg}}{1} \times \frac{1 \text{ mL}}{5 \text{ mg}} = 0.75 \text{ mL}$$

So, you would administer 0.75 mL of the Valium IVP slowly.

Administration of Intravenous Medications Using a Volume Control Chamber

Pediatric intravenous medications are frequently administered using a volume control chamber (VCC). In order to avoid fluid overload, a VCC (burette, Volutrol, Buretrol, Soluset) is often used when administering pediatric intravenous fluids (see Figure 12.6).

NOTE

Know the facility's policy concerning the amount of fluid used to flush the VCC tubing.

A VCC is calibrated in 1 mL increments and has a capacity of 100–150 mL. It can be used as a primary or secondary line. When administering IVPB medications, the medication is added to the top injection port of the VCC. Fluid is then added from the IV bag to further dilute the medication. After the infusion is complete, additional IV fluid is added to the VCC to flush any remaining medication left in the tubing.

The following example illustrates the use of such a device.

Example 12.10

The physician orders Garamycin (gentamycin) 25 mg IVPB q8h for a child, who weighs 20 kg. The medication is supplied in 20 mg vials with a strength of 10 mg/mL.

(a) How many milliliters would you withdraw from the vials?

(b) Using a volume control chamber, how many milliliters of IV solution do you need to add to the volume control chamber to obtain the recommended concentration of 2 mg/mL?

(a) You want to convert the order of 25 mg to mL.

$$25 \text{ mg} \longrightarrow ? \text{ mL}$$

$$25 \text{ mg} \times \frac{? \text{ mL}}{? \text{ mg}} = ? \text{ mL}$$

Because the vial label says that the strength is 10 mg/mL, the unit fraction is $\frac{1 \text{ mL}}{10 \text{ mg}}$

$$\frac{25 \text{ mg}}{1} \times \frac{1 \text{ mL}}{10 \text{ mg}} = 2.5 \text{ mL}$$

So, you would withdraw 2.5 mL from the vial.

(b) The 2.5 mL (containing 25 mg of Garamycin) taken from the vial is added to the VCC and it then needs to be further diluted to a concentration of 2 mg/mL.

You must convert the 25 mg of Garamycin in the VCC to milliliters of solution of strength 2 mg/mL.

$$25 \text{ mg} \longrightarrow ? \text{ mL}$$

$$25 \text{ mg} \times \frac{? \text{ mL}}{? \text{ mg}} = ? \text{ mL}$$

Because the recommended concentration is 2 mg/mL, the unit fraction is $\frac{1 \text{ mL}}{2 \text{ mg}}$

$$\frac{25 \text{ mg}}{1} \times \frac{1 \text{ mL}}{2 \text{ mg}} = 12.5 \text{ mL of solution in the VCC}$$

Therefore, 10 mL (12.5–2.5 mL) of IV solution should be added to the VCC.

In summary, in Example 12.10, you would add the *2.5 mL from the vial of Garamycin* to the top injection port of a volume control chamber (●**Figure 12.6**) and then add an additional *10 mL of IV solution* from the bag to obtain the *12.5 mL,*which will contain the recommended *safe medication concentration.*

Volume Control Chamber

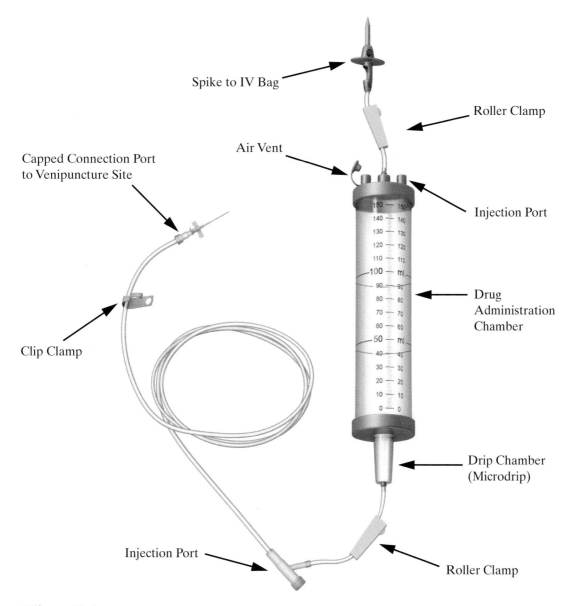

Spike to IV Bag

Roller Clamp

Air Vent

Capped Connection Port
to Venipuncture Site

Injection Port

Drug
Administration
Chamber

Clip Clamp

Drip Chamber
(Microdrip)

Injection Port

Roller Clamp

● **Figure 12.6**
Volume control chamber.

Example 12.11

Order: *Chloromycetin (chloramphenicol) 500 mg in 100 mL of* D$_5$W
IVPB q6h.

The recommended dose is 50–75 mg/kg/day divided every 6 hours. The
child weighs 34.6 kg.
Is the order in the safe dose range?

Method 1 Convert both the safe dose range and the prescribed dose to
mg/day.

First, use the minimum safe dose (50 mg/kg/day) to determine how many mg/day the patient should minimally receive as follows:

$$34.6 \ \cancel{kg} \times \frac{50 \ mg}{\cancel{kg} \times day} = 1,730 \ \frac{mg}{day} \qquad \text{Minimum}$$

Now, use the maximum safe dose (75 mg/kg/day) to determine how many mg/day the patient should maximally receive as follows:

$$34.6 \ \cancel{kg} \times \frac{75 \ mg}{\cancel{kg} \times day} = 2,595 \ \frac{mg}{day} \qquad \text{Maximum}$$

So, the safe dose range for this patient is 1,730–2,595 mg/day.
The ordered dose is 500 mg every 6 hours. Convert this to mg/day as follows:

$$\frac{500 \ mg}{6 \ \cancel{h}} \times \frac{24 \ \cancel{h}}{day} = 2,000 \frac{mg}{day}$$

The ordered dose is equivalent to 2,000 mg/day. This is within the safe dose range of 1,730–2,595 mg/day and the patient is receiving a safe dose.

Method 2 Convert the ordered dose of 500 mg every 6 hours, to mg/kg/day. Then compare this to the safe dose range of 50–75 mg/kg/day. This may be a mathematically more sophisticated approach, but it requires fewer calculations.

Realize that what you are looking for, mg/kg/day, is in the form of amount of drug/weight of patient/time.

An amount of drug (500 mg) is ordered for a (34.6 kg) patient over a period of time (6 hours). So, the order is 500 mg/34.6 kg/6 h.
You want to change this to mg/kg/day, which can be done in one line as follows:

$$\frac{500 \ mg}{34.6 \ kg \times \underset{1}{\cancel{6 \ h}}} \times \frac{\overset{4}{\cancel{24 \ h}}}{day} = 57.8 \frac{mg}{kg \times day}$$

The ordered dose is equivalent to 57.8 mg/kg/day. This is within the safe dose range of 50–75 mg/kg/day.

Calculating Daily Fluid Maintenance

The administration of pediatric intravenous medications requires careful and exact calculations and procedures. Infants and severely ill children are not able to tolerate extreme levels of hydration and are quite susceptible to dehydration, fluid overload, and drug overdose. Therefore, you must closely monitor the amount of fluid a child receives. The fluid a child requires over a 24-hour period is referred to as *daily maintenance fluid needs*. Daily maintenance fluid includes both oral and parenteral fluids. The amount of maintenance fluid required depends on the weight of the patient (see the formula in Table 12.1). The daily maintenance fluid does not include body fluid losses through vomiting, diarrhea, or fever. Additional fluids referred to as *replacement fluids* (usually Lactated Ringer's or 0.9% NaCl) are utilized to replace fluid losses and are based on each child's condition (e.g., if 20 mL are lost, then 20 mL of replacement fluids are usually added to the daily maintenance).

Table 12.1	**Daily Fluid Maintenance Formula**

Pediatric Daily Fluid Maintenance Formula		
For the *first*	*10 kg* of body weight:	*100 mL/kg*
For the *next*	*10 kg* of body weight:	*50 mL/kg*
For *each kg above*	*20 kg* of body weight:	*20 mL/kg*

Example 12.12

If the order is *half maintenance* for a child who weighs 25 kg, at what rate should the pump be set in mL/h?

Because the child weighs 25 kg, this weight would be divided into three portions following the formula in Table 12.1 as follows:

$$25 \text{ kg} = 10 \text{ kg} + 10 \text{ kg} + 5 \text{ kg}$$

For each of these three portions, the number of milliliters must be calculated. A table will be useful for organizing the calculations (Table 12.2). The daily "maintenance" was determined to be 1,600 mL. "Half maintenance" ($\frac{1}{2}$ of maintenance) is, therefore, $\frac{1}{2}$ of 1,600 mL, or 800 mL.

Now, you must change $\dfrac{800 \text{ mL}}{\text{day}}$ to $\dfrac{\text{mL}}{\text{h}}$.

$$\frac{800 \text{ mL}}{\text{day}} \times \frac{1 \text{ day}}{24 \text{ h}} = 33.3 \frac{\text{mL}}{\text{h}} = 33 \frac{\text{mL}}{\text{h}}$$

So, the pump would be set at 33 mL/h.

Table 12.2	**Daily Fluid Maintenance Computations for Example 12.12**				
1st Portion	10 kg	×	$\dfrac{100 \text{ mL}}{\text{kg}}$	=	1,000 mL
2nd Portion	10 kg	×	$\dfrac{50 \text{ mL}}{\text{kg}}$	=	500 mL
3rd Portion	5 kg	×	$\dfrac{20 \text{ mL}}{\text{kg}}$	=	100 mL
Total	25 kg				1,600 mL

Summary

In this chapter you used dimensional analysis to calculate oral and parenteral dosages for pediatric patients. Some dosages were based on body weight or BSA. Daily fluid maintenance needs were calculated. You also determined whether ordered dosages were in the safe dose range.

- Taking shortcuts in pediatric medication administration can be fatal.

- Check to see if the order is in the safe dose range.

- Consult a reliable source when in doubt about a pediatric medical order.

- Question the order or check your calculations if the ordered dose differs from the manufacturer's recommended dose.

- Amounts of medication used for children are small: No more than 1 mL should be given IM, and IV bags of no more than 500 mL should be hung.
- Pediatric dosages are generally rounded down.
- Because accuracy is crucial in pediatric infusions, electronic control devices or volume control chambers should always be used.
- For a volume control chamber, a flush is always used to clear the tubing after the medication is infused.
- Know the facility policy regarding the inclusion of medication volume as part of the total infusion volume.
- Daily fluid maintenance depends on the weight of the child and includes both oral and parenteral fluids.

Case Study 12.1

A 4-year-old girl is admitted to the hospital with a diagnosis of cystic fibrosis and pneumonia. Her parents say that she has been very irritable, has had a chronic cough, decreased appetite, and diarrhea for almost a week. Chest auscultation revealed labored breathing with the presence of rhonchi in the right upper lobe (RUL) of the lung, and inspection revealed mild circumoral cyanosis. She is small in stature for a child of her age (38 inches tall) and underweight (30 pounds). She is allergic to milk products. Vital signs are: T 102 °F; BP 88/64; P 100; R 26. Throat culture returned positive for Group A streptococcus. Her orders include the following:

- Bed rest
- Diet as tolerated, encourage PO fluids
- Peptamin Junior Supplement 600 mL HS via pump to GT over 6 hours
- Fluids 1,800 mL/m² day
- Ventolin (albuterol) 1 mg with Intal (cromolyn sodium) $\frac{1}{2}$ ampule (20 mg in a 2 mL ampule) q8h via nebulizer q6h

- Pulmozyme (deoxyribonuclease) $\frac{1}{2}$ ampule (2.5 mg in a 1 mL ampule) q12h via nebulizer
- Tobramycin $\frac{1}{2}$ ampule (300 mg in a 5 mL ampule) q12h via nebulizer for 28 days
- CPT and postural drainage q 4h following nebulization therapy
- Penicillin G 600,000 units in 50 mL D₅W IVPB q6h
- Tylenol (acetaminophen) 180 mg PO q4h prn temp over 101°
- Vitamin ADEK 2 mL once daily in A.M.

1. Calculate the child's 24-hour fluid requirement.
2. The recommended dose for penicillin G is 150,000 units /kg /day divided in equal doses every 4–6 hours. Is the ordered dose safe?
3. The penicillin G is available in a 5,000,000 units vial (● **Figure 12.7** for a portion of package insert). How many milliliters of diluent will you use to obtain a concentration of 750,000 units/mL, and how many mL of penicillin G will you withdraw from the vial?

● **Figure 12.7**
Portion of penicillin G package insert.

(Reg. Trademark of Pfizer Inc. Reproduced with permission.)

Buffered
PFIZERPEN®
(penicillin G potassium)
for Injection

Reconstitution
The following table shows the amount of solvent required for solution of various concentrations:

Approx. Desired Concentration (units/mL)	Approx. Volume (mL) 1,000,000 units	Solvent for Vial of 5,000,000 units	Infusion Only 20,000,000 units
50,000	20.0	–	–
100,000	10.0	–	–
250,000	4.0	18.2	75.0
500,000	1.8	8.2	33.0
750,000	–	4.8	–
1,000,000	–	3.2	11.5

http://www.pfizer.com/pfizer/download/uspi_pfizerpen.pdf

4. Calculate the setting in mL/h on the infusion pump to administer the penicillin G if it were given over 30 minutes.

5. If the usual dose range of albuterol is 0.1 to 0.15 mg/kg per dose, is the albuterol dose safe for this child?

6. How many milligrams of Pulmozyme is the patient receiving per dose?

7. How many milligrams of the cromolyn sodium will you administer with the albuterol?

8. If the Ventolin is supplied 1.25 mg/3 mL, what is the total amount of solution (in milliliters) in the nebulizer containing the combination of the Ventolin and the Intal?

9. How many milliliters of Pulmozyme will you administer?

10. How many milligrams of Tobramycin will you administer?

11. The label on the acetaminophen elixir states 160 mg/5 ml. Mark the liquid administration devices in ● Figure 12.8 to show how much you would administer.

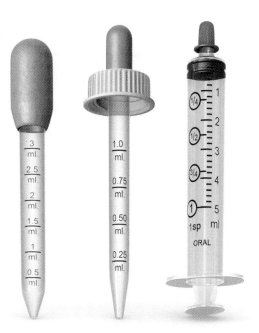

● Figure 12.8
Droppers and syringe for liquid medication administration.

Practice Sets

The answers to *Try These for Practice*, *Exercise*, and *Cumulative Review Exercises* appear in Appendix A at the end of the book. Ask your instructor for the answers to the *Additional Exercises*.

Try These for Practice

Test your comprehension after reading the chapter.

1. The following order has been given for a child who weighs 45 kilograms:
Humulin R insulin 0.1 unit/kg subcutaneously b.i.d. ac breakfast and dinner
How many units will this child receive of this insulin in 24 h? _____

Workspace

2. Order: *Retrovir (azidothymidine) 90 mg IVPB q6h*. The patient is a two-year-old child with BSA of 0.62 m². If the recommended safe dose range is 100–180 mg/m² q6h, is the prescribed dose safe?

3. The order is *Amoxil (amoxicillin) 250 mg PO*. The label reads 125 mg/5 mL. How many milliliters would you administer?

4. Read the information on the label in ●**Figure 12.9**. How many milliliters of codeine would you administer to a child who weighs 40 kg when the order is 0.3 mg/kg PO q4h?

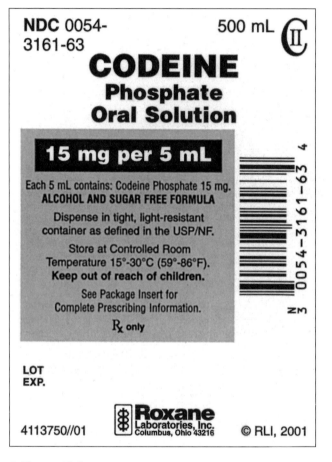

●**Figure 12.9**
Drug label for codeine.
(Courtesy of Roxane Laboratories Inc.)

5. Order: IV D5/$\frac{1}{3}$NS at maintenance and one half for a 42 kg child. How many mL/h does the child need?

Exercises

Reinforce your understanding in class or at home.

1. The prescriber ordered gentamicin 50 mg IVPB q8h for a child who weighs 40 lb. The recommended dosage is 6–7.5 mg/kg/day divided in three equal doses. Is the prescribed dose within the safe range?

2. The prescriber ordered Vancocin (vancomycin) 10 mg/kg q12h, IV for a neonate who weighs 4,000g. What is the dose in milligrams?

3. The prescriber ordered methotrexate 2.9 mg PO weekly for a child who is 42 inches tall and weighs 50 pounds. The package insert states that the recommended dosage is 7.5–30 mg/m^2 q1–2 weeks. Is the order a safe dose?

4. Order: *Panadol (acetaminophen) 10 mg/kg PO q4h prn* for a child who weighs 32 kg. How many milligrams will you administer?

5. A manufacturer recommends giving 350 mg/m^2/day to a maximum of 450 mg/m^2/day for a drug. A child has a BSA of 1.2 m^2. Calculate the safe dose range (in milligrams per day) for this child.

6. Order: *Ceclor (cefaclor) suspension 30 mg/kg/day q8h*. The child weighs 77 pounds. The label reads 187 mg/mL. How many milliliters will you administer?

7. Order: *1,000 mL D5/RL infuse at 65 mL/h*. The drop factor is 60 mcgtt/mL. Calculate the infusion rate in microdrops per minute.

8. Order: *Zantac (ranitidine) 30 mg IV q8h*. The patient weighs 52 pounds. The package insert states that the recommended dose in pediatric patients is for a total dose of 2–4 mg/kg/day, to be divided and administered every 6 to 8 hours, up to a maximum of 50 mg per dose. Is the prescribed dose safe?

9. Order: IV D5/0.33% NS.
   (a) The child weighs 55 lb. If the child is NPO, what is the daily IV fluid maintenance?
   (b) What is the rate of flow in mL/h?

10. A child has a BSA of 0.82 m^2. The recommended dose of a drug is 2 million units/m^2. How many units will you administer?

11. Order: Claforan (cefotamine sodium) 1.2 g IV q8h. The safe dose range for the solution concentration is 20–60 mg/mL to infuse over 15 to 30 minutes. What is the minimal amount of IV fluid needed to safely dilute this dosage? [HINT: The minimal amount of IV fluid is the maximal safe concentration.]

12. Calculate the daily fluid maintenance for an infant who weighs 7 lb.

13. Order: Retrovir (zidovudine) 160 mg/m^2 q8h PO. The child has a BSA of 1.1 m^2. Read the label in ● **Figure 12.10**. How many milliliters will you prepare?

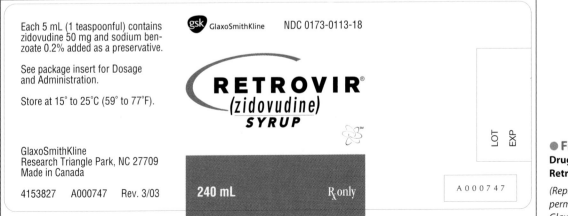

Each 5 mL (1 teaspoonful) contains zidovudine 50 mg and sodium benzoate 0.2% added as a preservative.

See package insert for Dosage and Administration.

Store at 15° to 25°C (59° to 77°F).

GlaxoSmithKline
Research Triangle Park, NC 27709
Made in Canada

4153827   A000747   Rev. 3/03

gsk GlaxoSmithKline   NDC 0173-0113-18

RETROVIR®
(zidovudine)
SYRUP

LOT EXP

A000747

240 mL   R only

● **Figure 12.10**
Drug label for Retrovir.

(Reproduced with permission of GlaxoSmithKline.)

14. Order: D5/$\frac{1}{2}$NS with KCl 20 mEq per liter, infuse at 30 mL/ h. The child is 60 cm and weighs 9.1 kg.
    (a) How many mEq of KCl would you add to a 500 mL IV bag?
    (b) The label on the KCl reads 2 mEq/mL. How many milliliters will you add to the IV?
    (c) How many mEq/h will the child receive?
    (d) The recommended dosage for children is up to 3 mEq/kg/day. Is the ordered dose safe?

15. Order: Erythromycin 125 mg PO q4h. The child weighs 14.5 kg. The usual dosage is 30–50 mg/kg/day in equally divided doses. The label reads Erythromycin 200 mg/5 mL.
    (a) Is the ordered dose safe?
    (b) How many milliliters would you administer?

16. Order: Vancocin (vancomycin) 40 mg/kg/d IV q6h to infuse over 90 minutes in 200 mL NS. The child weighs 41 kg. The Vancocin has a concentration of 50 mg/mL. What will you set the pump at in mL/h?

17. A medication of 100 mg in 1 mL is diluted to 15 mL and administered IVP over 20 minutes. How many mg/min is the patient receiving?

18. A drug is labeled 250 mg/5 mL. The drug is added to 40 mL of IV fluids and is to infuse over 60 minutes. What is the rate of flow in microdrops per minute?

19. Order: Pediaprophen (ibuprofen) 20 mg/kg/dose. The label reads 100 mg/2.5 mL. The child weighs 35 pounds. How many milliliters will you administer?

20. Order: Ampicillin 125 mg PO q6h. A child weighs 22 pounds. The package insert states that the recommended dose is 50 mg/kg/24 h. Is the prescribed dose safe?

Additional Exercises

Now, test yourself!

1. The antiretroviral medication didanosine (Videx) has been prescribed for a child with a BSA 0.9 m^2. The order is 120 mg PO per m^2 b.i.d. and the concentration is 10 mg/mL. How many milliliters will you administer to the child? _____

2. Physician's order:

   lamivudine (Epivir) 4 mg/kg PO b.i.d.

   The label reads 10 mg/mL. How many milliliters will you prepare for an infant who weighs 16 pounds? _____

3. Physician's order:

   digoxin (Lanoxin) 35 mcg/kg IV push as a loading dose, divided into 3 doses in 24 h

   The label reads 100 mg/mL, and the infant weighs 7 pounds. How many milliliters will you prepare for this infant? _____

4. Order:

   Rocaltrol (calcitriol) 0.01 mcg/kg PO daily

   The label reads 1 mcg/mL. How many milliliters will you prepare for a child who weighs 35 kg?

5. Physician's order:

   Diamox (acetazolamide) 8 mg/kg IV push q6h

   The label reads 500 mg in 5 mL. How many milliliters will you prepare for a child with acute angle-closure glaucoma who weighs 56 pounds? _____

6. Physician's order: Vistaril (hydroxyzine pamoate) 20 mg IM q4h prn nausea. The safe dose is 0.5–1 mg/kg/dose q 4–6h as needed. Is the prescribed dose safe for a 44-pound child? _____

7. The order for hepatitis A vaccine, inactivated (Havrix), is 720 Elisa units (EL. units) subcut. The label reads 1,440 EL. units/mL. How many milliliters will you prepare? _____

8. The physician ordered 120 mg of guaifenesin PO q4h prn. The label reads 100 mg in 5 mL. How many milliliters will you prepare?

9. The order for Regular insulin is 0.1 units per kilogram IV bolus stat. The child weighs 18 kg. How many units will you administer? _____

10. Physician's order:

    Add 100 units of Regular insulin to 100 milliliters of normal saline. Infuse at a rate of 0.1 units per kilogram per hour IV.

    The child weighs 50 pounds; how many milliliters per hour will the child receive? _____

11. Lorabid (loracarbef) has been prescribed for a 2-year-old child with acute otitis media. The order is 30 milligrams per kilogram PO, q12h and the child weighs 21 pounds. The oral suspension is labeled 100 mg in 5 mL. How many milliliters will you give this child? _____

12. Biaxin (clarithromycin) 7.5 mg/kg q12h PO has been ordered for a child with a weight of 23 kg. The label reads 125 milligrams in 5 milliliters. How many milliliters will you prepare? _____

13. Physician's order:

    Apply 0.025% vitamin A acid (tretinoin) solution to affected skin once daily at hour of sleep.

    How many milligrams of vitamin A acid are in 4 mL of solution? _____

14. The BSA of a child is 0.5 m^2, and the order is 400 mg/m^2 of a drug PO. The label reads 250 mg in 5 mL. How many milliliters will you prepare for this child? _____

15. The normal dose range for erythromycin, is 30–50 mg/kg PO in divided doses q6h. The physician ordered 250 mg PO q6h for a child who weighs 30 kg. Is this a safe dose for this child? _____

16. Prescriber's order:

    Mefoxin (cefoxitin) 35 mg/kg IVPB 60 minutes before surgery. The postoperative order is 35 mg/kg q6h for 24h

    The child weighs 35 kg. What is the total amount in grams that the child will receive preoperatively and postoperatively? _____

17. Order:

    150 mg Vantin (cefpodoxime) PO q12h

    The label reads 50 mg/5 mL. How many milliliters will you prepare? _____

18. The prescriber ordered 1.0 g of Rocephin (ceftriaxone) IVPB stat. The label on the vial reads 1 g in 10 mL of D/5/W. Add to 90 mL D_5W. Infuse total amount in 30 minutes. Calculate the amount in microdrops per minute. _____

19. Order: D5/0.22 NaCl at maintenance for a 19 kg child. How many mL/d does the child need?

20. Ampicillin 25 mg/kg PO q.i.d. has been prescribed for a child who weighs 42 pounds. The label reads 250 mg = 5 mL. Calculate the dose in milliliters for this child. _____

Cumulative Review Exercises

Review your mastery of earlier chapters.

1. How many milligrams PO of ethambutol HCl (Myambutal), an antitubercular drug, would you administer if the prescribed dose is 15 milligrams per kilogram and the child weighs 35 kg? _____

2. How many units of Regular insulin subcutaneously would you prepare for a child who weighs 30 kg if the order is 1 unit per kilogram? _____

3. The order reads:

   Cefixime 8 mg/kg PO once daily
   (a) How many milligrams of this antibiotic would you administer to a child whose weight is 25 kg?
   (b) Each tablet contains 0.2 g
   How many tablets will you administer? _____

4. The order reads:

   50 units of Lente insulin subcutaneously ac breakfast

   The vial is labeled 100 units per milliliter. How many units would you administer to the patient? _____

5. The prescriber has ordered 10 million units of penicillin G IVPB q12h. The 20-million-unit vial of powder has these instructions: add 40 mL of sterile water. How many milliliters equal 10,000,000 units? _____

6. The order is for 300 mg of ranitidine PO. The label indicates that each capsule contains 150 mg.
   (a) How many capsules equal the prescribed dose? _____
   (b) Calculate the dose in grams.

7. The order reads:

   Inocor (inamrinone) 0.75 mg/kg IV bolus

   How many milligrams will you prepare of this inotropic drug if the patient weighs 180 lbs? _____

8. The prescriber ordered 900 mL of 5% D/W IV in 5 h. Calculate the flow rate in drops per minute when the drop factor is 20 drops per milliliter. _____

9. The order reads:

   cimetidine 300 mg IVPB in 50 mL of 5% D/W. Infuse in 20 minutes

   Calculate the flow rate in milliliters per minute for this histamine-2 receptor antagonist drug. _____

10. The prescriber ordered 1,000 mL 5% D/W at 17 gtt/min IV. The infusion began at 9:00 P.M. At what time will this solution be completed? The drop factor is 15 drops per milliliter. _____

11. 0.002 g = gr _____

12. How many tablets of naproxen would you administer PO to an adult with a BSA of 1.9 square meters if the order is 200 mL/m^2 and each tablet contains 375 mg? _____

13. Describe how to prepare 100 mL of a 1:3 solution from a 1:2 solution. _____

14. The order is verapamil 80 mg PO q8h. Each tablet contains 40 mg. How many tablets will you administer of this calcium channel blocker drug? _____

15. The order for a child with a BSA of 1.2 m^2 reads: Zithromax 175 mg/m^2 PO. Read the label in ●Figure 12.11 and determine how many milliliters the child will receive. _____

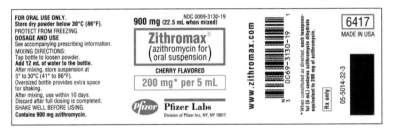

●**Figure 12.11**
Drug label for Zithromax.

(Reg. Trademark of Pfizer Inc. Reproduced with permission.)

Comprehensive
Self-Tests

Comprehensive Self-Test 1

Answers to *Comprehensive Self-Tests* 1–4 can be found in Appendix A at the back of the book.

1. Calculate the dosage of calcium EDTA for a patient who has a BSA of 1.47 m². The recommended dose is 500 mg/m².

2. Order: Tikosyn 1 mg PO q8h. Read the label in ● **Figure S.1** to determine how many capsules you will give the patient.

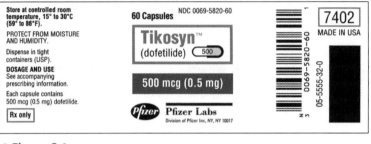

● **Figure S.1**
Drug label for Tikosyn.   *(Reg. Trademark of Pfizer Inc. Reproduced with permission.)*

3. How would you prepare 400 mL of 10% Clorox solution from a 100% solution?

4. Kineret (anakinra) 100 mg subcut daily has been prescribed for a patient with rheumatoid arthritis. The prefilled syringe is labeled 100 mg/mL. Calculate the dose in grams.

5. An IV of 1,000 mL D5W is infusing at a rate of 40 gtt/min. How long will it take to finish if the drop factor is 20 gtt/mL?

6. Calculate the number of grams of dextrose in 250 mL of D5W.

7. Order: Humulin Regular insulin U-100 6 units and Humulin NPH insulin 14 units subcutaneous ac breakfast. Read the labels in ● **Figure S.2** and place an arrow on the syringe indicating the total amount of insulin you will give.

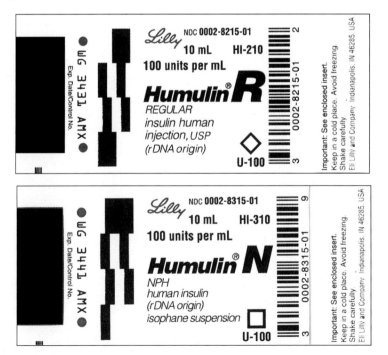

● **Figure S.2**
Drug labels for Humulin R and Humulin N and syringe.

(Copyright Eli Lilly and Company. Used with permission.)

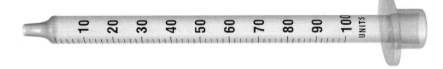

8. The prescriber ordered Cordarone (amiodarone HCl) 400 mg PO b.i.d. Each tablet contains 200 mg. How many tablets will you give the patient?

9. The prescriber ordered Cefobid (cefoperazone) 1g IVPB q12h to infuse in 30 minutes. The label on the premixed IV bag reads cefoperazone 50 mL, 50 mg/mL.
   (a) Calculate the flow rate in milliliters per hour.
   (b) How many milligrams will the patient receive?

10. Your patient is to receive morphine sulfate 5 mg subcutaneously stat. The 20 mL multiple dose vial is labeled morphine 15 mg/mL. Calculate the dose and place an arrow on the syringe indicating the dose.

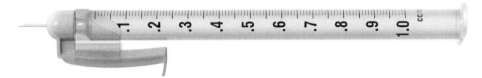

11. How will you prepare 200 mL of 1/3 strength Isocal from $\frac{1}{2}$ strength Isocal?

12. A prescriber ordered a premixed solution of nitroglycerine 25 mg in 250 mL D5W to be titrated at a rate of 5 mcg/min, increase q 5–10 min until pain subsides. The medication is to be infused via pump.
    How many mL/h will you set the pump to begin the infusion?

13. Order: Humulin R insulin 100 units in 100 mL NS, infuse at 0.1 unit/kg/h. The patient weighs 68 kg. How many units per hour is the patient receiving?

14. The prescriber ordered Claforan (cefotaxime) 750 mg IM q12h. The 1 g vial of Claforan is in a powder form. The package insert states for IM injection, add 3 mL of sterile water for injection for an approximate volume of 3.4 mL containing 300 mg/mL. How many milliliters will you give the patient?

15. Rebif (interferon beta-1a) 44 mcg subcutaneous three times a week is prescribed for a patient with multiple sclerosis. How many milligrams will the patient receive in one week?

16. Order: Lanoxin (digoxin) elixir 0.15 mg PO q12h. The child weighs 70 lb and the recommended maintenance dose is 7–10 mcg/kg/day.
    (a) What is the minimum daily maintenance dosage in mg/day?
    (b) What is the maximum daily maintenance dosage in mg/day?
    (c) Is the dose ordered safe?

17. Vibramycin (doxycycline hyclate) 4.4 mg/kg IVPB daily is ordered for a child who weighs 80 pounds. The premixed IV solution bag is labeled Vibramycin 200 mg/250 mL D5W to infuse in 4 hours.
    (a) How many milligrams of Vibramycin will the patient receive?
    (b) Calculate the flow rate in mL/h.

18. Order: Levaquin (levofloxacin) 500 mg in 100 mL D5W IVPB daily for 14 days to infuse in 1 h. Calculate the flow rate in drops per minute if the drop factor is 15 gtt/mL.

19. Calculate the BSA of a child who is 44 inches and weighs 72 pounds.

20. Order: heparin 5,000 units subcutaneous q12h. The multidose vial label reads 10,000 units/mL. How many milliliters will you give the patient?

21. Order: D10W 1,000 mL to infuse at 75 mL/h. The drop factor is 20 gtt/mL.
    (a) What is the rate of flow in $\dfrac{\text{mL}}{\text{min}}$?
    (b) How many drops per minute will you set the IV to infuse?
    (c) How long will it take for the infusion to be complete?

22. Calculate the total daily fluid maintenance for a child who weighs 45 kg.

23. Order: Keflex (cephalexin) oral suspension 50 mg/kg PO q6h. The label reads 125 mg/5 mL. The patient weighs 33 pounds. How many milliliters will you give?

24. Read the label in ● Figure S.3.

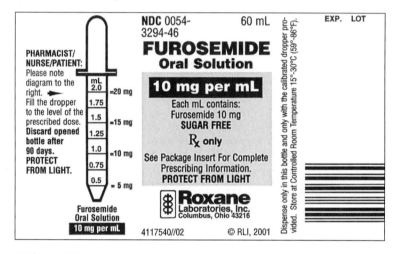

● Figure S.3
Drug label for furosemide.   (Courtesy of Roxane Laboratories Inc.)

    (a) How many milligrams of furosemide are in 1 mL?
    (b) How many milliliters of furosemide are in the bottle?

25. The prescriber ordered ReoPro (abciximab) 0.125 mcg/kg IV in 250 mL NS to be infused in 12 hours for a patient who weighs 75 kg. The abciximab label reads 2 mg/mL.
    (a) How many milligrams will the patient receive?
    (b) Calculate the flow rate in milliliters per hour.

Comprehensive Self-Test 2

1. A patient has an IV of 250 mL D5RL with 25,000 units of heparin infusing at 20 mL/h. How many units of heparin is the patient receiving each hour?

2. Order:

Alkeran (melphalan HCl) 16 mg/m² IV q2 weeks for four doses infuse in 20 min

    The package insert states to rapidly inject 10 mL of supplied diluent into a 50 mg vial and shake vigorously until a clear solution results (5 mg/mL). The patient has a BSA of 1.2 m².
    (a) How many milligrams contain the dose?
    (b) How many milliliters of Alkeran will you add to 100 mL of NS?
    (c) Determine the flow rate in mL/h.

3. A patient is receiving Zantac (ranitidine HCl) 150 mg PO b.i.d. The label reads 150 mg tablets. How many tablets will the patient receive in 24 hours?

4. Order:

> Lanoxicaps (digoxin solution in capsules) 0.1 mg PO b.i.d.

The label on the bottle reads 50 mcg/capsule. How many capsules will you give the patient?

5. Order:

> protamine sulfate 22 mg IVP over 10 min

The label reads 50 mg/5 mL. Dilute with 20 mL of NS or D5W. How many milliliters of protamine sulfate will you prepare?

6. Order:

> Garamycin (gentamicin sulfate) 9 mg IM q12h

The package insert states that the recommended dose for neonates is 2.5 mg/kg q 12–24h. The label on the vial reads Pediatric Injectable Garamycin 10 mg/mL. The infant weighs 10 lb.
(a) Is the dose safe?
(b) How many milliliters will you give?

7. An IV of D5/NS (1,000 mL) is infusing at 50 mL/h. The infusion started at 1300h; what time will it finish?

8. The prescriber ordered Dilantin (phenytoin sodium) 250 mg/m^2 in three divided doses for a child who has a BSA of 1.25 m^2. The bottle is labeled 125 mg/5 mL oral suspension. How many milliliters will you give for each dose?

9. Order:

> Lasix (furosemide) 20 mg IM stat

The label reads 40 mg/4 mL.
(a) How many milliliters will you give the patient?
(b) Place an arrow on the syringe that indicates the dose.

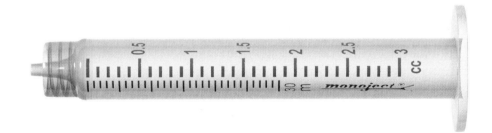

10. The recommended dose of Cleocin (clindamycin) pediatric oral solution is 8 to 25 mg/kg/day in three to four equally divided doses. A child weighs 60 pounds.
(a) Calculate the minimum safe daily dose.
(b) Calculate the maximum safe daily dose.

11. Calculate how many grams of sodium chloride are in 250 mL of a 0.9% NaCl solution.

12. A patient has an IV infusing at 25 gtt/min. How many mL/h is the patient receiving? The drop factor is 15 gtt/mL.

13. Calculate the total volume and hourly IV flow rate for a 10-pound infant who is receiving maintenance fluids.

14. Order:

   nitroprusside sodium 50 mg in 250 mL D$_5$W infuse at 1 mL/h

   The recommended dosage range is 0.1 to 5 mcg/kg/min. The patient weighs 154 pounds. Is this a safe dose?

15. Prepare 200 mL of a 10% boric acid solution from a 50% boric acid solution.

16. Your patient has an IV of Humulin R insulin 50 units in 500 mL of NS infusing at 12 units per hour. Calculate the flow rate in mL/h.

17. Order:

   Ticar (ticarcillin disodium) 1g IM q6h

   The package insert states to reconstitute each 1g vial with 2 mL of sterile water for injection. Each 2.5 mL = 1g. How many milliliters will you administer?

18. Order:

   Indocin SR (indomethacin) 150 mg PO t.i.d. for 7 days

   The label reads Indocin SR 75 mg capsules.
   (a) How many capsules will you give the patient for each dose?
   (b) Calculate the entire 7 day dosage in grams.

19. Order:

   Colace (docusate sodium) syrup 100 mg via PEG t.i.d.

   The label reads 50 mg/15 mL. How many mL will you give?

20. Order:

   theophylline 0.8 mg/kg/h IV via pump

   The premixed IV bag is labeled theophylline 800 mg in 250 mL D$_5$W. The patient weighs 185 pounds. How many mL/h will you set the pump?

21. Order:

   Kefzol (cefalozin) 1 g in 50 mL D$_5$W IV PB q6h, infuse in 20 minutes

   Read the information on the label in ●Figure S.4.

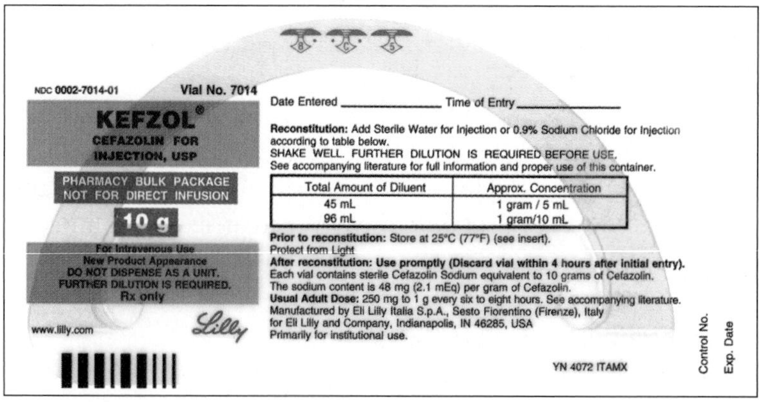

●Figure S.4
Drug label for Kefzol.

(Copyright Eli Lilly and Company. Used with permission.)

(a) How many milliliters of diluent will you add to the vial so that 1 g of Kefzol = 5 mL?
(b) Calculate the flow rate in milliliters per minute; the drop factor is 60 mcgtt/mL.

22. The nurse has prepared 7 mg of dexamethasone for IV administration. The label on the vial reads 10 mg/mL. How many milliliters did the nurse prepare?

23. Order:

    Cogentin (benztropine mesylate) 2 mg IM stat and then 1 mg IM daily

    The label reads 2 mg/2 mL.
    (a) How many milliliters will you administer daily?
    (b) What size syringe will you use?

24. Order:
    $\frac{2}{3}$ strength Sustacal 900 mL via PEG, give over 8h

    How will you prepare this solution?

25. An IV of 250 mL NS is infusing at 25 mL/h. The infusion began at 1800h. What time will it be completed?

Comprehensive Self Test-3

1. An IV is infusing at 35 gtt/min. How many milliliters will the patient receive in 6 hours? The drop factor is 10 gtt/mL.

2. Order:
                Augmentin (amoxicillin clavulanate potassium)
                200 mg oral suspension PO q12h

    The label reads 125 mg/5 ml. How many milliliters will you administer?

3. The prescriber ordered neomycin sulfate 8.75 mg/kg PO q6h for an infant with infectious diarrhea. The vial is labeled 125 mg/5 mL. The infant weighs 8 pounds. How many milliliters will you administer?

4. Order:

        heparin 40,000 units in 1,000 mL NS, infuse at 40 mL/h

    The normal heparinizing range is 20,000–40,000 units q24h. Calculate the units/h and determine if the dose is safe.

5. Order:
                Amicar (aminocaproic acid) 3g/m^2 IV,
                add to 250 mL NS and infuse via pump over 1h

    The patient weighs 30 pounds and is 32 inches tall.
    (a) How many mg/kg is the child receiving?
    (b) At what rate will you set the pump in mL/h?

6. A prescriber ordered Amphojel (aluminum hydroxide) 10 mL q2h prn. The label reads 675 mg/5 mL. What is the maximum dose in milligrams that the patient may receive in 24 hours?

7. A patient is to receive 3,500 units of heparin subcutaneously. The label reads 10,000 units/mL.
    (a) How many milliliters will you administer?
    (b) What type of syringe will you use?

8. Order:
                Epivir (lamivudine) oral solution 150 mg PO b.i.d.

    The recommended safe dose is 4 mg/kg b.i.d. Is this a safe dose for a child who weighs 42 pounds?

9. Order:

> Mandol (cefamandole nafate)750 mg IM q8h

The instructions on the 1g vial state reconstitute with 3 mL of sterile water for injection. The resulting solution is 285 mg/mL.
(a) How many milliliters will you administer?
(b) What size syringe will you use?

10. Order:

> potassium chloride 40 mEq PO daily

The label reads potassium chloride 20 mEq per 15 mL. How many milliliters will you administer?

11. Calculate the hourly IV flow rate and total daily IV fluid volume for a child who is NPO, weighs 15 pounds, and is receiving maintenance fluids.

12. Order:

> Novolin R regular insulin 24 units and Novolin N NPH
> insulin 17 units subcutaneous ac breakfast

Draw an arrow on the syringe indicating the dose of each of the insulins.

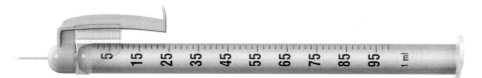

13. A patient who is 160 cm tall and weighs 60 kg is to receive Intron A (interferon alpha-2b) 20,000 units/m^2. How many units contain this dose?

14. Order:

> Unipen (nafcillin sodium) oral solution 500 mg PO q4h

The label reads 250 mg/5 mL. How many milliliters will you give the patient?

15. A patient is receiving an IV of 1,000 mL of D5W with 15 mEq of KCL for 24 hours. Calculate the flow rate in mL/h. The drop factor is 10 gtt/mL.

16. A patient is receiving TPN 1,500 mL at a rate of 65 mL/h via pump. The infusion began at 0600. What time will it be finished?

17. Order:

> Myambutol (ethambutol HCl)15 mg/kg PO daily

The label reads 400 mg tablets. How many tablets will you give the patient who weighs 178 pounds?

18. A patient is receiving Zyloprim (allopurinol) 300 mg PO daily. What is the total number of grams per day?

19. Order:

> Pitocin (oxytocin) 20 units IV in LR 1,000 mL via pump.
> Start at 1 milliunit/min, increase by 1 milliunit q 15-30 min
> to a maximum of 20 milliunits/min.

What rate will you set the infusion pump in mL/h to begin the infusion?

20. Calculate how many grams of sodium chloride are contained in 1,000 mL of D$_5$1/3 NS.

21. Order:

    heparin 750 units subcutaneously daily

    The vial is labeled 1,000 units/mL. What size syringe will you use?

22. A patient has an IV of 0.9% sodium chloride infusing at 75 mL/h.

    The drop factor is 60 gtt/mL. Calculate the flow rate in drops per minute.

23. Order:

    Decadron (dexamethasone) 1.5 mg PO daily

    The label reads 0.75 mg tablets. How many tablets will you give?

24. Calculate the body surface area for a child who is 28 inches tall and weighs 30 pounds.

25. Calculate the daily fluid maintenance needs for a child who weighs 13.6 kg.

Comprehensive Self-Test 4

1. Order: Adriamycin PFS (doxorubicin HCl) 80 mg IV once q21days. The package insert states that the recommended dose for use as a single agent is 60–75 mg/m^2 repeat every 3 weeks. Is this a safe dose for a patient who weighs 39 kg and is 51 inches tall?

2. Order:

    Biaxin (clarithromycin) oral suspension 7.5 mg/kg PO q12h

    The label reads 250 mg/5 mL. How many milliliters will you give a child who weighs 40 pounds?

3. Order:

    nitroglycerine 0.6 mg SL stat

    The label reads 0.3 mg tablets. How many tablets will you give the patient?

4. A patient has an IV of 1,000 mL LR infusing at 125 mL/h. How many hours will it take to infuse?

5. Calculate the daily fluid maintenance needs for an infant who weighs 2,500 g.

6. Order:

    Dilaudid-HP (hydromorphone HCl) 4 mg IM stat

    The label reads 10 mg/mL.
    (a) How many milliliters will you administer?
    (b) What size syringe will you use?

7. Order:

    Synthroid (levothroxine sodium) 50 mcg PO daily

    How many milligrams is the patient receiving?

8. Order:

    Procardia (nifedipine) 20 mg PO t.i.d.

Read the label in ● **Figure S.5** and calculate how many capsules of this calcium channel blocker drug the patient is receiving daily.

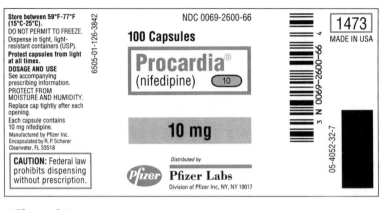

● **Figure S.5**
Drug label for Procardia.   *(Reg. Trademark of Pfizer Inc. Reproduced with permission.)*

9. Order:

atropine sulfate 0.4 mg IM on call to OR

The label reads 1 mg/mL. How many milliliters will you give the patient?

10. Order:

Sandostatin (octreotide acetate) 200 mcg subcutaneously q.i.d

The label reads 1 mg/mL. How many milliliters will you administer?

11. Order:

Normodyne (labetalol HCl) 20 mg IVP slowly over 2 min

The label reads 5 mg/mL. How many milliliters of this antihypertensive drug will the patient receive per minute?

12. Order:

lidocaine 1% drip 2 mg/min IV via pump

The label reads D_5W 250 mL with lidocaine 1%. Calculate the pump setting in mL/h.

13. Order:

Zantac (ranitidine) 50 mg in 100 mL D_5W IVPB q8h, infuse in 20 min

The label reads 25 mg/mL. Calculate the flow rate in milliliters per minute.

14. Prepare 3,000 mL of a 1% Neosporin solution from a 5% Neosporin solution.

15. Order:

Pfizerpen (penicillin G potassium) 350,000 units IM b.i.d.

The label reads 500,000 units/1.8 mL.
(a) How many milliliters will you give the patient?
(b) What size syringe will you use?

16. Calculate the amount of dextrose and sodium chloride in 500 mL of $D5/\frac{1}{3}$ NS.

17. An infusion of D_5W has 800 milliliters left in the bag. The flow rate is 31 drops per minute, and the drop factor is 15 gtt/mL. How long will it take for the remainder of this IV fluid to infuse?

18. Order:

     Mutamycin (mitomycin-C) 20 mg/m² IV once q6weeks.

     Calculate the dose for a patient who has a BSA of 1.62 m².

19. Calculate the total daily fluid maintenance for a child who weighs 26 pounds.

20. Order:

     Tagamet (cimetidine) 250 mg IVPB q6h

     The recommended dose is 5 to 10 mg/kg q6h. Is this a safe dose for a child who weighs 80 pounds?

21. Order:

     Humulin R regular insulin 300 units in 150 mL NS infuse at 10 mL/h.

     How many units/h is the patient receiving?

22. Order:

     heparin 5,000 units subcutaneous q12h

     The label reads 10,000 units/mL. How many milliliters will you give the patient?

23. Order: Ancef (cefazolin) 500 mg IM q8h. The directions for the 1 g vial state: reconstitute with 2.5 mL of sterile water for injection and 330 mg/mL. How many milliliters will you give the patient?

24. Order:

     Proventil (albuterol) syrup 4 mg daily.

     The label reads Proventil (albuterol sulfate) syrup 2 mg per 5 mL. How many milliliters will you administer?

25. A prescriber ordered Vancocin (vancomycin HCl) 500 mg PO q6h for a child who weighs 110 pounds. The package insert states that the recommended child's dose is 40 mg/kg/d in three or four divided doses. Is the prescribed dose safe?

Appendices

Appendix A

Diagnostic Test of Arithmetic

1. $\frac{3}{8}$

2. 0.285

3. 6.5

4. 0.83

5. 31.5

6. 3.8

7. 0.0639

8. 500

9. 2

10. $\frac{1}{4}$ and 0.25

11. $2\frac{1}{3}$

12. $\frac{1}{25}$

13. $\frac{9}{20}$

14. 0.025

15. $\frac{18}{7}$

Chapter 1

Try These for Practice

1. 0.3125

2. 74.4

3. 0.4 and $\frac{2}{5}$

4. $\frac{1}{3}$

5. 2

Exercises

1. $0.85 = \dfrac{85 \div 5}{100 \div 5} = \dfrac{17}{20}$

2. $2.7 = 2\dfrac{7}{10}$

3. $\dfrac{\overset{5}{\cancel{40}}}{1} \times \dfrac{1}{2} \times \dfrac{9}{\underset{2}{\cancel{16}}} = \dfrac{45}{4} = 11\dfrac{1}{4}$

4. $2\dfrac{3}{5} \div \dfrac{2}{1} = \dfrac{13}{5} \times \dfrac{1}{2} = \dfrac{13}{10} = 1\dfrac{3}{10}$

5. $\dfrac{15}{1} \div \dfrac{11}{3} = \dfrac{15}{1} \times \dfrac{3}{11} = \dfrac{45}{11} = 4\dfrac{1}{11}$

6. $9.6 \div \dfrac{3}{7} = \dfrac{9.6}{1} \times \dfrac{7}{3} = \dfrac{67.2}{3} = 22.4 = 22\dfrac{2}{5}$

7. $\dfrac{\overset{14}{\cancel{42}}}{1} \times \dfrac{1}{\underset{3150}{\cancel{9450}}} \times \dfrac{3}{0.02} = \dfrac{42}{63} = \dfrac{2}{3}$

8.
$$
\begin{array}{r}
.125 \\
8\overline{)1.000} \approx 0.12 \\
\underline{8} \\
20 \\
\underline{16} \\
40 \\
\underline{40} \\
0
\end{array}
$$

9.
$$
\begin{array}{r}
.56 \\
25\overline{)14.00} \quad 0.56 \\
\underline{12\,5} \\
1\,50 \\
\underline{1\,50} \\
0
\end{array}
$$

10. $5\dfrac{3}{10} = 5.3$

11.
$$
\begin{array}{r}
.005 \\
200\overline{)1.000} \quad 0.005 \\
\underline{1\,000} \\
0
\end{array}
$$

12.
$$
\begin{array}{r}
.013 \\
75\overline{)1.000} \approx 0.01 \\
\underline{75} \\
250 \\
\underline{225} \\
25
\end{array}
$$

13. $\dfrac{870}{1000} = 8\underset{\smile\smile\smile}{7\,0} = 0.87$ 14. $\dfrac{2.73}{100} = \underset{\smile\smile}{273} = 0.0273$

15. $\begin{array}{r} 2.05 \\ 7\overline{)14.36} \\ 14 \\ \hline 0\ 3 \\ 0 \\ \hline 36 \\ 35 \\ \hline 1 \end{array} \approx 2.0$ 16. $\begin{array}{r} .7 \\ 0.9\overline{)0.63} \\ 63 \\ \hline 0 \end{array}$ 0.7

.

17. $\begin{array}{r} .7 \\ 0.09\,\overline{)0.063} \\ 63 \\ \hline 0 \end{array}$ 0.7   18. $5\tfrac{1}{2}\% = 5.5\% = \underset{\curvearrowleft\curvearrowleft}{5.5} = 0.055$

19. $55\% = \underset{\curvearrowleft\curvearrowleft}{55} = 0.55$ 20. $\begin{array}{r} 4.6\underline{3} \\ \times\ 6.2\underline{1} \\ \hline 4\ 63 \\ 92\ 6 \\ 2778 \\ \hline 28.7523 \end{array} \approx 28.75$ 21. $0.0\underset{\curvearrowright\curvearrowright}{0\,4} = 0.4$

22. $2.\underset{\curvearrowright\curvearrowright\curvearrowright}{3\ 4\ 5\ 6} = 2{,}345.6$ 23. $\begin{array}{r} 28.33 \\ 0.03\overline{).8500} \\ 6 \\ \hline 25 \\ 24 \\ \hline 10 \\ 9 \\ \hline 10 \\ 9 \\ \hline 1 \end{array} \approx 28.3$

24. $\begin{array}{r} 70.833 \\ 0.12\overline{)8.50000} \\ 8\ 4 \\ \hline 10 \\ 0 \\ \hline 100 \\ 96 \\ \hline 40 \\ 36 \\ \hline 40 \\ 36 \\ \hline 4 \end{array} \approx 70.83$ 25. $0.72 \times \dfrac{1}{0.7} = \dfrac{0.72}{0.7} \Rightarrow \begin{array}{r} 1.02 \\ .7\overline{).720} \\ 7 \\ \hline 02 \\ 0 \\ \hline 20 \\ 14 \\ \hline 6 \end{array} \approx 1.0$

$\dfrac{0.72 \times 100}{0.7 \times 100} = \dfrac{72}{70} = 1\tfrac{2}{70}$

$1\tfrac{2}{70}$ and 1.0

26. $\dfrac{\frac{2}{3}}{\frac{3}{8}} = 2 \div \dfrac{3}{8} = \dfrac{2}{1} \times \dfrac{8}{3} = \dfrac{16}{3} = 5\dfrac{1}{3}$

$\begin{array}{r} 5.33 \\ 3\overline{)16.00} \end{array} \approx 5.3$

$\underline{15}$

$1\,0$

$\underline{9}$

10

$\underline{9}$

1

$\qquad\qquad 5\dfrac{1}{3}$ and 5.3

27. $\dfrac{\frac{2}{5}}{\frac{100}{100}} \times \dfrac{\cancel{500}}{6} = \dfrac{\frac{2}{\cancel{5}} \times \frac{\cancel{5}}{1}}{6} = \dfrac{2}{6} = \dfrac{1}{3}$

$\begin{array}{r} .33 \\ 3\overline{)1.00} \end{array} \approx 0.3$

$\underline{9}$

10

$\underline{9}$

1

$\qquad\qquad \dfrac{1}{3}$ and 0.3

28. $\dfrac{26 \times \frac{5}{13}}{\frac{9}{100}} = \dfrac{26}{1} \times \dfrac{5}{13} \div \dfrac{9}{100} = \dfrac{\overset{2}{\cancel{26}}}{1} \times \dfrac{5}{\underset{1}{\cancel{13}}} \times \dfrac{100}{9} = \dfrac{1{,}000}{9}$

$\begin{array}{r} 111 \\ 9\overline{)1{,}000} \end{array} \Rightarrow 111\dfrac{1}{9}$

$\underline{9}$

10

$\underline{9}$

10

$\underline{9}$

1

$\begin{array}{r} .11 \\ 9\overline{)1.00} \end{array} \quad 111\dfrac{1}{9} \approx 111.11 \approx 111.1$

$\underline{9}$

10

$\underline{9}$

1

$\qquad\qquad\qquad 111\dfrac{1}{9}$ and 111.1

29. $10.3\% = \underset{\curvearrowleft\curvearrowleft}{10.3} = 0.103 \approx 0.1$

$0.103 = \dfrac{103}{1{,}000}$

$\dfrac{103}{1{,}000}$ and 0.1

30. $99.5\% = \underset{\curvearrowleft\curvearrowleft}{99.5} = 0.995 \approx 1.0$

$0.995 = \dfrac{995 \div 5}{1{,}000 \div 5} = \dfrac{191}{200}$

$\dfrac{191}{200}$ and 1.0

Chapter 2

Try These for Practice

1. PO (orally)

2. 1,000

3. 125 mg

4. Gleevec

5. lopinavir 80 mg
   and ritonavir 20 mg

Exercises

1. lopinavir/ritonavir

2. Singulair

3. 60 mL

4. 400 mg per tablet

5. 40 mg per tablet

6. (a) Anusol supp
   (b) 6 A.M.
   (c) 4
   (d) Bonivar, Humulin N, Humulin R
   (e) December 16

7. (a) digoxin, Lasix
   (b) Reglan
   (c) 10 mg PO
   (d) transdermal
   (e) Omnicef

8. (a) 2 mg to 10 mg, 3 or 4 times daily
   (b) periodic blood counts and liver function tests
   (c) 5 mg/5 mL
   (d) 0054-3185-44

9. (a) 9 A.M.–0900h
       3 P.M.–1500h
       Noon–1200h
       6 P.M.–1800h
       8:15 P.M.–2015h
       2:30 A.M.–0230h
       4:45 P.M.–1645h
       6 A.M.–0600h
       Midnight–0000h

Chapter 3

Try These for Practice

1. 270 min

2. 115 oz

3. 252 h

4. 6 qt/h

5. 1.1 lb/wk

Exercises

1. $\dfrac{1.5 \; \cancel{\text{min}}}{1} \times \dfrac{60 \text{ sec}}{1 \; \cancel{\text{min}}} = 90 \text{ sec}$ 2. $\dfrac{11 \; \cancel{\text{yr}}}{\underset{1}{\cancel{2}}} \times \dfrac{\overset{6}{\cancel{12}} \text{ mon}}{1 \; \cancel{\text{yr}}} = 66 \text{ mon}$

3. $\dfrac{17 \; \cancel{\text{d}}}{\underset{1}{\cancel{4}}} \times \dfrac{\overset{6}{\cancel{24}} \text{ h}}{1 \; \cancel{\text{d}}} = 102 \text{ h}$ 4. $\dfrac{\overset{5}{\cancel{40}} \; \cancel{\text{oz}}}{1} \times \dfrac{1 \text{ lb}}{\underset{2}{\cancel{16}} \; \cancel{\text{oz}}} = \dfrac{5 \text{ lb}}{2} = 2\dfrac{1}{2} \text{ lb}$

5. $\dfrac{3 \; \cancel{\text{h}}}{\underset{1}{\cancel{4}}} \times \dfrac{\overset{15}{\cancel{60}} \text{ min}}{1 \; \cancel{\text{h}}} = 45 \text{ min}$ 6. $\dfrac{\overset{17}{\cancel{51}} \; \cancel{\text{mon}}}{1} \times \dfrac{1 \text{ yr}}{\underset{4}{\cancel{12}} \; \cancel{\text{mon}}} = \dfrac{17 \text{ yr}}{4} = 4\dfrac{1}{4} \text{ yr}$

7. $3 \; \cancel{\text{qt}} \times \dfrac{2 \text{ pt}}{1 \; \cancel{\text{qt}}} = 6 \text{ pt}$ 8. $3 \; \cancel{\text{lb}} \times \dfrac{16 \text{ oz}}{\cancel{\text{lb}}} = 48 \text{ oz}$

9. $\dfrac{\cancel{12} \; \cancel{\text{in}}}{\text{sec}} \times \dfrac{1 \text{ ft}}{\cancel{12} \; \cancel{\text{in}}} = 1\dfrac{\text{ft}}{\text{sec}}$ 10. $\dfrac{\overset{1}{\cancel{30}} \text{ pt}}{\text{min}} \times \dfrac{1 \; \cancel{\text{min}}}{\underset{2}{\cancel{60}} \text{ sec}} = \dfrac{1 \text{ pt}}{2 \text{ sec}} = \dfrac{1}{2}\dfrac{\text{pt}}{\text{sec}}$

11. 8 lb 10 oz = 8 lb + 10 oz

$\dfrac{8 \; \cancel{\text{lb}}}{1} \times \dfrac{16 \text{ oz}}{1 \; \cancel{\text{lb}}} = 128 \text{ oz} + 10 \text{ oz} = 138 \text{ oz}$

12. 6 ft 4 in = 6 ft + 4 in

$6 \; \cancel{\text{ft}} \times \dfrac{12 \text{ in}}{1 \; \cancel{\text{ft}}} = 72 \text{ in} + 4 \text{ in} = 76 \text{ in}$

13. $\dfrac{4 \; \cancel{\text{yard}}}{1} \times \dfrac{3 \; \cancel{\text{ft}}}{1 \; \cancel{\text{yard}}} \times \dfrac{12 \text{ in}}{1 \; \cancel{\text{ft}}} = 144 \text{ in}$

14. $\dfrac{\overset{7}{\cancel{42}} \; \cancel{\text{in}}}{1} \times \dfrac{1 \text{ ft}}{\underset{2}{\cancel{12}} \; \cancel{\text{in}}} = \dfrac{7 \text{ ft}}{2} = 3\dfrac{1}{2} \text{ ft}$

15. $2700.0 \; \cancel{\text{sec}} \times \dfrac{\cancel{\text{min}}}{60 \; \cancel{\text{sec}}} \times \dfrac{\text{h}}{60 \; \cancel{\text{min}}} = \dfrac{27 \text{ h}}{36} = \dfrac{3}{4} \text{ h}$

16. $\dfrac{\overset{3}{\cancel{6}} \; \cancel{\text{pt}}}{\cancel{\text{h}}} \times \dfrac{1 \text{ qt}}{\underset{1}{\cancel{2}} \; \cancel{\text{pt}}} \times \dfrac{24 \; \cancel{\text{h}}}{\text{day}} = 72 \dfrac{\text{qt}}{\text{day}}$

17. $\dfrac{\overset{1}{\cancel{6}} \; \cancel{\text{qt}}}{\cancel{\text{day}}} \times \dfrac{2 \text{ pt}}{1 \; \cancel{\text{qt}}} \times \dfrac{1 \; \cancel{\text{day}}}{\underset{\underset{2}{12}}{\cancel{24}} \text{ h}} = \dfrac{1 \text{ pt}}{2 \text{ h}}$

18. $\overset{240}{\cancel{1680}} \; \cancel{\text{h}} \times \dfrac{\cancel{\text{day}}}{24 \; \cancel{\text{h}}} \times \dfrac{\text{week}}{\underset{1}{\cancel{7}} \; \cancel{\text{days}}} = 10 \text{ week}$

19. $\dfrac{1,209,600.0 \; \cancel{\text{sec}}}{1} \times \dfrac{1 \; \cancel{\text{min}}}{60 \; \cancel{\text{sec}}} \times \dfrac{1 \; \cancel{\text{h}}}{60 \; \cancel{\text{min}}} \times \dfrac{1 \; \cancel{\text{day}}}{24 \; \cancel{\text{h}}} \times \dfrac{1 \text{ week}}{7 \; \cancel{\text{days}}} = 2 \text{ week}$

20. $\dfrac{5 \; \cancel{\text{cases}}}{1} \times \dfrac{24 \; \cancel{\text{cans}}}{\cancel{\text{case}}} \times \dfrac{12 \; \cancel{\text{oz}}}{\cancel{\text{can}}} \times \dfrac{1 \text{ cup}}{\cancel{60} \; \cancel{\text{oz}}} = 24 \text{ cups}$

Chapter 4

Try These for Practice

1. (a) 1,000 mL   (c) 1,000 cc   (e) 1,000 mg

   (b) 1 cc   (d) 1,000 g   (f) 1,000 mcg

(g) 1,000 micrograms   (k) 8 oz   (o) 16 oz

(h) 2 pt   (l) 2 T   (p) dr 8

(i) 16 oz   (m) 3 t   (q) minims 60

(j) 8 oz   (n) 60 gtt

2. 0.01 g   3. 5,000 mcg   4. 1.8 L

5. 3 pt

Exercise

1. $\dfrac{400 \text{ mg}}{1} \times \dfrac{1 \text{ g}}{1{,}000 \text{ mg}} = \dfrac{4}{10} \text{ g} = 0.4 \text{ g}$

2. $\dfrac{0.003 \text{ g}}{1} \times \dfrac{1{,}000 \text{ mg}}{1 \text{ g}} = 3 \text{ mg}$

3. $\dfrac{0.07 \text{ g}}{1} \times \dfrac{1{,}000 \text{ mg}}{1 \text{ g}} = 70 \text{ mg}$

4. $\dfrac{3 \text{ L}}{1} \times \dfrac{1{,}000 \text{ mL}}{1 \text{ L}} = 3{,}000 \text{ mL}$

5. $\dfrac{2500 \text{ mL}}{1} \times \dfrac{1 \text{ L}}{1{,}000 \text{ mL}} = \dfrac{25}{10} \text{ L} = 2.5 \text{ L}$

6. $\dfrac{600 \text{ mcg}}{1} \times \dfrac{1 \text{ mg}}{1{,}000 \text{ mcg}} = \dfrac{6}{10} \text{ mg} = 0.6 \text{ mg}$

7. $\dfrac{1.7 \text{ L}}{1} \times \dfrac{1{,}000 \text{ mL}}{1 \text{ L}} = 1{,}700 \text{ mL}$

8. $\dfrac{9 \text{ qt}}{2} \times \dfrac{2 \text{ pt}}{1 \text{ qt}} = 9 \text{ pt}$

9. $\dfrac{2.5 \text{ kg}}{1} \times \dfrac{1{,}000 \text{ g}}{1 \text{ kg}} = 2{,}500 \text{ g}$

10. $\dfrac{4 \text{ T}}{1} \times \dfrac{3 \text{ t}}{1 \text{ T}} = 12 \text{ t}$

11. $\dfrac{5 \text{ T}}{1} \times \dfrac{1 \text{ oz}}{2 \text{ T}} = \dfrac{5}{2} \text{ oz} = 2\dfrac{1}{2} \text{ oz}$

12. $\dfrac{\overset{2}{32} \text{ oz}}{1} \times \dfrac{1 \text{ pt}}{\underset{1}{16} \text{ oz}} = 2 \text{ pt}$

13. $\dfrac{40 \text{ mg}}{1} \times \dfrac{1{,}000 \text{ mcg}}{1 \text{ mg}} = 40{,}000 \text{ mcg}$

14. $\dfrac{520 \text{ mcg}}{1} \times \dfrac{1 \text{ mg}}{1{,}000 \text{ mcg}} = \dfrac{52}{100} \text{ mg} = 0.52 \text{ mg}$

15. $\dfrac{50 \text{ mg}}{1} \times \dfrac{1 \text{ g}}{1{,}000 \text{ mg}} = \dfrac{5}{100} \text{ g} = 0.05 \text{ g}$

16. $\dfrac{8 \text{ h}}{1} \times \dfrac{\frac{1}{2} \text{ pt}}{2 \text{ h}} \times \dfrac{1 \text{ qt}}{2 \text{ pt}} = \dfrac{4}{4} \text{ qt} = 1 \text{ qt}$

17. $\dfrac{100 \text{ mg}}{1} \times \dfrac{1 \text{ g}}{1{,}000 \text{ mg}} = \dfrac{1}{10} = 0.1 \text{ g}$

18. $\dfrac{3,4\cancel{00}\ \cancel{g}}{1} \times \dfrac{1\ kg}{1,0\cancel{00}\ \cancel{g}} = \dfrac{34}{10}\ kg = 3.4\ kg$

19. $\dfrac{\cancel{dr}\ \overset{3}{\cancel{12}}}{1} \times \dfrac{oz\ 1}{\underset{2}{\cancel{dr}\ \cancel{8}}} = oz\ \dfrac{3}{2} = oz\ 1\tfrac{1}{2}$

20. $\dfrac{\cancel{dr}\ 3}{\underset{1}{\cancel{2}}} \times \dfrac{minims\ \overset{30}{\cancel{60}}}{\cancel{dr}\ 1} = minims\ 90$

Cumulative Review Exercises

1. 7,800 mg
2. 250 mcg
3. 4,500 mL

4. dr 224
5. 1.2 L
6. 7,600 g

7. 0.75 L
8. 15 t
9. 1,000 mg

10. 0.25 g
11. 650 mcg
12. 6 t

13. 15 mL
14. 0.25 L
15. 32 mg

Chapter 5

Try These for Practice

1. (a) 1 cc
   (b) 1,000 mL
   (c) 1,000 g
   (d) 1 g
   (e) 1 mg
   (f) 8 oz
   (g) 2 T
   (h) 3 t

   (i) 16 oz
   (j) 12 in
   (k) 2 pt
   (l) 16 oz
   (m) dr 8
   (n) minims 60
   (o) 1 t = minims 60 = 5 mL
   (p) 2 T = dr 8 = 30 mL

   (q) 1 glass = oz 8 = $\tfrac{1}{2}$ pt
   (r) 60 mg
   (s) gr 15
   (t) 2.2 lb
   (u) 2.5 cm

2. 0.025 g
3. 110 lb
4. 1 t

5. 300 mg

Exercises

1. $\dfrac{4,5\cancel{00}\ \cancel{mcg}}{1} \times \dfrac{mg}{1,0\cancel{00}\ \cancel{mcg}} = \dfrac{45}{10}\ mg = 4.5\ mg$

2. $1.5\ \cancel{L} \times \dfrac{1,000\ mL}{1\ \cancel{L}} = 1,500\ mL$

3. $\dfrac{4\ \cancel{t}}{1} \times \dfrac{5\ mL}{\cancel{t}} = 20\ mL$

4. $\dfrac{\overset{3}{\cancel{15}}\ \cancel{mL}}{1} \times \dfrac{t}{\underset{1}{\cancel{5}\ \cancel{mL}}} = 3\ t$

5. $\dfrac{45\ \cancel{kg}}{1} \times \dfrac{2.2\ lb}{\cancel{kg}} = 99\ lb$

6. $\dfrac{110\ \cancel{lb}}{1} \times \dfrac{kg}{2.2\ \cancel{lb}} = \dfrac{110}{2.2}\ kg = 50\ kg$

7. $\dfrac{\overset{3}{\cancel{48} \cancel{\text{oz}}}}{1} \times \dfrac{\text{pt}}{\underset{1}{\cancel{16} \cancel{\text{oz}}}} = 3 \text{ pt}$

8. $\dfrac{3 \cancel{\text{oz}}}{1} \times \dfrac{2 \text{ T}}{1 \cancel{\text{oz}}} = 6 \text{ T}$

9. $\dfrac{10 \cancel{\text{cm}}}{1} \times \dfrac{1 \text{ in}}{2.5 \cancel{\text{cm}}} = \dfrac{10}{2.5} \text{ in} = 4 \text{ in}$

10. $\dfrac{6 \cancel{\text{in}}}{1} \times \dfrac{2.5 \text{ cm}}{1 \cancel{\text{in}}} = 15 \text{ cm}$

11. $\dfrac{6 \cancel{\text{ft}}}{1} \times \dfrac{12 \text{ in}}{1 \cancel{\text{ft}}} = 72 \text{ in} + 2 \text{ in} = 74 \text{ in}$

$\dfrac{74 \cancel{\text{in}}}{1} \times \dfrac{2.5 \text{ cm}}{1 \cancel{\text{in}}} = 185 \text{ cm}$

12. $10 \text{ mg} = 1 \text{ mL}$

$\dfrac{1 \cancel{\text{mL}}}{1} \times \dfrac{1 \text{ oz}}{30 \cancel{\text{mL}}} = \dfrac{1}{30} \text{ oz}$

13. $\dfrac{165 \cancel{\text{lb}}}{1} \times \dfrac{\text{kg}}{2.2 \cancel{\text{lb}}} = \dfrac{165}{2.2} \text{ kg} = 75 \text{ kg}$

14. $2 \cancel{\text{t}} \times \dfrac{5 \text{ mL}}{1 \cancel{\text{t}}} = 10 \text{ mL}$

15. $\dfrac{\overset{5}{\cancel{25} \cancel{\text{mg}}}}{1} \times \dfrac{\text{gr } 1}{\underset{12}{\cancel{60} \cancel{\text{mg}}}} = \text{gr} \dfrac{5}{12}$

16. $10 \text{ mg} = 5 \text{ mL}$

$\dfrac{5 \cancel{\text{mL}}}{1} \times \dfrac{1 \text{ t}}{5 \cancel{\text{mL}}} = 1 \text{ t}$

17. $\dfrac{12 \cancel{\text{oz}}}{1} \times \dfrac{30 \text{ mL}}{1 \cancel{\text{oz}}} = 360 \text{ mL}$

18. $\dfrac{32 \cancel{\text{mcg}}}{1} \times \dfrac{1 \text{ mg}}{1{,}000 \cancel{\text{mcg}}} = \dfrac{32}{1{,}000} \text{ mg} = 0.032 \text{ mg}$

19. $\dfrac{120 \cancel{\text{sprays}}}{\text{container}} \times \dfrac{32 \cancel{\text{mcg}}}{1 \cancel{\text{spray}}} \times \dfrac{1 \text{ mg}}{1{,}000 \cancel{\text{mcg}}} = \dfrac{384}{100} \dfrac{\text{mg}}{\text{container}} = 3.84 \dfrac{\text{mg}}{\text{container}}$

20. $\dfrac{3 \cancel{\text{tab}}}{1} \times \dfrac{10 \cancel{\text{mg}}}{1 \cancel{\text{tab}}} \times \dfrac{\text{gr } 1}{60 \cancel{\text{mg}}} = \text{gr} \dfrac{3}{6} = \text{gr} \dfrac{1}{2}$

Cumulative Review Exercises

1. 125 mcg

2. 9 mg

3. 5,650 g

4. 100 mcg

5. 60 mg

6. 4,500 mg

7. 7,750 mL

8. 600 mcg

9. 1.25 L

10. gr $\frac{1}{2}$

11. gr $2\frac{1}{2}$

12. 0.15 g

13. 0.01 g

14. 100 tab

15. 0.09 g

Chapter 6

Case Study

1. 650 mL + 150 mL + 200 mL = 1,000 mL

   1,500 mL − 1,000 mL = 500 mL

2. (a) $\dfrac{3 \text{ cups}}{\underset{1}{\cancel{2}}} \times \dfrac{\overset{4}{\cancel{8} \text{ oz}}}{1 \text{ cup}} \times \dfrac{30 \text{ mL}}{1 \text{ oz}} = 360$ mL

   (b) $\dfrac{3 \text{ cups}}{\underset{1}{\cancel{2}}} \times \dfrac{\overset{195}{\cancel{390} \text{ mg}}}{\text{cup}} \times \dfrac{g}{1,000 \text{ mg}} = \dfrac{585}{1,000}$ g = 0.585 g

   (c) 2 g − 0.59 g = 1.41 g

3. (a) $\overset{4}{\cancel{80} \text{ mg}} \times \dfrac{1 \text{ tab}}{\underset{1}{\cancel{20} \text{ mg}}} = 4$ tab (for stat dose)

   (b) $\overset{3}{\cancel{60} \text{ mg}} \times \dfrac{1 \text{ tab}}{\underset{1}{\cancel{20} \text{ mg}}} = 3$ tab (12 h later)

   4 tab + 3 tab = 7 tab within first 20 hours.

4. $5 \text{ days} \times \dfrac{20 \text{ mEq}}{\text{day}} = 100$ mEq

5. (a) t.i.d. means 3 times per day.

   (b) $\dfrac{2 \text{ days}}{1} \times \dfrac{3 \text{ doses}}{\text{day}} \times \dfrac{\overset{5}{\cancel{100} \text{ mg}}}{\text{dose}} \times \dfrac{5 \text{ mL}}{\underset{1}{\cancel{20} \text{ mg}}} = 150$ mL

6. $3 \text{ mg} \times \dfrac{\text{tab}}{1 \text{ mg}} = 3$ tab

7. $0.25 \text{ mg} \times \dfrac{1,000 \text{ mcg}}{1 \text{ mg}} = 250$ mcg

   one 200-mcg tab and one 50-mcg tab.

8. $7 \text{ days} \times \dfrac{125 \text{ mg}}{\text{day}} = 875$ mg

   $\overset{35}{\cancel{875} \text{ mg}} \times \dfrac{\text{tab}}{\underset{10}{\cancel{250} \text{ mg}}} = \dfrac{35}{10}$ tab = $3\dfrac{1}{2}$ tab

Practice Reading labels

1. $0.05 \text{ g} \times \dfrac{1,000 \text{ mg}}{\text{g}} \times \dfrac{\text{tab}}{50 \text{ mg}} = \dfrac{50}{50}$ tab = 1 tab

2. $2\cancel{00} \text{ mg} \times \dfrac{\text{tab}}{1\cancel{00} \text{ mg}} = 2$ tab

3. $0.04 \text{ g} \times \dfrac{1,000 \text{ mg}}{\text{g}} \times \dfrac{\text{cap}}{20 \text{ mg}} = \dfrac{4}{2}$ cap = 2 cap

4. $\overset{2}{\cancel{40} \text{ mg}} \times \dfrac{5 \text{ mL}}{\underset{1}{\cancel{20} \text{ mg}}} = 10$ mL

5. $0.666 \ \cancel{g} \times \dfrac{1{,}000 \ \cancel{mg}}{1 \ \cancel{g}} \times \dfrac{tab}{333 \ \cancel{mg}} = \dfrac{666}{333} \ tab = 2 \ tab$

6. $\overset{2}{\cancel{800}} \ \cancel{mg} \times \dfrac{tab}{\underset{1}{\cancel{400}} \ \cancel{mg}} = 2 \ tab$

7. $\overset{2}{\cancel{12}} \ \cancel{mg} \times \dfrac{cap}{\underset{1}{\cancel{6}} \ \cancel{mg}} = 2 \ cap$

8. $\overset{1}{\cancel{20}} \ \cancel{mg} \times \dfrac{mL}{\underset{4}{\cancel{80}} \ \cancel{mg}} = \dfrac{1}{4} \ mL = 0.25 \ mL$

9. $0.6 \ \cancel{g} \times \dfrac{1{,}000 \ \cancel{mg}}{\cancel{g}} \times \dfrac{tab}{300 \ \cancel{mg}} = \dfrac{600}{300} \ tab = 2 \ tab$

10. $\overset{2}{\cancel{100}} \ \cancel{mg} \times \dfrac{5 \ mL}{\underset{1}{\cancel{50}} \ \cancel{mg}} = 10 \ mL$

11. $\overset{1}{\cancel{125}} \ \cancel{mcg} \times \dfrac{mL}{\underset{2}{\cancel{250}} \ \cancel{mcg}} = \dfrac{1}{2} \ mL = 0.5 \ mL$

12. $0.2 \ \cancel{mg} \times \dfrac{1{,}0\cancel{0}0 \ \cancel{mcg}}{\cancel{mg}} \times \dfrac{1 \ cap}{10\cancel{0} \ \cancel{mcg}} = 2 \ cap$

13. $0.4 \ \cancel{g} \times \dfrac{1{,}0\cancel{0}0 \ \cancel{mg}}{\cancel{g}} \times \dfrac{tab}{2\cancel{0}0 \ \cancel{mg}} = \dfrac{4}{2} \ tab = 2 \ tab$

14. $5 \ \cancel{mg} \times \dfrac{tab}{2.5 \ \cancel{mg}} = \dfrac{5}{2.5} \ tab = 2 \ tab$

15. $\overset{4}{\cancel{16}} \ \cancel{mg} \times \dfrac{tab}{\underset{1}{\cancel{4}} \ \cancel{mg}} = 4 \ tab$

16. $\overset{4}{\cancel{80}} \ \cancel{mg} \times \dfrac{cap}{\underset{1}{\cancel{20}} \ \cancel{mg}} = 4 \ cap$

17. $0.05 \ \cancel{mg} \times \dfrac{\cancel{5} \ mL}{\cancel{5} \ \cancel{mg}} = 0.05 \ mL$

18. $5 \ \cancel{mg} \times \dfrac{1 \ cap}{2.5 \ \cancel{mg}} = \dfrac{5}{2.5} \ cap = 2 \ cap$

19. $0.1 \ \cancel{mg} \times \dfrac{1{,}0\cancel{0}0 \ \cancel{mcg}}{\cancel{mg}} \times \dfrac{1 \ mL}{10\cancel{0} \ \cancel{mcg}} = 1 \ mL$

20. $0.08 \ \cancel{g} \times \dfrac{1{,}0\cancel{0}0 \ \cancel{mg}}{\cancel{g}} \times \dfrac{tab}{4\cancel{0} \ \cancel{mg}} = \dfrac{8}{4} \ tab = 2 \ tab$

21. $13\cancel{0} \ \cancel{mg} \times \dfrac{mL}{8\cancel{0} \ \cancel{mg}} = \dfrac{13}{8} \ mL \approx 1.6 \ mL$

22. $\overset{3}{\cancel{75}} \ \cancel{mg} \times \dfrac{cap}{\underset{1}{\cancel{25}} \ \cancel{mg}} = 3 \ cap$

23. $\overset{2}{\cancel{8}} \ \cancel{mg} \times \dfrac{tab}{\underset{1}{\cancel{4}} \ \cancel{mg}} = 2 \ tab$

24. $\overset{8}{\cancel{400}} \ \cancel{mcg} \times \dfrac{mL}{\underset{5}{\cancel{250}} \ \cancel{mcg}} = \dfrac{8}{5} \ mL = 1.6 \ mL$

25. $\overset{2}{\cancel{300}}$ $\cancel{mg} \times \dfrac{tab}{\underset{1}{\cancel{150}\ \cancel{mg}}} = 2\ tab$

26. $2\ \cancel{g} \times \dfrac{\overset{2}{\cancel{1,000}}\ \cancel{mg}}{\cancel{g}} \times \dfrac{cap}{\underset{1}{\cancel{500}\ \cancel{mg}}} = 4\ cap$

27. $150\ \cancel{mg} \times \dfrac{tab}{25\ \cancel{mg}} = 6\ tab$

28. $0.25\ \cancel{mg} \times \dfrac{tab}{0.125\ \cancel{mg}} = \dfrac{0.25}{0.125} \times \dfrac{1,000}{1,000} = \dfrac{250}{125} = 2\ tab$

29. $\overset{3}{\cancel{75}}\ \cancel{mg} \times \dfrac{tab}{\underset{1}{25\ \cancel{mg}}} = 3\ tab$

30. $\overset{4}{\cancel{100}}\ \cancel{mg} \times \dfrac{5\ mL}{\underset{1}{25\ \cancel{mg}}} = 20\ mL$

31. $0.5\ \cancel{g} \times \dfrac{\overset{4}{\cancel{1,000}}\ \cancel{mg}}{\cancel{g}} \times \dfrac{tab}{\underset{1}{250\ \cancel{mg}}} = 2\ tab$

32. $\overset{3}{\cancel{900}}\ \cancel{mg} \times \dfrac{tab}{\underset{1}{\cancel{300}\ \cancel{mg}}} = 3\ tab$

33. $2500\ \cancel{mcg} \times \dfrac{\cancel{mg}}{1000\ \cancel{mcg}} \times \dfrac{tab}{2.5\ \cancel{mg}} = \dfrac{25}{25}\ tab = 1\ tab$

34. $4\ \cancel{mg} \times \dfrac{5\ mL}{4\ \cancel{mg}} = 5\ mL$

35. $10\ \cancel{mg} \times \dfrac{tab}{2.5\ \cancel{mg}} = \dfrac{10}{2.5}\ tab = 4\ tab$

36. $\overset{2}{\cancel{4}}\ \cancel{mg} \times \dfrac{tab}{\underset{1}{\cancel{2}\ \cancel{mg}}} = 2\ tab$

37. $400\ \cancel{mg} \times \dfrac{5\ mL}{100\ \cancel{mg}} = 20\ mL$

38. $20\ \cancel{mg} \times \dfrac{tab}{2.5\ \cancel{mg}} = \dfrac{20 \times 10}{2.5 \times 10} = \dfrac{200}{25} = 8\ tab$

39. $0.6\ \cancel{g} \times \dfrac{1,000\ \cancel{mg}}{\cancel{g}} \times \dfrac{tab}{600\ \cancel{mg}} = \dfrac{6}{6}\ tab = 1\ tab$

40. $200\ \cancel{mg} \times \dfrac{tab}{100\ \cancel{mg}} = 2\ tab$

41. $10\ \cancel{mg} \times \dfrac{tab}{2.5\ \cancel{mg}} = \dfrac{10}{2.5}\ tab = 4\ tab$

42. $5\ \cancel{mg} \times \dfrac{tab}{2.5\ \cancel{mg}} = \dfrac{5}{2.5}\ tab = 2\ tab$

43. $\overset{2}{\cancel{80}}\ \cancel{mg} \times \dfrac{tab}{\underset{1}{\cancel{40}\ \cancel{mg}}} = 2\ tab$

44. $\overset{3}{\cancel{75}}\ \cancel{mg} \times \dfrac{cap}{\underset{1}{25\ \cancel{mg}}} = 3\ cap$

45. $1,\cancel{000}\text{ mg} \times \dfrac{5\text{ mL}}{2\cancel{00}\text{ mg}} = \dfrac{50}{2}\text{ mL} = 25\text{ mL}$

46. $5\cancel{0}\text{ mg} \times \dfrac{\text{tab}}{1\cancel{0}\text{ mg}} = 5\text{ tab}$

47. $\overset{2}{\cancel{500}}\text{ mg} \times \dfrac{\text{tab}}{\underset{1}{\cancel{250}}\text{ mg}} = 2\text{ tab}$

48. $\overset{2}{\cancel{16}}\text{ mg} \times \dfrac{\text{tab}}{\underset{1}{\cancel{8}}\text{ mg}} = 2\text{ tab}$

49. $\cancel{75}\text{ mg} \times \dfrac{\text{tab}}{\cancel{75}\text{ mg}} = 1\text{ tab}$

50. $0.5\cancel{\text{ g}} \times \dfrac{\overset{2}{\cancel{1,000}}\text{ mg}}{\cancel{\text{g}}} \times \dfrac{\text{tab}}{\underset{1}{\cancel{500}}\text{ mg}} = 1\text{ tab}$

51. $\cancel{20}\text{ mg} \times \dfrac{\text{tab}}{\cancel{20}\text{ mg}} = 1\text{ tab}$

52. $\overset{3}{\cancel{375}}\text{ mg} \times \dfrac{5\text{ mL}}{\underset{1}{\cancel{125}}\text{ mg}} = 15\text{ mL}$

53. $8\cancel{\text{ mg}} \times \dfrac{\text{mL}}{10\cancel{\text{ mg}}} = \dfrac{8}{10}\text{ mL} = 0.8\text{ mL}$

54. $2\cancel{0}\text{ mg} \times \dfrac{1\text{ tab}}{1\cancel{0}\text{ mg}} = 2\text{ tab}$

55. $\overset{3}{\cancel{75}}\text{ mg} \times \dfrac{5\text{ mL}}{\underset{1}{\cancel{25}}\text{ mg}} = 15\text{ mL}$

56. $\overset{4}{\cancel{80}}\text{ mg} \times \dfrac{\text{tab}}{\underset{1}{\cancel{20}}\text{ mg}} = 4\text{ tab}$

57. $\overset{2}{\cancel{100}}\text{ mg} \times \dfrac{\text{tab}}{\underset{1}{\cancel{50}}\text{ mg}} = 2\text{ tab}$

58. $0.4\cancel{\text{ g}} \times \dfrac{1,\cancel{000}\text{ mg}}{\cancel{\text{g}}} \times \dfrac{\text{tab}}{4\cancel{00}\text{ mg}} = \dfrac{4}{4}\text{ tab} = 1\text{ tab}$

59. $0.08\cancel{\text{ g}} \times \dfrac{1,\cancel{000}\text{ mg}}{\cancel{\text{g}}} \times \dfrac{\text{cap}}{8\cancel{0}\text{ mg}} = \dfrac{8}{8}\text{ cap} = 1\text{ cap}$

60. $0.8\cancel{\text{ g}} \times \dfrac{1,\cancel{000}\text{ mg}}{\cancel{\text{g}}} \times \dfrac{\text{cap}}{1\cancel{00}\text{ mg}} = 8\text{ cap}$

Try These for Practice

1. (a) 3 tablets
   (b) 0.06 g

2. 86 mg   3. 30 mL   4. 6 capsules

5. One 50 mg and two 15 mg tablets

Exercises

1. $40 \text{ mg} \times \dfrac{\text{g}}{1,000 \text{ mg}} \times \dfrac{\text{tab}}{0.02 \text{ g}} = \dfrac{4}{2} \text{ tab} = 2 \text{ tab}$

2. $500 \text{ mcg} \times \dfrac{\text{mg}}{1,000 \text{ mcg}} \times \dfrac{\text{mL}}{0.05 \text{ mg}} = \dfrac{50}{5} \text{ mL} = 10 \text{ mL}$

3. $4 \text{ weeks} \times \dfrac{7 \text{ days}}{\text{week}} \times \dfrac{40 \text{ mg}}{\text{day}} \times \dfrac{\text{cap}}{10 \text{ mg}} = 112 \text{ cap}$

4. $\overset{3}{75} \text{ mg} \times \dfrac{\text{tab}}{\underset{1}{25} \text{ mg}} = 3 \text{ tab per dose} \times 3 \text{ doses per day} = 9 \text{ tab}$

5. $7 \text{ days} \times \dfrac{200 \text{ mg}}{\text{day}} \times \dfrac{\text{tab}}{200 \text{ mg}} = 7 \text{ tab}$

6. $40 \text{ kg} \times \dfrac{50 \text{ mg}}{\text{kg}} \times \dfrac{\text{tab}}{500 \text{ mg}} = \dfrac{20}{5} = 4 \text{ tab daily which is 2 tab per dose}$

7. $600 \text{ mg} \times \dfrac{5 \text{ mL}}{100 \text{ mg}} = 30 \text{ mL}$

8. $0.015 \text{ g} \times \dfrac{1,000 \text{ mg}}{\text{g}} \times \dfrac{\text{tab}}{7.5 \text{ mg}} = \dfrac{15}{7.5} \text{ tab} = 2 \text{ tab}$

9. $\dfrac{\overset{6}{150} \text{ mg}}{\text{day}} \times \dfrac{\text{tab}}{\underset{1}{25} \text{ mg}} = \dfrac{6 \text{ tab}}{\text{day}}$ in three divided doses means give 2 tablets per dose

10. $25 \text{ mg} \times \dfrac{5 \text{ mL}}{10 \text{ mg}} = \dfrac{125}{10} \text{ mL} = 12.5 \text{ mL}$

11. $\dfrac{\overset{1}{25} \text{ mg}}{\text{day}} \times \dfrac{\text{tab}}{\underset{2}{50} \text{ mg}} = \dfrac{1}{2} \text{ tab per day or } 1\dfrac{1}{2} \text{ tab in 3 days}$

12. $7.5 \text{ mg} \times \dfrac{\text{tab}}{15 \text{ mg}} = \dfrac{7.5}{15} \text{ tab} = \dfrac{1}{2} \text{ tab per dose.}$ Since there are 3 doses per day, the patient receives $1\dfrac{1}{2}$ tablets daily.

13. $\overset{3}{75} \text{ mg} \times \dfrac{\text{cap}}{\underset{1}{25} \text{ mg}} = 3 \text{ cap}$

14. $\dfrac{2 \text{ tab}}{\text{dose}} \times \dfrac{4 \text{ dose}}{\text{day}} \times \dfrac{300 \text{ mg}}{\text{tab}} = 2,400 \text{ mg per day}$

15. $\overset{2}{4} \text{ mg} \times \dfrac{\text{cap}}{\underset{1}{2} \text{ mg}} = 2 \text{ cap}$

16. $0.25 \text{ g} \times \dfrac{1,000 \text{ mg}}{\text{g}} \times \dfrac{\text{tab}}{500 \text{ mg}} = \dfrac{250}{500} \text{ tab} = \dfrac{1}{2} \text{ tab}$

17. Patient receives Coumadin on Mon., Wed., Fri., and Sun.

$\dfrac{6.5 \text{ mg}}{\text{dose}} \times \dfrac{4 \text{ dose}}{\text{wk}} = 26 \text{ mg per week}$

18. $200 \text{ mg} \times \dfrac{5 \text{ mL}}{100 \text{ mg}} = 10 \text{ mL}$

19. $5 \text{ ft} \times \dfrac{12 \text{ in}}{\text{ft}} = 60 \text{ in} + 6 \text{ in} = 66 \text{ in}$

$\text{BSA} = \sqrt{\dfrac{66 \times 140}{3{,}131}} \approx 1.72 \text{ m}^2$

$1.72 \text{ m}^2 \times \dfrac{60 \text{ mg}}{\text{m}^2} \approx 103 \text{ mg}$

(b) $103 \text{ mg} \times \dfrac{\text{tab}}{50 \text{ mg}} = \dfrac{103}{50} \text{ tab} = 2.06 \approx 2 \text{ tab}$

20. 500 mg on day 1 and 250 mg on next 4 days means
500 mg + 1,000 mg = 1,500 mg in total

Cumulative Review Exercises

1. 1 tab
2. 10 mL
3. gr 3

4. 400 mg
5. 2,500 mL
6. 3,494 g

7. 2 cups
8. 10 mL
9. 2 cap

10. 4 tab
11. 3 tab
12. 3 tab

13. 0.2 g
14. 2 tab
15. 5 mL

Chapter 7

Case Study 7.1

1. $75 \text{ mg} \times \dfrac{\text{mL}}{100 \text{ mg}} = \dfrac{75}{100} \text{ mL} = 0.75 \text{ mL}$

the 1 mL syringe

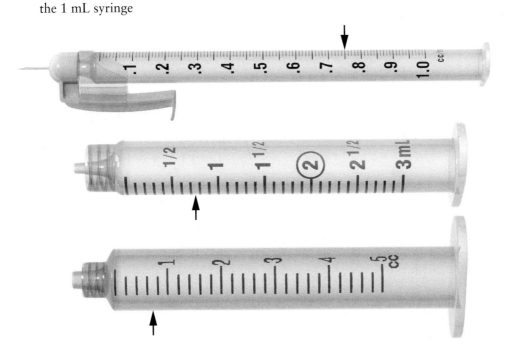

2. 75 mg/mL

Demerol: $\cancel{75\ mg} \times \dfrac{mL}{\cancel{75\ mg}} = 1$ mL of Demerol

$\cancel{25\ mg} \times \dfrac{mL}{\cancel{25\ mg}} = 1$ mL of Phenergan

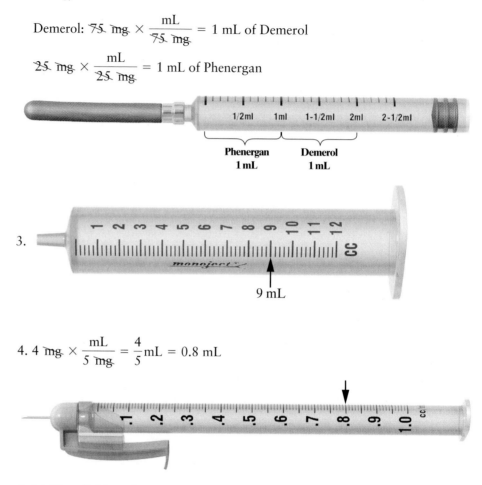

3.

9 mL

4. $4\ \cancel{mg} \times \dfrac{mL}{5\ \cancel{mg}} = \dfrac{4}{5} mL = 0.8$ mL

5. (a) Vistaril 25 mg/mL

(b) $75\ \cancel{mg} \times \dfrac{mL}{100\ \cancel{mg}} = \dfrac{75}{100} mL = 0.75$ mL Demerol

(c) $\cancel{25\ mg} \times \dfrac{mL}{\cancel{25\ mg}} = 1$ mL Vistaril

Using a 3 mL syringe remove 0.75 mL of Demerol and then remove 1 mL of Vistaril for a total volume of 1.75 mL

(d)

6. (a) $1\ \cancel{g} \times \dfrac{\overset{20}{\cancel{1,000}}\ \cancel{mg}}{1\ \cancel{g}} \times \dfrac{mL}{\underset{1}{\cancel{50}}\ \cancel{mg}} = 20$ mL of Merrem

(b)

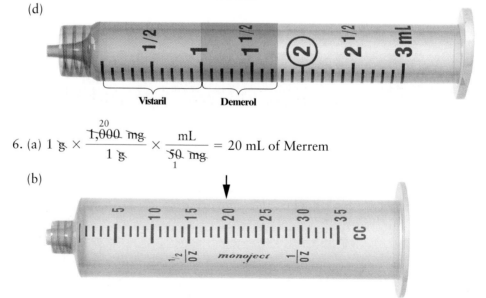

7. (a) 13 units + 6 units = 19 units

(b)

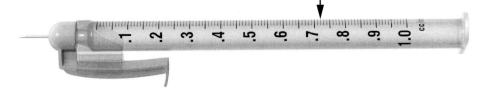

Humulin
N
13 units

Humulin
R
6 units

Try These for Practice

1. 1 mL tuberculin syringe; 0.72 mL

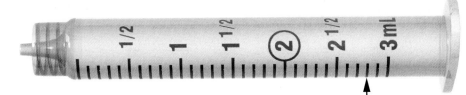

2. 12 mL syringe; 6.8 mL

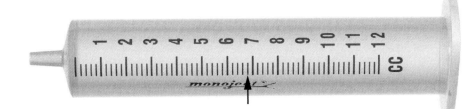

3. 3 mL syringe; 2.8 mL

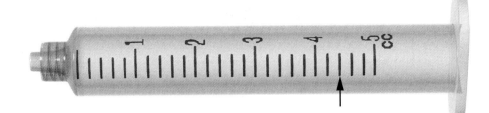

4. 5 mL syringe; 4.4 mL

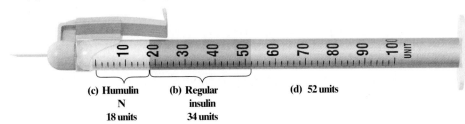

5. (a) 100 unit insulin syringe

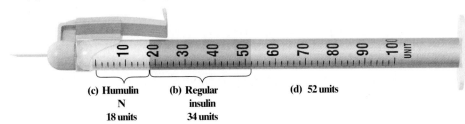

(c) Humulin
N
18 units

(b) Regular
insulin
34 units

(d) 52 units

Exercises

1. 1 mL tuberculin syringe; 0.62 mL

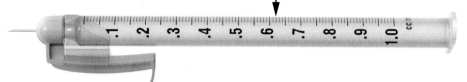

2. 30 unit Lo-Dose insulin syringe; 28 units

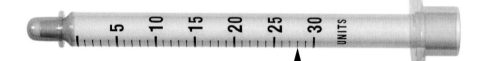

3. 5 mL syringe; 3.6 mL

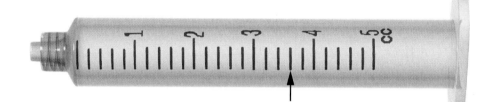

4. 3 mL syringe; 1.4 mL

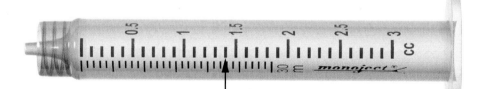

5. 35 mL syringe; 13 mL

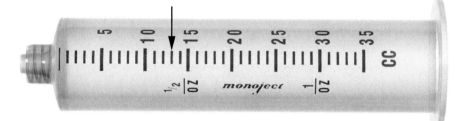

6. 12 mL syringe; 9.6 mL

7. 50 unit Lo-Dose insulin syringe; 32 units

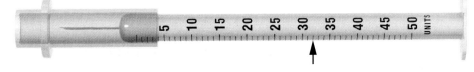

8. 100 unit insulin syringe; 56 units

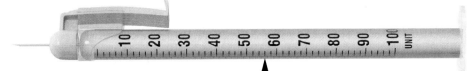

9. 1 mL tuberculin syringe; 0.37 mL

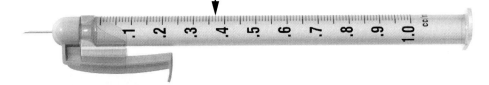

10. 100 unit insulin syringe; 51 units

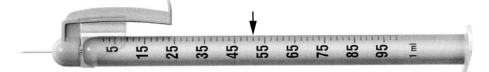

11. 12 mL syringe; 6.6 mL

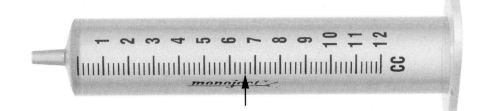

12. 1 mL tuberculin syringe; 0.72 mL

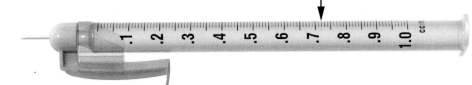

13. 12 mL syringe; 8.2 mL

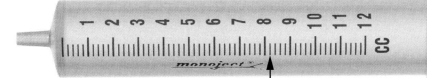

14. 35 mL syringe; 27 mL

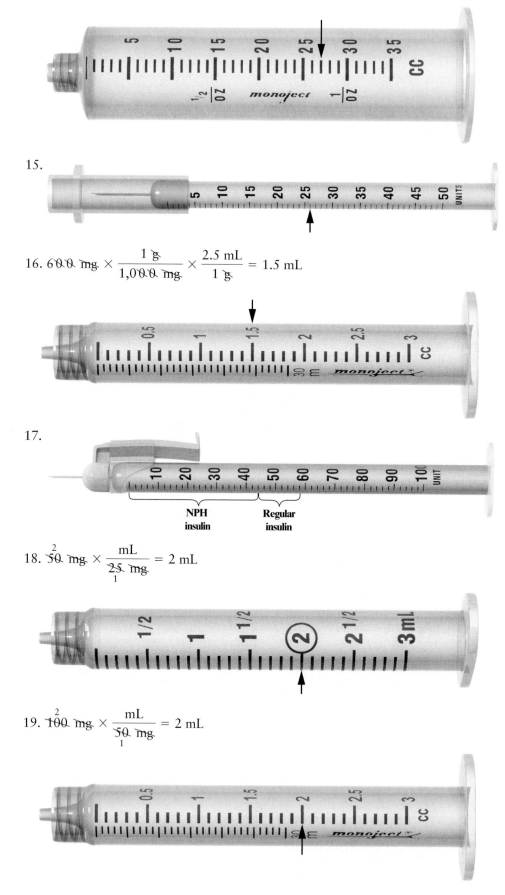

15.

16. $600.0 \text{ mg} \times \dfrac{1 \text{ g}}{1,000.0 \text{ mg}} \times \dfrac{2.5 \text{ mL}}{1 \text{ g}} = 1.5 \text{ mL}$

17.

NPH insulin   **Regular insulin**

18. $\overset{2}{50} \text{ mg} \times \dfrac{\text{mL}}{\underset{1}{25} \text{ mg}} = 2 \text{ mL}$

19. $\overset{2}{100} \text{ mg} \times \dfrac{\text{mL}}{\underset{1}{50} \text{ mg}} = 2 \text{ mL}$

20. $0.2 \text{ mg} \times \dfrac{\text{mL}}{0.4 \text{ mg}} = \dfrac{0.2}{0.4} \text{ mL} = 0.5 \text{ mL}$

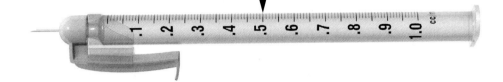

Cumulative Review Exercises

1. 50 mg

2. 1.6 L

3. 28 capsules

4. 6 times per day

5. 0.8 mL

6. 5 mL

7. 4 oz

8. 120 mL

9. gr $\frac{1}{150}$

10. 0.3 mg

11. 3 cap

12. 3 tab

13. 1 cap

14. 1.5 mL

15. 0.025 mg

Chapter 8

Case Study 8.1

1. 0.5 mL—use 1 mL tuberculin syringe

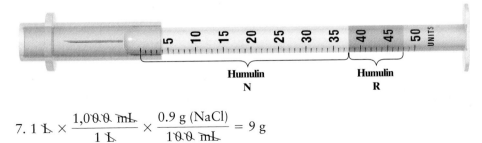

2. 180 mg = 120 mg + 60 mg

Use one 120 mg and one 60 mg tablet for each dose. Administer the two tablets daily.

3. $\overset{1}{\cancel{20}} \text{ mEq} \times \dfrac{15 \text{ mL}}{\underset{2}{\cancel{40}} \text{ mEq}} = 7.5 \text{ mL}$

4. Administer one 75 mg tablet.

5. $\overset{2}{\cancel{1,000}} \text{ mg} \times \dfrac{\text{tab}}{\underset{1}{\cancel{500}} \text{ mg}} = 2 \text{ tab}$

6. Withdraw 10 units of Humulin R insulin, then into the same syringe withdraw 38 units of Humulin N insulin for a total of 48 units.

7. $1 \text{ \cancel{L}} \times \dfrac{1,0\cancel{00} \text{ \cancel{mL}}}{1 \text{ \cancel{L}}} \times \dfrac{0.9 \text{ g (NaCl)}}{10\cancel{0} \text{ \cancel{mL}}} = 9 \text{ g}$

Try These for Practice

1. $\dfrac{\text{Drug}}{\text{Solution}} = \dfrac{\overset{1}{\cancel{80}}\ \text{mg}}{\underset{4}{\cancel{320}}\ \text{mL}} \times \dfrac{1\ \text{g}}{1{,}000\ \cancel{\text{mg}}} = \dfrac{1\ \text{g}}{4{,}000\ \text{mL}}$

$\dfrac{1}{4{,}000} = 0.00025 = 0.025\%$

2. $1\ \cancel{\text{L}} \times \dfrac{1{,}000\ \cancel{\text{mL}}}{1\ \cancel{\text{L}}} \times \dfrac{10\ \cancel{\text{g}}}{100\ \cancel{\text{mL}}} \times \dfrac{1\ \text{tab}}{5\ \cancel{\text{g}}} = 20\ \text{tab}$

Take 20 tablets and dissolve with water, then add more water to the level of 1 L.

3. $20\ \cancel{\text{g}} \times \dfrac{\overset{4}{\cancel{100}}\ \text{mL}}{\underset{1}{\cancel{25}}\ \cancel{\text{g}}} = 80\ \text{mL}$

4. $\dfrac{200\ \text{mL} \times \dfrac{5\ \text{g}}{100\ \text{mL}}}{\dfrac{20\ \text{g}}{100\ \text{mL}}} = \text{Amount of stock}$

$\overset{10}{\cancel{200}}\ \text{mL} \times \dfrac{5\ \cancel{\text{g}}}{\cancel{100}\ \cancel{\text{mL}}} \times \dfrac{\cancel{100}\ \cancel{\text{mL}}}{\underset{1}{\cancel{20}}\ \cancel{\text{g}}} = 50\ \text{mL}$

Take 50 mL of the stock solution and add water to the level of 200 mL.

5. $\dfrac{\overset{1}{\cancel{500}}\ \cancel{\text{mcg}}}{2\ \text{mL}} \times \dfrac{1\ \text{mg}}{\underset{2}{\cancel{1{,}000}}\ \cancel{\text{mcg}}} = \dfrac{1\ \text{mg}}{4\ \text{mL}} = 0.25\ \text{mg/mL}$

Exercises

1. $\dfrac{\text{Drug}}{\text{Solution}} = \dfrac{\overset{1}{\cancel{15}}\ \text{mL}}{\underset{50}{\cancel{750}}\ \text{mL}} = \dfrac{1}{50}$

The strength is 1:50 or 2%

2. $\dfrac{\text{Drug}}{\text{Solution}} = \dfrac{\overset{}{\cancel{60}}\ \text{g}}{2\ \cancel{\text{L}}} \times \dfrac{1\ \cancel{\text{L}}}{1{,}000\ \text{mL}} = \dfrac{3\ \text{g}}{100\ \text{mL}}$

The strength is 3:100 or 3%

3. $\overset{}{\cancel{300}}\ \cancel{\text{mL}} \times \dfrac{0.9\ \text{g}}{\cancel{100}\ \cancel{\text{mL}}} = 2.7\ \text{g}$

Take 2.7 g of sodium chloride crystals, dissolve with water then add more water to the level of 300 mL.

4. $120\ \cancel{\text{mL}} \times \dfrac{\overset{5}{\cancel{25}}\ \text{mg}}{\underset{1}{\cancel{5}}\ \cancel{\text{mL}}} = 600\ \text{mg}$

5. $20\ \cancel{\text{mg}} \times \dfrac{\overset{1}{\cancel{5}}\ \text{mL}}{\underset{5}{\cancel{25}}\ \cancel{\text{mg}}} = 4\ \text{mL}$

6. $\overset{}{\cancel{400}}\ \cancel{\text{mL (solution)}} \times \dfrac{50\ \text{mL (drug)}}{\cancel{100}\ \cancel{\text{mL (solution)}}} = 200\ \text{mL (drug)}$

Take 200 mL of the pure drug and add water to the level of 400 mL.

7. $\overset{3}{\cancel{18}}\ \cancel{\text{g}} \times \dfrac{100\ \text{mL}}{\underset{1}{\cancel{6}}\ \cancel{\text{g}}} = 300\ \text{mL}$

8. $300 \text{ mg} \times \dfrac{\text{g}}{1,000 \text{ mg}} \times \dfrac{100 \text{ mL}}{4 \text{ g}} = \dfrac{30}{4} \text{ mL} = 7.5 \text{ mL}$

9. $\dfrac{20 \text{ mg}}{\text{mL}} \times \dfrac{1 \text{ g}}{1,000 \text{ mg}} = \dfrac{2 \text{ g}}{100 \text{ mL}}$

   $\dfrac{2}{100} = 2\%$

10. $\dfrac{500 \text{ mL} \times \dfrac{1 \text{ g}}{4 \text{ mL}}}{\dfrac{1 \text{ g}}{3 \text{ mL}}} = \text{Amount of stock}$

    $\overset{125}{500} \text{ mL} \times \dfrac{1 \text{ g}}{\underset{1}{4} \text{ mL}} \times \dfrac{3 \text{ mL}}{1 \text{ g}} = 375 \text{ mL}$

    Take 375 mL of the stock solution and add water to the level of 500 mL.

11. $\dfrac{1,000 \text{ mL} \times \dfrac{0.45 \text{ g}}{100 \text{ mL}}}{\dfrac{0.9 \text{ g}}{100 \text{ mL}}} = \text{Amount of stock}$

    $1,000 \text{ mL} \times \dfrac{0.45 \text{ g}}{100 \text{ mL}} \times \dfrac{100 \text{ mL}}{0.9 \text{ g}} = \dfrac{450}{0.9} \text{ mL} = 500 \text{ mL}$

    Take 500 mL of the stock solution and add water to the level of 1 L.

12. $\dfrac{\text{Drug}}{\text{Solution}} = \dfrac{120 \text{ mL}}{600 \text{ mL}} = \dfrac{1}{5},\ 1{:}5 \text{ or } 20\%$

13. $\dfrac{\text{Drug}}{\text{Solution}} = \dfrac{\overset{2}{2,000} \text{ mg}}{1 \text{ L}} \times \dfrac{1 \text{ L}}{\underset{1}{1,000} \text{ mL}} \times \dfrac{1 \text{ g}}{1,000 \text{ mg}} = \dfrac{2 \text{ g}}{1,000 \text{ mL}}$

    $\dfrac{2}{1,000} = \dfrac{1}{500},\ 1{:}500 \text{ or } 0.2\%$

14. $800 \text{ mL} \times \dfrac{10 \text{ g}}{100 \text{ mL}} \times \dfrac{\text{tab}}{20 \text{ g}} = 4 \text{ tab}$

    Take 4 tablets, dissolve with water, and add more water to the level of 800 mL.

15. $12 \text{ mL} \times \dfrac{5 \text{ mg}}{5 \text{ mL}} = 12 \text{ mg}$

16. $35 \text{ mg} \times \dfrac{5 \text{ mL}}{5 \text{ mg}} = 35 \text{ mL}$

17. $1,200 \text{ mL} \times \dfrac{25 \text{ g}}{100 \text{ mL}} = 300 \text{ g}$

    Take 300 g of the pure drug, dissolve with water; then add more water to the level of 1,200 mL.

18. $\dfrac{10 \text{ mg}}{\text{mL}} \times \dfrac{\text{g}}{1,000 \text{ mg}} = \dfrac{1 \text{ g}}{100 \text{ mL}}$

    $\dfrac{1}{100} = 1\%$

19. $\dfrac{200 \text{ mL} \times \dfrac{25 \text{ g}}{100 \text{ mL}}}{\dfrac{35 \text{ g}}{100 \text{ mL}}} = \text{Amount of stock}$

$$200 \text{ mL} \times \frac{\overset{5}{\cancel{25} \text{ g}}}{\cancel{100 \text{ mL}}} \times \frac{\cancel{100 \text{ mL}}}{\underset{7}{\cancel{35} \text{ g}}} = \frac{1,000}{7} \text{ mL} \approx 143 \text{ mL}$$

Take 143 mL of the stock solution and add water to the level of 200 mL.

20. $\dfrac{2,000 \text{ mL} \times \dfrac{1 \text{ g}}{5 \text{ mL}}}{\dfrac{1 \text{ g}}{2 \text{ mL}}}$ = Amount of stock

$$\overset{400}{\cancel{2,000}} \text{ mL} \times \frac{1 \cancel{\text{ g}}}{\underset{1}{\cancel{5 \text{ mL}}}} \times \frac{2 \cancel{\text{ mL}}}{1 \cancel{\text{ g}}} = 800 \text{ mL}$$

Take 800 mL of the stock solution and add water to the level of 2 L.

Cumulative Review Exercises

1. 12.5 g or 12,500 mg   2. 60 mL   3. 50 mL of H_2O
                                                      and 150 mL of Isocal

4. 0.5 mg   5. 16 oz   6. gr $\frac{1}{1,000}$

7. 0.6 mg   8. gr $1\frac{2}{3}$ or gr $1\frac{1}{2}$ 9. 66 in

10. 0.0004 mg   11. 250 mcg   12. 0.2 mg

13. 3.6 g   14. 2 tab   15. 15 mL

Chapter 9

Case Study 9.1

1. $2 \cancel{\text{ mg}} \times \dfrac{\text{mL}}{5 \cancel{\text{ mg}}} = \dfrac{2}{5} \text{ mL} = 0.4 \text{ mL}$

   1 mL tuberculin

2. $5,\cancel{000} \cancel{\text{ units}} \times \dfrac{\text{mL}}{20,\cancel{000} \cancel{\text{ units}}} = 0.25 \text{ mL}$

   1 mL tuberculin

3. $5 \cancel{\text{ mg}} \times \dfrac{\text{mL}}{1 \cancel{\text{ mg}}} = 5 \text{ mL}$

4. $150 \cancel{\text{ lb}} \times \dfrac{\cancel{\text{ kg}}}{2.2 \cancel{\text{ lb}}} \times \dfrac{7.5 \text{ mg}}{\cancel{\text{ kg}}} = 511 \text{ mg}$

5. $\dfrac{\cancel{30 \text{ mg}}}{\cancel{\text{dose}}} \times \dfrac{\text{mL}}{\cancel{30 \text{ mg}}} \times \dfrac{4 \cancel{\text{ dose}}}{\text{day}} = 4 \text{ mL in 24h}$

6. $\dfrac{\cancel{400 \text{ mg}}}{\cancel{\text{day}}} \times \dfrac{250 \text{ mL}}{\cancel{400 \text{ mg}}} \times 5 \cancel{\text{ days}} = 1,250 \text{ mL}$

7. $0.5 \cancel{\text{ mg}} \times \dfrac{\text{cap}}{0.5 \cancel{\text{ mg}}} = 1 \text{ cap}$

8. $\overset{2}{\cancel{10}} \cancel{\text{ mg}} \times \dfrac{\text{tab}}{\underset{1}{\cancel{5 \text{ mg}}}} = 2 \text{ tab}$

9. (a) 5 mg
   (b) 1 tab

10. $20 \cancel{\text{ mg}} \times \dfrac{\text{tab}}{10 \cancel{\text{ mg}}} = 2 \text{ tab}$

Try These for Practice

1. (a) $\overset{3}{\cancel{750}} \text{ mg} \times \dfrac{1 \cancel{g}}{\underset{4}{\cancel{1,000} \cancel{mg}}} \times \dfrac{3 \text{ mL}}{1 \cancel{g}} = \dfrac{9}{4} \text{ mL} = 2.25 \text{ mL} \approx 2.3 \text{ mL}$

 (b) 3 mL syringe

2. (a) $75 \text{ mg} \times \dfrac{2 \text{ mL}}{100 \text{ mg}} = \dfrac{6}{4} \text{ mL} = 1.5 \text{ mL}$

 (b) 3 mL syringe

3. (a) $135 \cancel{\text{lb}} \times \dfrac{\cancel{\text{kg}}}{2.2 \cancel{\text{lb}}} \times \dfrac{0.05 \text{ mg}}{\cancel{\text{kg}}} = 3.1 \text{ mg}$

 (b) $3.1 \cancel{\text{mg}} \times \dfrac{2 \text{ mL}}{2 \cancel{\text{mg}}} = 3.1 \text{ mL}$

4. (a) $8,\cancel{000} \cancel{\text{units}} \times \dfrac{\text{mL}}{10,\cancel{000} \cancel{\text{units}}} = 0.8 \text{ mL}$

 (b) 1 mL tuberculin

5. (a) $1 \cancel{g} \times \dfrac{\text{tab}}{0.5 \cancel{g}} = 2 \text{ tab}$

 (b) $2 \cancel{g} \times \dfrac{2.5 \text{ mL}}{1 \cancel{g}} = 5 \text{ mL}$

Exercises

1. $75\cancel{0} \cancel{\text{mg}} \times \dfrac{\text{mL}}{25\cancel{0} \cancel{\text{mg}}} = 3 \text{ mL}$

2. $1.5 \cancel{g} \times \dfrac{1,000 \cancel{\text{mg}}}{1 \cancel{g}} \times \dfrac{\text{mL}}{375 \cancel{\text{mg}}} = 4 \text{ mL}$

3. (a) $155 \cancel{\text{lb}} \times \dfrac{\cancel{\text{kg}}}{2.2 \cancel{\text{lb}}} \times \dfrac{0.49 \cancel{\text{mcg}}}{\cancel{\text{kg}}} \times \dfrac{1 \text{ mL}}{40 \cancel{\text{mcg}}} = 0.86 \text{ mL}$

 (b) 1 mL tuberculin

4. (a) $1,2\cancel{00} \cancel{\text{mg}} \times \dfrac{1 \text{ g}}{1,0\cancel{00} \cancel{\text{mg}}} = 1.2 \text{ g}$ (use the 2 g vial)

 (b) $1,20\cancel{0} \text{ mg} \times \dfrac{\text{mL}}{33\cancel{0} \text{ mg}} = 3.6 \text{ mL}$

5. $\overset{1}{\cancel{500}} \cancel{\text{mg}} \times \dfrac{1 \cancel{g}}{\underset{2}{\cancel{1,000} \cancel{\text{mg}}}} \times \dfrac{2.5 \text{ mL}}{1 \cancel{g}} = 1.25 \text{ mL} \approx 1.3 \text{ mL}$

6. (a) $1.4 \cancel{\text{mg}} \times \dfrac{\text{mL}}{2 \cancel{\text{mg}}} = 0.7 \text{ mL}$

 (b) 1 mL tuberculin

7. $\overset{2}{\cancel{50}} \cancel{\text{mg}} \times \dfrac{\text{vial}}{\underset{1}{\cancel{25} \cancel{\text{mg}}}} = 2 \text{ vials}$

8. (a) $6,\cancel{000} \cancel{\text{units}} \times \dfrac{\text{mL}}{20,\cancel{000} \cancel{\text{units}}} = 0.3 \text{ mL}$

 (b) 1 mL tuberculin

9. $60 \cancel{\text{mg}} \times \dfrac{\text{mL}}{40 \cancel{\text{mg}}} = 1.5 \text{ mL}$

10. (a) $5 \cancel{\text{mg}} \times \dfrac{\text{mL}}{15 \cancel{\text{mg}}} = 0.33 \text{ mL}$

 (b) 1 mL tuberculin

11. $30 \text{ mg} \times \dfrac{\text{mL}}{40 \text{ mg}} = 0.75 \text{ mL}$

12. $3 \text{ mg} \times \dfrac{\text{mL}}{4 \text{ mg}} = 0.75 \text{ mL}$

13. 320 is between 281 and 340. Give 6 units.

14. (a) $3{,}500 \text{ units} \times \dfrac{\text{mL}}{5{,}000 \text{ units}} = 0.7 \text{ mL}$

    (b) 1 mL tuberculin

15. (a) 25 units

    (b) 30 unit Lo-Dose insulin

16. $650{,}000 \text{ units} \times \dfrac{\text{mL}}{1{,}000{,}000 \text{ units}} = 0.65 \text{ mL}$

17. (a) $0.2 \text{ mg} \times \dfrac{\text{mL}}{0.4 \text{ mg}} = 0.5 \text{ mL}$

    (b) 1 mL tuberculin

18. (a) $12.5 \text{ mg} \times \dfrac{\text{mL}}{50 \text{ mg}} = 0.25 \text{ mL}$

    (b) 1 mL tuberculin

19. (a) $\overset{8}{40} \text{ mg} \times \dfrac{\text{mL}}{\underset{5}{25} \text{ mg}} = 1.6 \text{ mL}$

    (b) 3 mL

20. (a) 18.2 mL

    (b) 8.2 mL

    (c) 5,000,000 units

    (d) $2{,}000{,}000 \text{ units} \times \dfrac{\text{mL}}{1{,}000{,}000 \text{ units}} = 2 \text{ mL}$

Add 3.2 mL of diluent to the vial and administer 2 mL of the reconstituted solution to the patient.

Cumulative Review Exercises

1. quinapril HCl	2. PO	3. Pfizer-Parke Davis
4. 8 tab	5. 2 tab	6. Celexa
7. 10 mg/5 mL	8. 10 mL	9. 12 doses
10. 2 cap	11. 0.4 mL	12. 3 mg
13. 540 mL	14. 196 lb	15. 2,500 mL

Chapter 10

Case Study 10.1

1. $\dfrac{1{,}000 \text{ mL}}{8 \text{ h}} = 125 \text{ mL/h}$

2. $\dfrac{125 \text{ mL}}{\text{h}} \times \dfrac{1 \text{ h}}{60 \text{ min}} \times \dfrac{15 \text{ gtt}}{\text{mL}} = 31 \text{ gtt/min}$

3. $\begin{array}{r} 1900 \\ +0800 \\ \hline 2700 \end{array}$ $\begin{array}{r} 2700 \\ -2400 \\ \hline 0300 \end{array}$ 0300 hours

4. $1{,}000 \text{ mL} \times \dfrac{5 \text{ g}}{100 \text{ mL}} = 50 \text{ g dextrose}$

$$1{,}000 \text{ mL} \times \frac{0.45 \text{ g}}{100 \text{ mL}} = 4.5 \text{ g NaCl}$$

5. $\dfrac{100 \text{ mL}}{60 \text{ min}} \times \dfrac{60 \text{ min}}{\text{h}} = \dfrac{100 \text{ mL}}{\text{h}}$

6. (a) $800 \text{ mL} \times \dfrac{3 \text{ mL}}{4 \text{ mL}} = 600 \text{ mL needed}$

$$600 \text{ mL} \times \frac{\text{oz}}{30 \text{ mL}} \times \frac{\text{can}}{10 \text{ oz}} = 2 \text{ cans}$$

(b) $\dfrac{800 \text{ mL}}{7 \text{ h}} = 114 \text{ mL/h}$

7. $0.5 \text{ mg} \times \dfrac{1 \text{ mL}}{1 \text{ mg}} = 0.5 \text{ mL}$

8. $200 \text{ mg} \times \dfrac{\text{mL}}{10 \text{ mg}} = 20 \text{ mL}$

9. $100 \text{ mg} \times \dfrac{\overset{1}{15} \text{ mL}}{\underset{4}{60} \text{ mg}} = 25 \text{ mL}$

Try These for Practice

1. $\dfrac{500 \text{ mL}}{8 \text{ h}} \times \dfrac{1 \text{ h}}{60 \text{ min}} \times \dfrac{10 \text{ gtt}}{\text{mL}} = 10 \text{ gtt/min}$

2. $\dfrac{575 \text{ mL}}{4 \text{ h}} \times \dfrac{1 \text{ h}}{\underset{4}{60} \text{ min}} \times \dfrac{\overset{1}{15} \text{ gtt}}{\text{mL}} = 36 \text{ gtt/min}$

3. $\dfrac{500 \text{ mL}}{4 \text{ h}} = 125 \text{ mL/h}$

4. $\dfrac{27 \text{ gtt}}{\text{min}} \times \dfrac{\text{mL}}{\underset{1}{15} \text{ gtt}} \times \dfrac{\overset{4}{60} \text{ min}}{\text{h}} = 108 \text{ mL/h}$

5. $\dfrac{400 \text{ mL}}{6 \text{ h}} = 67 \text{ mL/h}$

Exercises

1. $\dfrac{750 \text{ mL}}{8 \text{ h}} \times \dfrac{1 \text{ h}}{60 \text{ min}} \times \dfrac{10 \text{ gtt}}{\text{mL}} = 16 \text{ gtt/min}$

2. $\dfrac{375 \text{ mL}}{3 \text{ h}} = 125 \text{ mL/h}$

3. $\dfrac{50 \text{ mL}}{\text{h}} \times \dfrac{1 \text{ h}}{60 \text{ min}} \times \dfrac{10 \text{ gtt}}{\text{mL}} = 8 \text{ gtt/min}$

4. $1{,}000 \text{ mL} \times \dfrac{\text{h}}{125 \text{ mL}} = 8 \text{ hours}$

5. $\dfrac{500 \text{ mL}}{3 \text{ h}} = 167 \text{ mL/h} = 167 \text{ mcgtt/min}$

6. (a) $\dfrac{1{,}500 \text{ mL}}{12 \text{ h}} \times \dfrac{1 \text{ h}}{\underset{3}{60} \text{ min}} \times \dfrac{\overset{1}{20} \text{ gtt}}{\text{mL}} = 42 \text{ gtt/min}$

(b) $\dfrac{1{,}200 \text{ mL}}{9 \text{ h}} \times \dfrac{1 \text{ h}}{\underset{3}{60} \text{ min}} \times \dfrac{\overset{1}{20} \text{ gtt}}{\text{mL}} = 44 \text{ gtt/min}$

(c) 25% of 42 = .25 × 42 = 10.5 gtt/min

44 − 42 = 2 gtt/min

Since 2 gtt/min is less than 10.5 gtt/min, the adjustment is within the guidelines.

7. $\dfrac{750 \ \cancel{mL}}{8 \ \cancel{h}} \times \dfrac{1 \ \cancel{h}}{\cancel{60} \ min} \times \dfrac{\overset{1}{\cancel{15}} \ gtt}{\cancel{mL}} = 23 \ gtt/min$

8. $750 \ \cancel{mL} \times \dfrac{h}{125 \ \cancel{mL}} = 6 \ h$ It will finish at 6 P.M. the same day.

9. $\dfrac{1{,}000 \ mL}{24 \ h} = 42 \ mL/h$

10. $\dfrac{90 \ \cancel{mL}}{\cancel{h}} \times \dfrac{1 \ \cancel{h}}{\underset{3}{\cancel{60}} \ min} \times \dfrac{\overset{1}{\cancel{20}} \ gtt}{\cancel{mL}} = 30 \ gtt/min$

11. $\dfrac{1{,}000 \ mL}{6 \ h} = 167 \ mL/h$

12. $500 \ \cancel{mL} \times \dfrac{h}{40 \ \cancel{mL}} = 12.5 \ h$

13. $\dfrac{750 \ mL}{24 \ h} = 31 \ mL/h$

14. $\dfrac{500 \ \cancel{mL}}{3.25 \ \cancel{h}} \times \dfrac{1 \ \cancel{h}}{\underset{2}{\cancel{60}} \ min} \times \dfrac{\overset{1}{\cancel{15}} \ gtt}{\cancel{mL}} = 38 \ gtt/min$

15. $\dfrac{90 \ mL}{45 \ \cancel{min}} \times \dfrac{60 \ \cancel{min}}{h} = 120 \ mL/h$

16. $\overset{10}{\cancel{350}} \ \cancel{mL} \times \dfrac{15 \ \cancel{gtt}}{\cancel{mL}} \times \dfrac{\cancel{min}}{\underset{1}{\cancel{35}} \ \cancel{gtt}} \times \dfrac{h}{60 \ \cancel{min}} = 2.5h = 2\frac{1}{2} \ h$

17. 32 mcgtt/min = 32 mL/h

$6 \ \cancel{h} \times \dfrac{32 \ mL}{\cancel{h}} = 192 \ mL$

18. $\dfrac{350 \ \cancel{mL}}{5 \ \cancel{h}} \times \dfrac{1 \ \cancel{h}}{\underset{4}{\cancel{60}} \ min} \times \dfrac{\overset{}{\cancel{15}} \ gtt}{\cancel{mL}} = 18 \ gtt/min$

19. $\dfrac{\overset{2}{\cancel{30}} \ \cancel{gtt}}{\cancel{min}} \times \dfrac{mL}{\underset{1}{\cancel{15}} \ \cancel{gtt}} \times \dfrac{60 \ \cancel{min}}{h} = 120 \ mL/h$

20. $500 \ \cancel{mL} \times \dfrac{10 \ \cancel{gtt}}{\cancel{mL}} \times \dfrac{\cancel{min}}{20 \ \cancel{gtt}} \times \dfrac{h}{60 \ \cancel{min}} = 4.17 \ h$

$0.17 \ h \times \dfrac{60 \ min}{h} = 10 \ min$ It will finish in 4 hours and 10 minutes.

Cumulative Review Exercises

1. 4.5 mg	2. 40 mL/h	3. 156 mL/h
4. 17 gtt/min	5. 2.11 m²	6. 1 cap
7. 80 mL/h	8. 3 mL	9. 1 cap
10. 63 mL/h	11. 12 t	12. gr $\frac{1}{10}$
13. 600 mcgtt	14. 8 oz	15. 30 mL

Chapter 11

Case Study 11.1

1. $\dfrac{1{,}000 \text{ mL}}{8 \text{ h}} = 125 \text{ mL/h}$

2. $6 \text{ mg} \times \dfrac{\text{mL}}{8 \text{ mg}} = 0.75 \text{ mL}$

3. $0.25 \text{ mg} \times \dfrac{1 \text{ mL}}{1 \text{ mg}} = 0.25 \text{ mL}$

4. $250 \text{ mg} \times \dfrac{\text{mL}}{350 \text{ mg}} = 0.71 \text{ mL}$

5. $\dfrac{105 \text{ mL}}{1 \text{ h}} \times \dfrac{1 \text{ h}}{\overset{\;}{\underset{4}{60}} \text{ mm}} \times \dfrac{\overset{1}{15} \text{ gtt}}{\text{mL}} = 26 \text{ gtt/min}$

6. $500 \text{ mg} \times \dfrac{4.8 \text{ mL}}{500 \text{ mg}} = 4.8 \text{ mL} + 250 \text{ mL} \Rightarrow 255 \text{ mL}$

   $\dfrac{255 \text{ mL}}{90 \text{ min}} \times \dfrac{60 \text{ min}}{\text{h}} = 170 \text{ mL/h (at most)}$

7. (a) $4 \text{ g} \times \dfrac{1{,}000 \text{ mL}}{40 \text{ g}} = 100 \text{ mL}$

   $\dfrac{100 \text{ mL}}{\underset{1}{20} \text{ min}} \times \dfrac{\overset{3}{60} \text{ min}}{\text{h}} = 300 \text{ mL/h}$

   (b) $\dfrac{1 \text{ g}}{\text{h}} \times \dfrac{1{,}000 \text{ mL}}{40 \text{ g}} = 25 \text{ mL/h}$

8. $\dfrac{0.5 \text{ mU}}{\text{min}} = \dfrac{1 \text{ unit}}{1{,}000 \text{ mU}} \times \dfrac{1{,}000 \text{ mL}}{10 \text{ unit}} \times \dfrac{60 \text{ min}}{\text{h}} = 3 \text{ mL/h}$

9. $\dfrac{9 \text{ mL}}{\text{h}} \times \dfrac{10 \text{ unit}}{1{,}000 \text{ mL}} \times \dfrac{1{,}000 \text{ mU}}{1 \text{ unit}} = 90 \text{ mU/h}$

10. $1 \text{ mg} \times \dfrac{\text{mL}}{2 \text{ mg}} = 0.5 \text{ mL}$

Try These for Practice

1. 25 gtt/min
2. 25 mL/h
3. 60 mg/h
4. 11 mcgtt/min
5. 12 mL/h

Exercises

1. $\dfrac{10 \text{ mEq}}{\text{h}} \times \dfrac{\overset{5}{100} \text{ mL}}{\underset{1}{20} \text{ mEq}} \times 50 \dfrac{\text{mL}}{\text{h}} = 50 \text{ mcgtt/min}$

2. $\dfrac{2 \text{ mcg}}{\text{min}} \times \dfrac{\text{mg}}{1{,}000 \text{ mcg}} \times \dfrac{250 \text{ mL}}{8 \text{ mg}} \times \dfrac{60 \text{ min}}{\text{h}} = 4 \text{ mL/h}$

3. $\dfrac{40 \text{ mL}}{\text{h}} \times \dfrac{1 \text{ h}}{60 \text{ min}} \times \dfrac{1 \text{ g}}{500 \text{ mL}} \times \dfrac{\overset{2}{1{,}000} \text{ mg}}{1 \text{ g}} = 1.3 \text{ mg/min}$

4. $91 \text{ kg} \times \dfrac{3 \text{ mcg}}{\text{kg} \cdot \text{min}} \times \dfrac{60 \text{ min}}{\text{h}} \times \dfrac{\text{mg}}{1{,}000 \text{ mcg}} \times \dfrac{250 \text{ mL}}{400 \text{ mg}} = 10 \dfrac{\text{mL}}{\text{h}}$

5. $\dfrac{500 \text{ mL}}{\underset{3}{90} \text{ min}} \times \dfrac{\overset{2}{60} \text{ min}}{\text{h}} = 333 \dfrac{\text{mL}}{\text{h}}$

6. $550 \text{ mL} \times \dfrac{\text{h}}{25 \text{ mL}} = 22 \text{ h}$

7. $\dfrac{1{,}000 \text{ units}}{\text{h}} \times \dfrac{1{,}000 \text{ mL}}{24{,}000 \text{ units}} = 42 \dfrac{\text{mL}}{\text{h}}$

8. $\dfrac{1 \text{ mL}}{\text{min}} \times \dfrac{60 \text{ min}}{\text{h}} \times \dfrac{50 \text{ units}}{500 \text{ mL}} = 6 \text{ units/h}$

9. $\dfrac{40 \text{ mL}}{15 \text{ min}} \times \dfrac{20 \text{ gtt}}{\text{mL}} = 53 \text{ gtt/min}$

10. $\dfrac{\text{drug}}{\text{weight} \times \text{time}} : \dfrac{20 \text{ mL}}{75 \text{ kg} \cdot \text{h}} \times \dfrac{50 \text{ mg}}{250 \text{ mL}} \times \dfrac{1{,}000 \text{ mcg}}{1 \text{ mg}} \times \dfrac{1 \text{ h}}{60 \text{ min}}$
    $= 0.89 \text{ mcg/kg/min}$

11. (a) 4 mg

    (b) $4 \text{ mg} \times \dfrac{2 \text{ mL}}{5 \text{ mg}} = 1.6 \text{ mL}$

    (c) 1.6 mL/min

12. $\dfrac{100 \text{ mL}}{60 \text{ min}} \times \dfrac{15 \text{ gtt}}{\text{mL}} = 25 \text{ gtt/min}$

13. $\dfrac{4 \text{ mcg}}{\text{min}} \times \dfrac{1 \text{ mg}}{1{,}000 \text{ mcg}} \times \dfrac{500 \text{ mL}}{2 \text{ mg}} \times \dfrac{60 \text{ min}}{\text{h}} = 60 \text{ mL/h}$

14. $\dfrac{20 \text{ mL}}{\text{h}} \times \dfrac{500 \text{ mg}}{1{,}000 \text{ mL}} = 10 \text{ mg/h}$

15. $82 \text{ kg} \times \dfrac{3 \text{ mcg}}{\text{kg} \cdot \text{min}} \times \dfrac{1 \text{ mg}}{1{,}000 \text{ mcg}} \times \dfrac{250 \text{ mL}}{50 \text{ mg}} \times \dfrac{60 \text{ min}}{\text{h}} = 74 \text{ mL/h}$

16. $2.33 \text{ m}^2 \times \dfrac{75 \text{ mg}}{\text{m}^2} \times \dfrac{1 \text{ mL}}{50 \text{ mg}} = 3.5 \text{ mL}$

17. $1{,}000 \text{ mL} \times \dfrac{20 \text{ gtt}}{\text{mL}} \times \dfrac{\text{min}}{22 \text{ gtt}} \times \dfrac{\text{h}}{60 \text{ min}} = 15.15 \text{ h}$

    $0.15 \text{ h} \times \dfrac{60 \text{ min}}{\text{h}} = 9 \text{ min}$

    It will take 15 h and 9 min to finish and will finish at 1:04 A.M. the next day.

18. $\dfrac{70 \text{ mL}}{30 \text{ min}} \times \dfrac{\overset{2}{60} \text{ min}}{\text{h}} = 140 \text{ mL/h}$

19. $\dfrac{1{,}200 \text{ units}}{\text{h}} \times \dfrac{500 \text{ mL}}{40{,}000 \text{ units}} = 15 \text{ mL/h}$

20. $\dfrac{\text{drug}}{\text{weight} \times \text{time}} : \dfrac{18 \text{ mcg}}{150 \text{ lb} \times \text{min}} \times \dfrac{2.2 \text{ lb}}{\text{kg}} = 0.26 \text{ mcg/kg/min}$

Cumulative Review Exercises

1. 4.4 mL	2. 2 tab	3. 3 mL
4. 1.7 mL	5. 10 mL	6. 10 mL
7. 2 tab	8. 20 mL	9. 2.4 L
10. gr $\frac{1}{100}$	11. 23 mcgtt/min	12. $2\frac{1}{2}$ qt
13. 0.5 mg	14. 3 t	15. $1\frac{1}{2}$ oz

Chapter 12

Case Study 12.1

1. $30 \text{ lb} \times \dfrac{1 \text{ kg}}{2.2 \text{ lb}} = 13.6 \text{ kg}$

$$
\left.
\begin{aligned}
10 \text{ kg} \times \dfrac{100 \text{ mL}}{\text{kg}} &= 1{,}000 \text{ mL} \\[6pt]
3.6 \text{ kg} \times \dfrac{50 \text{ mL}}{\text{kg}} &= 180 \text{ mL}
\end{aligned}
\right\} \; 1{,}180 \text{ mL}
$$

2. $13.6 \text{ kg} \times \dfrac{150{,}000 \text{ units}}{\text{kg} \cdot \text{day}} = 2{,}040{,}000 \text{ units/day (recommended)}$

$\dfrac{600{,}000 \text{ units}}{\text{dose}} \times \dfrac{4 \text{ doses}}{\text{day}} = 2{,}400{,}000 \text{ units/day (ordered)}$

The ordered dose is not safe.

3. 4.8 mL of diluent

$600{,}000 \text{ units} \times \dfrac{1 \text{ mL}}{750{,}000 \text{ units}} = 0.8 \text{ mL}$

4. $\dfrac{50.8 \text{ mL}}{30 \text{ min}} \times \dfrac{60 \text{ min}}{\text{h}} = 102 \, \dfrac{\text{mL}}{\text{h}}$

5. $30 \text{ lb} \times \dfrac{\text{kg}}{2.2 \text{ lb}} \times \dfrac{0.1 \text{ mg}}{\text{kg} \cdot \text{dose}} = 1.4 \text{ mg/dose (minimum)}$

$30 \text{ lb} \times \dfrac{\text{kg}}{2.2 \text{ lb}} \times \dfrac{0.15 \text{ mg}}{\text{kg} \cdot \text{dose}} = 2.0 \text{ mg/dose (maximum)}$

1 mg is too low. It is not a safe dose.

6. $\dfrac{1 \text{ ampule}}{2} \times \dfrac{2.5 \text{ mg}}{1 \text{ ampule}} = 1.25 \text{ mg}$

7. $\dfrac{1 \text{ ampule}}{2} \times \dfrac{20 \text{ mg}}{1 \text{ ampule}} = 10 \text{ mg}$

8. Ventolin: $\quad 1 \text{ mg} \times \dfrac{3 \text{ mL}}{1.25 \text{ mg}} = 2.4 \text{ mL}$

$\left.
\begin{aligned}
& \\
&\text{Intal:} \quad \dfrac{1 \text{ ampule}}{2} \times \dfrac{2 \text{ mL}}{\text{ampule}} = 1 \text{ mL}
\end{aligned}
\right\} \; 3.4 \text{ mL}$

9. $\dfrac{1 \text{ ampule}}{2} \times \dfrac{1 \text{ mL}}{\text{ampule}} = 0.5 \text{ mL}$

10. $\dfrac{1 \text{ ampule}}{2} \times \dfrac{300 \text{ mg}}{\text{ampule}} = 150 \text{ mg}$

11. $180 \text{ mg} \times \dfrac{5 \text{ mL}}{160 \text{ mg}} = 5.6 \text{ mL}$

Try These for Practice

1. $45 \text{ kg} \times \dfrac{0.1 \text{ unit}}{\text{kg}} = \dfrac{4.5 \text{ units}}{\text{dose}} \times \dfrac{2 \text{ doses}}{\text{day}} = 9 \text{ units per day}$

2. $0.62 \text{ m}^2 \times \dfrac{100 \text{ mg}}{\text{m}^2} = 62 \text{ mg (minimum)}$

$$0.62 \; \cancel{m^2} \times \frac{180 \; mg}{\cancel{m^2}} = 111 \; mg \; (maximum)$$

Since 90 is between 62 and 111, the dose is safe.

3. $250 \; \cancel{mg} \times \dfrac{5 \; mL}{125 \; \cancel{mg}} = 10 \; mL$

4. $40 \; \cancel{kg} \times \dfrac{0.3 \; \cancel{mg}}{\cancel{kg}} \times \dfrac{5 \; mL}{15 \; \cancel{mg}} = 4 \; mL$

5. $42 = 10 + 10 + 22$

$$\left.\begin{array}{c} 10 \; \cancel{kg} \times \dfrac{100 \; mL}{\cancel{kg}} = 1{,}000 \; mL \\[2mm] 10 \; \cancel{kg} \times \dfrac{50 \; mL}{\cancel{kg}} = 500 \; mL \\[2mm] 22 \; \cancel{kg} \times \dfrac{20 \; mL}{\cancel{kg}} = 440 \; mL \end{array}\right\} 1{,}940 \; mL \text{ is maintenance}$$

$1{,}940 \; mL \times 1.5 = 2{,}910 \; mL$ (maintenance and a half)

$$\dfrac{2{,}910 \; mL}{24 \; h} = 121 \; mL/h$$

Exercises

1. $40 \; \cancel{lb} \times \dfrac{kg}{2.2 \; \cancel{lb}} \times \dfrac{6 \; mg}{kg \cdot day} = 109 \; mg$ (minimum recommended)

$40 \; \cancel{lb} \times \dfrac{kg}{2.2 \; \cancel{lb}} \times \dfrac{7.5 \; mg}{kg \cdot day} = 136 \; mg$ (maximum recommended)

$\dfrac{50 \; mg}{\cancel{dose}} \times \dfrac{3 \; \cancel{doses}}{day} = 150 \; mg$

Since 150 mg is higher than the maximum recommended daily dose, the prescribed dose is not safe.

2. $4{,}000 \; \cancel{g} \times \dfrac{kg}{1{,}000 \; \cancel{g}} \times \dfrac{10 \; mg}{\cancel{kg}} = 40 \; mg$

3. $BSA = \sqrt{\dfrac{42 \times 50}{3{,}131}} = \sqrt{0.6707} = 0.81 \; m^2$

$\left.\begin{array}{c} 0.81 \; \cancel{m^2} \times \dfrac{7.5 \; mg}{\cancel{m^2}} = 6.0 \; mg \; (minimum) \\[3mm] 0.81 \; \cancel{m^2} \times \dfrac{30 \; mg}{\cancel{m^2}} = 24.3 \; mg \; (maximum) \end{array}\right\}$ recommended every 1–2 weeks

Since the ordered dose of 2.9 mg is below the recommended minimum dose, it is not safe.

4. $32 \; \cancel{kg} \times \dfrac{10 \; mg}{\cancel{kg}} = 320 \; mg$

5. $1.2 \; \cancel{m^2} \times \dfrac{350 \; mg}{m^2 \cdot day} = 420 \; mg/day$ (minimum)

$1.2 \; \cancel{m^2} \times \dfrac{450 \; mg}{m^2 \cdot day} = 540 \; mg/day$ (maximum)

The safe dose range for the child is 420–540 mg/day.

6. $77 \; \cancel{lb} \times \dfrac{kg}{2.2 \; lb} \times \dfrac{30 \; \cancel{mg}}{kg \cdot day} \times \dfrac{mL}{187 \; \cancel{mg}} = 5.6 \; mL/day$

$$\frac{5.6 \text{ mL}}{\text{day}} \times \frac{\text{day}}{3 \text{ doses}} = 1.8 \text{ mL per dose}$$

7. $\dfrac{65 \text{ mL}}{\text{h}} = 65 \text{ mcgtt/min}$

8. $52 \text{ lb} \times \dfrac{\text{kg}}{2.2 \text{ lb}} \times \dfrac{2 \text{ mg}}{\text{kg} \cdot \text{day}} = 47.2 \text{ mg/days (minimum)}$
$52 \text{ lb} \times \dfrac{\text{kg}}{2.2 \text{ lb}} \times \dfrac{4 \text{ mg}}{\text{kg} \cdot \text{day}} = 94.5 \text{ mg/days (maximum)}$ } recommended

$$\frac{30 \text{ mg}}{\text{dose}} \times \frac{3 \text{ doses}}{\text{day}} = 90 \text{ mg/day}$$

Since 90 is between 47.2 and 94.5 and since 30 is lens than 50, the prescribed dose is safe.

9. (a) $55 \text{ lb} \times \dfrac{\text{kg}}{2.2 \text{ lb}} = 25 \text{ kg} = (10 + 10 + 5) \text{ kg}$

$10 \text{ kg} \times \dfrac{100 \text{ mL}}{\text{kg}} = 1{,}000 \text{ mL}$
$10 \text{ kg} \times \dfrac{50 \text{ mL}}{\text{kg}} = 500 \text{ mL}$ } $1{,}600 \text{ mL (maintenance)}$
$5 \text{ kg} \times \dfrac{20 \text{ mL}}{\text{kg}} = 100 \text{ mL}$

(b) $\dfrac{1{,}600 \text{ mL}}{24 \text{ h}} = 66 \text{ mL/h}$

10. $0.82 \text{ m}^2 \times \dfrac{2{,}000{,}000 \text{ units}}{\text{m}^2} = 1{,}640{,}000 \text{ units}$

11. $1.2 \text{ g} \times \dfrac{1{,}000 \text{ mg}}{1 \text{ g}} \times \dfrac{\text{mL}}{60 \text{ mg}} = 20 \text{ mL}$

12. $7 \text{ lb} \times \dfrac{\text{kg}}{2.2 \text{ lb}} = 3.18 \text{ kg}$

$3.18 \text{ kg} \times \dfrac{100 \text{ mL}}{\text{kg}} = 318 \text{ mL}$

13. $1.1 \text{ m}^2 \times \dfrac{160 \text{ mg}}{\text{m}^2} \times \dfrac{5 \text{ mL}}{50 \text{ mg}} = 17.6 \text{ mL}$

14. (a) $500 \text{ mL} \times \dfrac{20 \text{ mEq}}{1{,}000 \text{ mL}} = 10 \text{ mEq}$

(b) $10 \text{ mEq} \times \dfrac{\text{mL}}{2 \text{ mEq}} = 5 \text{ mL}$

(c) $\dfrac{30 \text{ mL}}{\text{h}} \times \dfrac{10 \text{ mEq}}{505 \text{ mL}} = 0.59 \text{ mEq/h}$

(d) $9.1 \text{ kg} \times \dfrac{3 \text{ mEq}}{\text{kg} \cdot \text{day}} = 27.3 \text{ mEq/day (recommended)}$

$\dfrac{0.6 \text{ mEq}}{\text{h}} \times \dfrac{24 \text{ h}}{\text{day}} = 14.4 \text{ mEq/day (ordered)}$

Since 14.4 is less than 27.3, the ordered dose is safe.

15. (a) $14.5 \text{ kg} \times \dfrac{30 \text{ mg}}{\text{kg} \cdot \text{day}} = 435 \text{ mg/day (minimum)}$
$14.5 \text{ kg} \times \dfrac{50 \text{ mg}}{\text{kg} \cdot \text{day}} = 725 \text{ mg/day (maximum)}$ } recommended

$$\frac{125 \text{ mg}}{\text{dose}} \times \frac{6 \text{ dose}}{\text{day}} = 750 \text{ mg/day}$$

Since 750 is larger then 725, the ordered dose is not safe.

(b) 0 mL. Consult the prescriber.

16. $41 \text{ kg} \times \dfrac{40 \text{ mg}}{\text{kg} \cdot \text{d}} = 1,640 \text{ mg/d}$

$$\frac{1,640 \text{ mg}}{\text{day}} \times \frac{\text{day}}{4 \text{ doses}} = 410 \text{ mg/dose}$$

$$410 \text{ mg} \times \frac{\text{mL}}{50 \text{ mg}} = 8.2 \text{ mL}$$

$$\frac{208.2 \text{ mL}}{90 \text{ min}} \times \frac{60 \text{ min}}{\text{h}} = 138 \text{ mL/h}$$

17. $\dfrac{100 \text{ mg}}{20 \text{ min}} = 5 \text{ mg/min}$

18. $\dfrac{40 \text{ mL}}{60 \text{ min}} = \dfrac{40 \text{ mL}}{1 \text{ h}} = 40 \text{ mcgtt/min}$

19. $35 \text{ lb} \times \dfrac{\text{kg}}{2.2 \text{ lb}} \times \dfrac{20 \text{ mg}}{\text{kg} \cdot \text{dose}} \times \dfrac{2.5 \text{ mL}}{100 \text{ mg}} = 8.0 \text{ mL/dose}$

20. $22 \text{ lb} \times \dfrac{\text{kg}}{2.2 \text{ lb}} \times \dfrac{50 \text{ mg}}{\text{kg} \cdot \text{day}} = 500 \text{ mg/day}$ (recommended)

$$\frac{125 \text{ mg}}{\text{dose}} \times \frac{4 \text{ doses}}{\text{day}} = 500 \text{ mg/dose (ordered)}$$

The prescribed dose is safe.

Cumulative Review Exercises

1. 525 mg
2. 30 units
3. (a) 200 mg
   (b) 1 tab

4. 50 units
5. 20 mL
6. (a) 2 cap
   (b) 0.3 g

7. 61.4 mg
8. 60 gtt/min
9. 2.5 mL/min

10. 11:42 A.M. the next day
11. gr $\frac{3}{100}$
12. 1 tab

13. Take 66.7 mL of the 1:2 solution add diluent to 100 mL.
14. 2 tab
15. 5.2 mL

Answers for Comprehensive Self-Tests

Comprehensive Self-Test 1

1. 735 mg
2. 2 cap
3. Take 40 mL of the 100% solution and add water to the level of 400 mL.
4. 0.1 g
5. 8 h 20 min

6. 12.5 g

7.

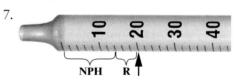

8. 2 tab

9. (a) 100 mL/h (b) 1,000 mg

10. 0.33 mL

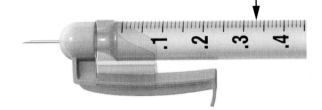

11. Take 133 mL of the $\frac{1}{2}$ strength Isocal and add water to the level of 200 mL.

12. 3 mL/h

13. 6.8 units/hour

14. 2.5 mL

15. 0.13 mL

16. (a) 0.22 mg/d   (b) 0.32 mg/d   (c) yes

17. (a) 160 mg   (b) 63 mL/h

18. 25 gtt/min

19. 1.00 m²

20. 0.5 mL

21. (a) 1.3 mL/min   (b) 25 gtt/min   (c) 13 h 20 min

22. 2,000 mL

23. 30 mL

24. (a) 10 mg   (b) 60 mL

25. (a) 0.009 mg   (b) 21 mL/h

Comprehensive Self-Test 2

1. 2,000 units

2. (a) 19.2 mg (b) 3.8 mL (c) 311 mL/h

3. 2 tab

4. 2 cap

5. 2.2 mL

6. (a) yes   (b) 1.1 mL

7. 0900h the next day

8. 12.5 mL

9. (a) 2 mL

(b)

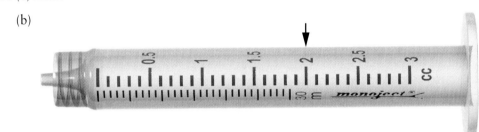

10. (a) 218 mg/d   (b) 681 mg/d

11. 2.25 g

12. 100 mL/h

13. 455 mL

14. yes

15. Take 40 mL of the 50% solution and add water to the level of 200 mL

16. 120 mL/h

17. 2.5 mL

18. (a) 2 cap (b) 3.15 g

19. 30 mL

20. 21 mL/h

21. (a) 45 mL   (b) 2.5 mL/min

22. 0.7 mL

23. (a) 1 mL   (b) 3 mL

24. Take 600 mL of Sustacal and add water to the level of 900 mL.

25. 0400 h the next day.

Comprehensive Self-Test 3

1. 1,260 mL

2. 8 mL

3. 1.2 mL

4. 1,600 units/hour and it is safe.

5. (a) 121 mg/kg   (b) 250 mL/h

6. 16,200 mg

7. (a) 0.35 mL   (b) tuberculin 1 mL

8. No

9. (a) 2.6 mL   (b) 3 mL

10. 30 mL

11. 28 mL/h and 681 mL

12.

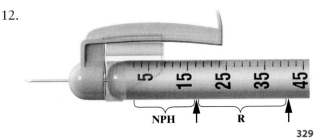

13. 32,962

14. 10 mL

15. 42 mL/h

16. 0505 h the next day

17. 3 tab

18. 0.3 g

19. 3 mL/h

20. 3 g

21. tuberculin 1 mL

22. 75 gtt/min

23. 2 tab

24. 0.51 m^2

25. 1,180 mL

Comprehensive Self-Test 4

1. yes

2. 2.7 mL

3. 2 tab

4. 8 h

5. 250 mL

6. (a) 0.4 mL (b) tuberculin 1 mL

7. 0.05 mg

8. 6 cap

9. 0.4 mL

10. 0.2 mL

11. 2 mL/min

12. 12 mL/h

13. 5 mL/min

14. Take 600 mL of the 5% solution and add water to the level of 3,000 mL.

15. (a) 1.3 mL   (b) 3 mL

16. 25 g of dextrose and 1.5 g of NaCl

17. 6 h 27 min

18. 32.4 mg

19. 1,090 mL

20. Yes

21. 20 units/hour

22. 0.5 mL

23. 1.5 mL

24. 10 mL

25. Yes

Appendix B

Common Abbreviations Used in Medical Documentation

To someone unfamiliar with prescriptive abbreviations, medication orders may look like a foreign language. To interpret prescriptive orders accurately and to administer drugs safely, a qualified person must have a thorough knowledge of common abbreviations. For instance, when the prescriber writes, "**Dilaudid (hydromorphone) 1.5 mg IM q4h prn**" the administrator knows how to interpret it as "Hydromorphone, 1.5 milligrams, intramuscular, every four hours, whenever necessary." For measurement abbreviations, refer to Appendix C.

Abbreviation	Meaning	Abbreviation	Meaning
ā	before (*abante*)	GT	gastrostomy tube
ac	before meals (*ante cibum*)	gtt	drop
ad lib	as desired (*ad libitum*)	h, hr	hour
A.M., am	morning	hs	hour of sleep; bedtime (*hora somni*)
amp	ampule		
aq	aqueous water	IC	intracardiac
b.i.d.	two times a day	ID	intradermal
BP	blood pressure	IM	intramuscular
c̄	with	IV	intravenous
C	Celsius; centigrade	USP	United States Pharmacopeia
cap	capsule	IVP	intravenous push
CBC	complete blood count	IVPB	intravenous piggyback
cc	cubic centimeter	IVSS	IV Soluset
CVP	central venous pressure	kg	kilogram
d	day	KVO	keep vein open
D/W	dextrose in water	L	liter
D5W or D5/W or D₅W	5% dextrose in water	LA	long acting
daw	dispense as written	lb	pound
dr	dram	LIB	left in bag, left in bottle
Dx	diagnosis	LOS	length of stay
elix	elixir	MAR	medication administration record
ER	extended release		
F	Fahrenheit	mcg	microgram
g	gram	mcgtt, μgtt	microdrop
gr	grain	mEq	milliequivalent

Abbreviation	Meaning	Abbreviation	Meaning
mg	milligram	q2h	every two hours
min	minute	q3h	every three hours
mL	milliliter	q4h	every four hours
mU	milliunit	q6h	every six hours
n, noct	night	q8h	every eight hours
NDC	national drug code	q12h	every 12 hours
NGT	nasogastric tube	q.i.d.	four times a day (quarter in die)
NKA	no known allergies	qn	every night (quaque noct)
NKDA	no known drug allergies	qs	quantity sufficient or sufficient amount (quantitas sufficiens)
NKFA	no known food allergies		
NPO	nothing by mouth (per ora)	R	respiration
NS	normal saline	R/O	rule out
NSAID	nonsteroidal anti-inflammatory drug	Rx	prescription, treatment
OTC	over the counter	s̄	without (sine)
oz	ounce	SIG	directions to the patient
p̄	after	SL	sublingual
PEG	percutaneous endoscopic gastrostomy tube	SR	sustained release
P	pulse	stat	immediately (statum)
pc	after meals (post cibum)	subcut	subcutaneous
PEJ	Percutaneous Endoscopic Jejunostomy	supp	suppository
PICC	peripherally inserted central catheter	susp	suspension
P.M., pm	afternoon, evening	T or tbs	tablespoon
PO	by mouth (per os)	t or tsp	teaspoon
POST-OP	after surgery	T	temperature
PR	by way of the rectum	t.i.d.	three times a day (ter in die)
PRE-OP	before surgery	tab	tablet
prn	when required or whenever necessary	TPN	total parenteral nutrition
Pt	patient	USP	United States Pharmacopeia
pt	pint	V/S	vital signs
q	every (quaque)	wt	weight
qh	every hour (quaque hora)		

Appendix C

Units of Measurement in Metric, Household, and Apothecary Systems

Abbreviations			
Volume	**Metric**		**Household**
milliliter	mL	microdrop	μgtt or mcgtt
liter	L	drop	gtt
cubic centimeter	cc	teaspoon	t or tsp
		tablespoon	T or tbs
Apothecary		fluid ounce	oz
fluid dram	dr	pint	pt
		quart	qt
Weight	**Metric**		**Household**
microgram	mcg	ounce	oz
milligram	mg	pound	lb
gram	g		
kilogram	kg		
Apothecary			
grain	gr		
Length	**Metric**		**Household**
centimeter	cm	inch	in
meter	m	foot	ft
Area	**Metric**		
square meter	m^2		

Appendix D

Celsius and Fahrenheit Temperature Conversions

Reading and recording a temperature is a crucial step in assessing a patient's health. Temperatures can be measured using either the Fahrenheit (F) scale or the Celsius or centigrade (C) scale. Celsius/Fahrenheit equivalency tables make it easy to convert Celsius to Fahrenheit, or vice versa. Still, it is useful to be able to make this conversion yourself.

You can use the following formulas to convert from one temperature scale to the other

$$C = \frac{F - 32}{1.8} \quad \text{and} \quad F = 1.8\,C + 32$$

For those unfamiliar with algebra, the following rules are equivalent to the algebraic formulas.

First rule: To convert to Celsius. Subtract 32 and then divide by 1.8.
Second rule: To convert to Fahrenheit. Multiply by 1.8 and then add 32.

NOTE

Temperatures are rounded to the nearest tenth.

Example D.1

Convert 102.5 °F to Celsius.

Using the first rule, we subtract 32.

$$\begin{array}{r} 102.5 \\ -32.0 \\ \hline 70.5 \end{array}$$

Then we divide by 1.8.

$$1.8\,\overline{)70.5000} \quad 39.17$$

So, 102.5 °F equals 39.2° C.

Example D.2

Convert 3° C to Fahrenheit.

Using the second rule, we first multiply by 1.8.

$$\begin{array}{r} 1.8 \\ \times 3 \\ \hline 5.4 \end{array}$$

Then we add 32.

$$\begin{array}{r} 5.4 \\ +32.0 \\ \hline 37.4 \end{array}$$

So, 3° C equals 37.4 °F

For those unfamiliar with the Celsius system, the following poem might be useful:

Thirty is hot
Twenty is nice
Ten is chilly
Zero is ice

Appendix E

Tables of Weight Conversions

Use the following tables to convert between the metric kilogram and the household pound.

Table E.1 Pounds to Kilograms					
lb	**kg**	**lb**	**kg**	**lb**	**kg**
2.2	1.0	120	54.5	240	109.1
5	2.3	125	56.8	245	111.4
10	4.5	130	59.1	250	113.6
15	6.8	135	61.4	255	115.9
20	9.1	140	63.6	260	118.2
25	11.4	145	65.9	265	120.5
30	13.6	150	68.2	270	122.7
35	15.9	155	70.5	275	125
40	18.2	160	72.7	280	127.3
45	20.5	165	75	285	129.5
50	22.7	170	77.3	290	131.8
55	25	175	79.5	295	134.1
60	27.3	180	81.8	300	136.4
65	29.5	185	84.1	305	138.6
70	31.8	190	86.4	310	140.9
75	34.1	195	88.6	315	143.2
80	36.4	200	90.9	320	145.5
85	38.6	205	93.2	325	147.7
90	40.9	210	95.5	330	150
95	43.2	215	97.7	335	152.3
100	45.5	220	100	340	154.5
105	47.7	225	102.3	345	156.8
110	50	230	104.5	350	159.1
115	52.3	235	106.8	355	161.4

Table E.2 Kilograms to Pounds

kg	lb	kg	lb	kg	lb
2	4.4	56	123.2	110	242
4	8.8	58	127.6	112	246.4
6	13.2	60	132	114	250.8
8	17.6	62	136.4	116	255.2
10	22	64	140.8	118	259.6
12	26.4	66	145.2	120	264
14	30.8	68	149.6	122	268.4
16	35.2	70	154	124	272.8
18	39.6	72	158.4	126	277.2
20	44	74	162.8	128	281.6
22	48.4	76	167.2	130	286
24	52.8	78	171.6	132	290.4
26	57.2	80	176	134	294.8
28	61.6	82	180.4	136	299.2
30	66	84	184.8	138	303.6
32	70.4	86	189.2	140	308
34	74.8	88	193.6	142	312.4
36	79.2	90	198	144	316.8
38	83.6	92	202.4	146	321.2
40	88	94	206.8	148	325.6
42	92.4	96	211.2	150	330
44	96.8	98	215.6	152	334.4
46	101.2	100	220	154	338.8
48	105.6	102	224.4	156	343.2
50	110	104	228.8	158	347.6
52	114.4	106	233.2	160	352
54	118.8	108	237.6	162	356.4

Appendix F

Ratio and Proportion Method for Dosage Calculation

There are methods other than Dimensional Analysis that can be used to calculate drug dosages.

Memorized formulas like

$$\text{Amount to administer} = \frac{\text{Desired dose}}{\text{Dose on hand}} \times \text{Quantity on hand}$$

were once popular.

Another technique uses a ratio and proportion approach, which is useful only in the simplest problems, and is illustrated in the following examples.

Example F.1

If each tablet contains 5 mg, how many tablets contain 15 mg?
The information in the example is summarized in the following table:

Known equivalent	1 tablet = 5 mg
Unknown equivalent	x tablets = 15 mg

The equivalents in the table are written as fractions (ratios) and are equated to form the following proportion:

$$\frac{1 \text{ tab}}{5 \text{ mg}} = \frac{x \text{ tab}}{15 \text{ mg}}$$

x is found by algebraically solving the proportion

$$\frac{1}{5} = \frac{x}{15}$$

Now, cross-multiply

$$\frac{1}{5} \diagdown \frac{x}{15}$$

$$5x = 15$$

Now, divide both sides by 5

$$\frac{5x}{5} = \frac{15}{5}$$

Cancel

$$\frac{\cancel{5}\, x}{\cancel{5}} = \frac{\overset{3}{\cancel{15}}}{\cancel{5}}$$

$$x = 3$$

So, 3 tablets contain 15 mg.

Example F.2

A vial label states: $\dfrac{75 \text{ mg}}{5 \text{ mL}}$. How many milliliters of this solution contains 10 milligrams of the drug?

The information in the example is summarized in the following table:

Known equivalent	75 mg = 5 mL
Unknown equivalent	10 mg = x mL

The equivalents in the table are written as fractions (ratios) and are equated to form the following proportion:

$$\frac{75 \text{ mg}}{5 \text{ mL}} = \frac{10 \text{ mg}}{x \text{ mL}}$$

x is found by algebraically solving the proportion

$$\frac{75}{5} = \frac{10}{x}$$

Now, cross-multiply

$$\frac{75}{5} \diagdown \frac{10}{x}$$

$$50 = 75x$$

Now, divide both sides by 75

$$\frac{50}{75} = \frac{75x}{75}$$

Cancel

$$\frac{\overset{2}{\cancel{50}}}{\underset{3}{\cancel{75}}} = \frac{\cancel{75}\,x}{\cancel{75}}$$

$$x = \frac{2}{3} \quad \text{or} \quad 0.67$$

So, 0.67 mL contains 10 mg of the drug.

Example F.3

If an IV containing 880 mL is to infuse in 8 hours, then how long will it take for 350 mL of this IV to infuse?

The information in the example is summarized in the following table:

Known equivalent	800 mL = 8 h
Unknown equivalent	350 mL = x h

The equivalents in the table are written as fractions (ratios) and are equated to form the proportion below:

$$\frac{880 \text{ mL}}{8 \text{ h}} = \frac{350 \text{ mL}}{x \text{ h}}$$

x is found by algebraically solving the proportion

$$\frac{880}{8} = \frac{350}{x}$$

Now, cross-multiply

$$\frac{880}{8} \diagtimes \frac{350}{x}$$

$$880x = 2,800$$

Now, divide both sides by 880

$$\frac{880x}{880} = \frac{2,800}{880}$$

Cancel

$$\frac{\cancel{880}\ x}{\cancel{880}} = \frac{2,800}{880}$$

$$x = \frac{2,800}{880} \quad \text{or} \quad 3.18$$

So, it will take about 3.18 hours for 350 mL to infuse.

To change 0.18 h to minutes, ratio and proportion could also be used.

Known equivalent	1 h = 60 min
Unknown equivalent	0.18 h = x min

The equivalents in the table are written as fractions (ratios) and are equated to form the proportion below:

$$\frac{1\ \text{h}}{60\ \text{min}} = \frac{0.18\ \text{h}}{x\ \text{min}}$$

x is found by algebraically solving the proportion

$$\frac{1}{60} = \frac{0.18}{x}$$

Now, cross-multiply

$$\frac{1}{60} \diagtimes \frac{0.18}{x}$$

$$10.8 = x$$

So, it will take about 3 hours and 11 minutes for 350 mL to infuse.

Index